KITCHENER PUBLIC LIBRARY

3 9098 02234343 7

W9-DHM-206

Autistic Spectrum Disorders in Children

edited by

Vidya Bhushan Gupta

*New York Medical College
and Columbia University
New York, New York, U.S.A.*

MARCEL

DEKKER

MARCEL DEKKER, INC.   NEW YORK · BASEL

Although great care has been taken to provide accurate and current information, neither the author(s) nor the publisher, nor anyone else associated with this publication, shall be liable for any loss, damage, or liability directly or indirectly caused or alleged to be caused by this book. The material contained herein is not intended to provide specific advice or recommendations for any specific situation.

Trademark notice: Product or corporate names may be trademarks or registered trademarks and are used only for identification and explanation without intent to infringe.

Library of Congress Cataloging-in-Publication Data
A catalog record for this book is available from the Library of Congress.

ISBN: 0-8247-5061-6

This book is printed on acid-free paper.

Headquarters
Marcel Dekker, Inc., 270 Madison Avenue, New York, NY 10016, U.S.A.
tel: 212-696-9000; fax: 212-685-4540

Distribution and Customer Service
Marcel Dekker, Inc., Cimarron Road, Monticello, New York 12701, U.S.A.
tel: 800-228-1160; fax: 845-796-1772

Eastern Hemisphere Distribution
Marcel Dekker AG, Hutgasse 4, Postfach 812, CH-4001 Basel, Switzerland
tel: 41-61-260-6300; fax: 41-61-260-6333

World Wide Web
http://www.dekker.com

The publisher offers discounts on this book when ordered in bulk quantities. For more information, write to Special Sales/Professional Marketing at the headquarters address above.

Copyright © 2004 by Marcel Dekker, Inc.   All Rights Reserved.

Neither this book nor any part may be reproduced or transmitted in any form or by any means, electronic or mechanical, including photocopying, microfilming, and recording, or by any information storage and retrieval system, without permission in writing from the publisher.

Current printing (last digit):

10 9 8 7 6 5 4 3 2 1

PRINTED IN THE UNITED STATES OF AMERICA

Foreword

For over 25 years, the Pediatric Habilitation series has brought to readers the latest information and significant emerging clinical approaches in the field of developmental disabilities in children. Focus has always been on those specific conditions demanding the greatest concern at the time. And developments have been regularly updated with new editions when there has been rapid change, as in the areas of cerebral palsy and attention deficit disorders.

Over this period of time there has been considerable shift in the disabilities encountered by health professionals, from the high-morbidity, low-frequency conditions, such as cerebral palsy and neural tube defects, to the low-morbidity, high-frequency attention deficit disorders, learning disabilities, and, more recently, the autistic spectrum disorders. These changes reflect advances in obstetric and neonatal care and consequences of genetic, environmental, and social factors. In addition, developmental disabilities in children are now seen as spectrum disorders that usually occur with closely related comorbid conditions, rather than as single and uniquely diagnosed entities that stand alone.

Since the inception of this series, nowhere has change been more striking and, indeed, more stressful than in the area of autistic spectrum disorders. Emerging data suggest a marked increase in incidence and prevalence, with a corresponding demand for accurate diagnosis and more effective long-term management. This comes at a time when accepted etiology of the autistic spectrum disorders has shifted dramatically from a psychiatric to a neurodevelopmental focus. Moreover, this field has been virtually flooded with literature dealing with etiology, diagnosis, therapy services, treatment, and pharmacological approaches. In addition, there has been a plethora of often confusing and conflicting claims concerning complementary and alternative medical treatments (CAM), to which both the health provider and lay public are constantly exposed. Finally, much more frequent literature reference is made to the family of the child with autistic spectrum disorder than in all other developmental disabilities. Yet neither the impact of this diagnosis on family functioning nor the unique role of the family in providing optimum care has been well delineated.

To provide for a comprehensive, multidisciplinary text that incorporates the emerging issues in this field, *Autistic Spectrum Disorders in Children* has been developed by a group of outstanding authorities and edited by Dr. Vidya Bhushan Gupta, who has made major contributions to the work. Like all the other books in the Pediatric Habilitation series, it is designed for a wide spectrum of providers, emphasizes the habilitation approach to care and management, and can lead to a better understanding of where further research is needed. It will clearly have an important role in helping to clarify and unify current understanding of the autistic spectrum disorders, and it is hoped this will result in a significant impact on clinical practice as well.

Alfred L. Scherzer

Preface

Only a few decades ago, autism was a medical curiosity, conjuring up visions of a child who walks on his toes like a ballerina, staring vacantly into space but is capable of performing complex mathematical operations at the speed of light. Its prevalence was reported to range from 0.7 to 4.5/10,000 children. Today, autism is being diagnosed in 5–6 of 1000 children and an epidemic is suspected. A debate is raging as to whether the prevalence of autism has truly increased or data merely reflect heightened awareness of the condition. It is now agreed that autism occurs along a spectrum, with only a few children manifesting the full range of symptoms. Inclusion of milder and atypical variants of autism, such as Asperger's and Rett's syndromes, under the rubric of pervasive developmental disorders, has also contributed to the increasing prevalence of autism. Nosology of the syndrome is still in flux, with terms such as autism, autistic spectrum disorder, pervasive developmental disorder, and mutlisystem disorder in vogue.

Our thinking about the origins of autism has undergone radical change. Long gone are Kannerian ideas of refrigerated mothers. Instead, autism is now regarded as a neurobiological disorder. However, as with any common disorder that does not have an incontrovertible candidate as its cause, autism has become a fertile ground for theories. There are theories about what part of an autistic brain is abnormal, the nature of the abnormality, and how the abnormality translates into abnormal behavior. No single area of the brain has been found to be consistently abnormal in children with autism, but abnormalities have been noticed in the cerebellum and the limbic system. The nature of the defect is uncertain—findings include fewer neurons, excessive but smaller neurons, and decreased dendritic branching. It is unclear as to how abnormal structure translates into abnormal behavior, through serotonin or some other neurotransmitter. What causes these neurobiological abnormalities? Is it an abnormal gene or an infectious, toxic, or immunological agent? Perhaps both interact; a toxic or infectious agent unmasks vulnerable genes, which then cause abnormal development of certain areas of the brain. This neurobiological abnormality, in turn, translates into abnormal behavior through abnormal neurotransmitter or electric discharge through critical neural networks. Perhaps many pathways lead independently or interactively to the constellation of symptoms that we call autism. While many of these theories are grounded in valid research, such as the cerebellar and serotonin theories, many are perpetuated by folklore and special interest groups, such as the MMR vaccination theory and the "yeast connection."

Management of autism, too, has undergone sweeping change in the last few decades. We have come a long way from institutions such as Vineland and Willowbrook, where children "who did not grow" used to be incarcerated for a lifetime. The emphasis today is on early detection and intervention. A substantial body of literature now suggests that if intensive interventions are started early in children with autism, many of them will be able to lead functional lives in the mainstream. Therefore, platitudes such as "he will outgrow this, he is just a little shy, give him some time," have given way to early intervention to improve the social and communication skills of these children. Better pharmacological agents are available to address maladaptive behaviors such as inattention, compulsive actions, and aggression.

There are many unanswered questions in the arena of autism and pervasive developmental disorders. How can the frontline clinicians detect the condition early? Is eliciting parental concerns or making informal observations during clinical encounters sufficient? Are generic developmental screens effective in diagnosing autism or should autism-specific screening tools such as CHAT be used? How should autism be confirmed once it is suspected? Few conditions in medicine can be pigeonholed into one discipline today. Autism sits on the mind–body cusp, a neurobiological disorder with behavioral symptomatology. Which professionals are competent to make the diagnosis—pediatricians, psychologists, neurologists, or psychiatrists—and which evaluations should be performed to develop a comprehensive management plan?

As a corollary to the myriad of theories about the causation of autism, a myriad of cures for autism are being promoted by both conventional and alternative schools of medicine. The purveyors of some of the unsubstantiated therapies are exploiting the desperation of parents for selfish ends.

A quantum change has occurred in physician–patient relations and the health care industry. Parents today are in the driver's seat directing the management of their child, instead of sitting in the backseat taking orders. While they demand that providers use the newer genetic and neuroimaging tools to diagnose and manage their children, the managed care organizations curtail their use to contain costs. Both the consumers and payers demand of the providers that they practice medicine according to the evidence-based guidelines developed by academic societies and use outcome research to guide their therapeutic decisions. The clinicians are caught in the crossfire of parental demand and payer oversight.

The idea for this book emerged in this radically changed environment. Autism in this book has been approached from a broad, multidisciplinary perspective, because many disciplines interact in the diagnosis and management of autism. Attempting to bridge the gap between science and strategy, some contributors have presented in depth the relevant scientific research available on the subject, while others have focused on practical guidelines to professionals to diagnose and manage children with autistic spectrum disorders in the context of current scientific research and the health care climate. We hope that this book will serve both the inquisitive, who want to explore the complex maze of autism, and the practical, who in the trenches provide services to children with autistic spectrum disorder.

I want to thank Dr. Alfred Scherzer, who inspired me to undertake this monumental task, and Dr. Raksha Gupta, my wife, who put up with my compulsive preoccupation with this book to the exclusion of almost everything else at home. I would also like to thank Moraima Suarez at Marcel Dekker for working so diligently with me.

Vidya Bhushan Gupta

Contents

Contributors

Pasquale J. Accardo, M.D.   James H. Franklin Professor of Developmental Research in Pediatrics, Department of Pediatrics, Virginia Commonwealth University, Richmond, Virginia, U.S.A.

Charlene Butler, Ed.D.   Special Education Consultant, Seattle School District, Seattle, Washington, U.S.A.

Laura Kresch Curran, B.A.   Center for Autism and Developmental Disabilities Epidemiology, Johns Hopkins Bloomberg School of Public Health, Baltimore, Maryland, U.S.A.

Kari A. Glasgow, O.T.R./L.   Occupational Therapist, Department of Rehabilitation, Children's Hospital, Richmond, Virginia, U.S.A

Vidya Bhushan Gupta, M.D., M.P.H.   Associate Professor of Clinical Pediatrics, Department of Pediatrics, New York Medical College, and Associate Research Scientist, Gertrude H. Sergievsky Center, Columbia University, New York, New York, U.S.A.

Chris Plauché Johnson, M.Ed., M.D.   Professor, Department of Pediatrics, University of Texas Health Science Center at San Antonio, San Antonio, Texas, U.S.A.

Tanya Karapurkar, M.P.H. Centers for Public Health Research and Evaluation, Batelle Memorial Institute, and Centers for Disease Control and Prevention, Atlanta, Georgia, U.S.A.

Nora L. Lee, B.S. Research Program Coordinator, Center for Autism and Developmental Disabilities Epidemiology, Johns Hopkins Bloomberg School of Public Health, Baltimore, Maryland, U.S.A.

Craig J. Newschaffer, Ph.D. Associate Professor, Department of Epidemiology, Johns Hopkins Bloomberg School of Public Health, Baltimore, Maryland, U.S.A.

Alfred L. Scherzer, Ed.D., M.D., F.A.A.P. Clinical Professor Emeritus of Pediatrics, Department of Pediatrics, Joan and Sanford I. Weill Medical College, Cornell University, New York, New York, U.S.A.

Elaine Dolgin Schneider, M.A., C.C.C. Speech Language Pathologist, Pediatric Neurological Associates, White Plains, New York, U.S.A.

Patricia M. Stevens, B.S./O.T.L. Occupational Therapist, Department of Rehabilitation, Children's Hospital, Richmond, Virginia, U.S.A.

John M. Suozzi, Ph.D. Clinical Psychologist, Department of Psychology, Children's Hospital, Richmond, Virginia, U.S.A.

Sallie Tidman, B.S., O.T./L. Community Rehabilitation Manager, Department of Rehabilitation, Children's Hospital, Richmond, Virginia, U.S.A.

Catherine Trapani, Ph.D. Director of Education, Marcus Institute, and Clinical Professor of Pediatrics, Emory University, Atlanta, Georgia, U.S.A.

Marshalyn Yeargin-Allsopp, M.D. Medical Epidemiologist, National Center on Birth Defects and Developmental Disabilities, Centers for Disease Control and Prevention, Atlanta, Georgia, U.S.A.

1

History, Definition, and Classification of Autistic Spectrum Disorders

Vidya Bhushan Gupta
New York Medical College and Columbia University, New York, New York, U.S.A.

I. ORIGINS

The term autism, meaning "living in self" (in Greek *aut* means self, and *ism* refers to a state), was coined by a Swiss psychiatrist, Eugen Bleuler, in 1911, to describe self-absorption due to poor social relatedness in schizophrenia (1). Leo Kanner (Fig. 1), in 1943, borrowed this term to describe 11 children who "were oblivious to other people, did not talk or who parroted speech, used idiosyncratic phrases, who lined up toys in long rows, and who remembered meaningless facts." In his classic paper, "Autistic Disturbances of Affective Contact," Kanner described the features of classic autism with uncanny detail (2). Describing the social isolation of his first case, Kanner said, "Donald got happiest when left alone, almost never cried to go with his mother, did not seem to notice his father's homecomings, and was indifferent to visiting relatives. The father made a special point of mentioning that Donald even failed to pay the slightest attention to Santa Claus in full regalia." His second child played abnormally, "He never was very good with cooperative play. He doesn't care to play with the ordinary things that other children play with, anything with wheels on." The third child said "no recognizable words, although he did make noises (3)." In 1956, Eisenberg and Kanner suggested two essential criteria for the disorder: inability to relate in the ordinary way to people and situations and failure to learn to speak or inability to convey meaning to others through language, both occurring from the beginning of life (4).

In 1944, Hans Asperger, a Viennese pediatrician, independently described a condition similar to that described by Leo Kanner and called it autistic psychopathy

1

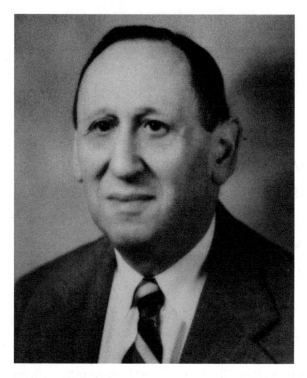

Figure 1   Leo Kanner, M.D., is credited with the first description of autism.

(5), because of "severe and characteristic difficulties of social integration." Like Kanner, he also noted peculiarities of the content and delivery of speech in these children. In addition, he commented on the oddity of gaze in these children: "His eye gaze was generally directed into the void and he darted short peripheral looks and glanced at people and objects only fleetingly." According to Uta Frith, Asperger's paper was ignored by the global academic community because it was written in German during the height of World War II (6).

II.   AUTISM AS A TYPE OF CHILDHOOD PSYCHOSIS

Use of the term "autism" by both Kanner and Asperger led to confusion about the relation of the newly described condition to schizophrenia. Although Kanner commented on the similarity of the clinical picture of autism with "some of the basic schizophrenic phenomena," he underscored the difference that autism was present since birth while schizophrenia occurred after years of normal development. Asperger, too, emphasized that while both autistic children and schizophrenics have "complete shutting off [of] relations between self and the outside world," the latter have a "gradual disintegration of personality" while the former have social withdrawal "from the start." To underscore this point, Asperger called the condition he described a psychopathy rather than psychosis.

Bender described a group of children similar to those described by Kanner in 1942, labeling them "childhood schizophrenics of the pseudodefective type (7)." Anthony (1958) described two types of autism, primary and secondary, both as subtypes of childhood psychosis (8). Primary autism described by him was similar to autism described by Kanner. In 1961, a group of British clinicians (the British Working Party, or BWP) gave nine points—the Nine Points—for the diagnosis of "schizophrenic children." The criteria included symptoms of autism described by Eisenberg and Kanner, but promoted the notion that autism was a type of childhood psychosis (9). These nine points were incorporated in the classification of childhood psychiatric disorders by the Group for the Advancement of Psychiatry (GAP) in 1966. Autism as described by Kanner (Kanner's syndrome) was included in the category of psychosis of infancy and early childhood (10).

Although clearly differentiated from childhood psychoses of late onset, autism continued to be labeled a childhood psychosis, albeit of early onset, until the early 1970s (11,12). Keeping in line with the then-prevalent views, DSM (*Diagnostic and Statistical Manual of the American Psychiatric Association*) I and II did not have a separate category of autism (13,14). In 1956, Eisenberg and Kanner challenged the view that childhood schizophrenia and autism were the same condition (4). In 1968, Ornitz and Ritvo, described autism as a specific syndrome with a cluster of symptoms, including abnormalities of perceptual integration (15). They clearly distinguished between the two conditions by their age of onset, autism occurring before the age of 30 months and schizophrenia later. Makita (16) and Rutter (17) made a case for separating autism from childhood schizophrenia. In his theoretical paper "Childhood Schizophrenia Reconsidered," Michael Rutter discussed the confusion between the terms "childhood schizophrenia" and "autism." He laid to rest the notion that autism was a type of childhood psychosis and argued that the term "childhood schizophrenia" be dropped forever, and that children with schizophrenia be simply called schizophrenic (17). Kolvin et al. (18) in England and Green et al. (19) in the United States restated the differences between autism and schizophrenia: early onset of autism, presence of positive symptoms such as hallucinations in schizophrenia, waxing and waning of symptoms in schizophrenia, and generally higher intelligence of children with schizophrenia. In 1978, Rutter gave criteria for autism that were incorporated in DSM-III under the category of infantile autism (20). These included (1) social delay or deviance that was not just a function of mental retardation, (2) communication problems, again not as a function of mental retardation, (3) unusual behaviors such as stereotypic movements and mannerisms, and (4) onset before the age of 30 months. In 1978, the professional advisory board of the National Society for Children and Adults with Autism defined autism as a behavioral disorder that had the following characteristics: signs and symptoms prior to the age of 30 months, characteristic disturbances of developmental rate/sequence, characteristic disturbances of responsiveness to sensory stimuli, characteristic disturbances of speech, language, and cognitive capacities, and characteristic disturbances of relating to people, events, and objects (21).

DSM-III followed through in resolving the confusion between autism and schizophrenia by including autism in the newly created category of pervasive developmental disorder (22). The term "pervasive" recognized that multiple domains of a child's functioning are affected by autism—social, communicative, and cognitive. DSM-III had four categories under pervasive developmental disorders: infantile autism, childhood-onset autism, atypical autism, and residual autism. Infantile autism and childhood-onset autism were differentiated by the age-of-onset criterion of 30 months. Because the age-of-onset criterion is dependent on age of recognition and not on the true age of onset, few cases of childhood-onset pervasive developmental disorder were described (23), DSM-IIIR replaced the category of infantile autism with autistic disorder, removed the category of childhood-onset pervasive developmental disorder, and extended the age of onset to 36 months (24). It included all cases that did not meet the full criteria of autistic disorder in the category of pervasive developmental disorder, not otherwise specified and eliminated the categories of atypical and residual autism. However, the criteria of DSM-IIIR were overinclusive and led to an overdiagnosis of autistic disorders (25) DSM-IV addressed the overinclusiveness of DSM-IIIR by reducing the criteria for autism from 16 to 12 and brought the classification more in line with the International Statistical Classification of Diseases and Related Health Problems (ICD-10) by creating independent categories of Asperger's syndrome, Rett's syndrome, and childhood disintegrative disorder (26). ICD-10, on the other hand, became closer to DSM-IV by finally moving pervasive developmental disorders from the category of childhood psychoses to an independent category (Table 1) (27). DSM-IV/ICD-10 criteria are more specific and have better interrater reliability than DSM-IIIR criteria, and diagnose autism (diagnosis made by expert clinicians) with a sensitivity of 0.79, specificity of 0.87, positive predictive validity of 0.87, negative predictive validity of 0.83, and interrater reliability of 0.70 (28).

Table 1 DSM-IV and ICD-10 Classification of Autism and Pervasive Developmental Disorders

Pervasive developmental disorders, DSM-IV (26)	Pervasive developmental disorders, ICD-10 (27)

Autistic disorder
PDD (NOS) including atypical autism
	Childhood autism
	Atypical autism
	    Atypicality in age of onset
	    Atypicality in symptomatology
	    Atypicality in both
	PDD, unspecified and residual

Asperger's syndrome Childhood disintegrative disorder Rett's syndrome	Asperger's syndrome Childhood disintegrative disorder Rett's syndrome Overactive disorder associated with MR and stereotyped movements

PDD (NOS), pervasive developmental disorder not otherwise specified; MR, mental retardation.

III. AUTISM: FROM A PSYCHOGENIC TO A NEUROBIOLOGICAL DISORDER

Families of the 11 children described by Kanner were "highly intelligent families, with few warm fathers and mothers who were preoccupied with abstractions of a scientific, literary, and artistic nature, and limited in genuine interest in people (3)." Like William John Little, who, more than a century ago, had implied that asphyxia caused cerebral palsy, based on a case series (29), Leo Kanner suggested that this family constellation "had contributed to the condition of the children." Although he noted that "these children came into the world with innate inability to form the usual, biologically provided affective contact with people," he wondered if "obsessiveness and lack of warm-heartedness in the family" somehow caused the condition. In 1949, Kanner described parents of children with autism as "refrigerators," who fail to provide emotional warmth to their children (8,30,31). However, the original sample of Kanner was self-selected, because only prosperous and intelligent parents might have had access to such a renowned psychiatrist (32). Alternatively, the parents were indeed abnormal, either by chance, or because they, too, suffered from a mild type of autism. The latter explanation is more plausible in view of the recent reports of a higher prevalence of autistic traits in first-degree relatives of children with autism.

Bruno Bettelheim, a psychoanalytically oriented author, whose views were shaped by his personal experiences of emotional trauma in a Nazi concentration camp, further promoted the psychogenic theory of autism, in his book *The Empty Fortress: Infantile Autism and the Birth of the Self* (33). The effects of maternal deprivation on the infant also suggested that mental disorders could be caused by lack of maternal availability and responsivity (34–36). For the next three decades autism was attributed to "refrigerator mothers" who did not show affection to their children. Widely publicized stories of feral children reinforced the view that autism was due to faulty nurture and not faulty nature (37). But the social skills of abandoned and neglected children often improve with nurturing care contrary to a little improvement in social relatedness of most autistic children despite intervention (38). Kasper Hauser, who was neglected and maltreated for many years, recovered and acquired some communication skills even after the age of 17 years (39). A follow-up of children who suffered severe psychosocial deprivation during the Ceausescu regime in Romania showed that with intervention many such children learned to communicate and make social approach, although deviant in quality (40). Moreover, abused or neglected children show unhealthy attachment to their caregivers, while autistic children are attached to primary caregivers (41).

The psychogenic theory of autism held sway until Bernard Rimland in his book *Infantile Autism* proposed that autism was neurogenic and not psychogenic (42). He argued that many autistic children were born to loving and caring parents and many perfectionist professional parents had normal offspring. Moreover, most autistic children did not acquire the disorder but were born with it. Kanner himself changed his views about his theory of "refrigerator mothers" when in 1969, at the National Association of Autistic Children, he declared, "Herewith I officially acquit of you people as parents" (43).

IV. AUTISM: A NEW DISORDER OR RECENTLY DISCOVERED OLD DISORDER?

Although autism was described as a distinct syndrome in 1943, it most certainly occurred before 1943. As early as 1867, Maudsley drew attention to severe mental disorders in young children with severe distortion of the developmental process (44). De Sanctis, in 1906, described a schizophrenia-like condition in prepubertal children under the term "dementia precocissima" (45). Disintegrative psychosis, a condition similar to autism, and according to some indistinguishable from autism, was first described in 1908 (46). In 1919, Lightner Witmer, considered the father of clinical psychology in the United States, described a 2 years and 7 months old boy, Don, who behaved like an autistic child (47). In the 1920s, a Russian child psychiatrist described children having characteristics similar to those described by Asperger (48).

Historians are now looking for signs of autism in two groups of individuals: low-functioning feral children who suffered severe psychosocial deprivation early in their lives, and highly accomplished individuals with poor social skills.

Although popular myth gives the impression that psychosocial deprivation explains most of the behaviors of the feral children, scientific examination suggests that many of these children had preexisting conditions such as mental retardation or autism (49). It is now believed that Victor, the Wild Boy of Aveyron, who was discovered in a jungle of Southern France in 1797 and was cared for and described by a French physician, Jean-Marc-Gaspard Itard, was abandoned by his parents during the French revolution because he was autistic. Like Fritz V of Asperger, he did not love anyone and could not show genuine affection (50–52). Feral children who are not autistic, such as Kasper Hauser, who was found in Germany in 1828, at the age of 16 years, recover partially and acquire communication skills even after many years of neglect and maltreatment (39,53).

Many famous individuals are now suspected to have Asperger's syndrome because they were socially aloof or inept. Among these are Henry Cavendish and Thomas Jefferson. Henry Cavendish was a famous British scientist of the eighteenth century, who "worked in complete solitude and rarely spoke to anyone" (54). Doubts are being raised if Thomas Jefferson's early aloofness, awkwardness, and ineptitude in social situations, and his fixations are compatible with the diagnosis of Asperger's syndrome (55). Rabson and Frith have written about Hugh Blair, an eighteenth-century Scottish landlord whose marriage was annulled on the ground of mental incapacity, but whose behavior as described in the court documents is suggestive of autism (56). Frith, in 1992, suggested that the fictional character of Sherlock Holmes was perhaps autistic (6), but others reached a different conclusion (57). Because making retrospective diagnoses, or "pathographies," based on scanty and unreliable old records is unreliable, the real diagnosis of these celebrities will never be known, but these reports underscore the fact that pervasive developmental disorders including autism and Asperger's syndrome occurred even prior to Kanner's description.

V. NOSOLOGY

Originally, Eugen Bleuler used the word autism to describe a state of extreme social withdrawal in schizophrenia (1). Kanner and Asperger borrowed the term as an adjective to describe a constellation of symptoms that included not only social withdrawal but communication difficulties and rigid and stereotypic behavior (2). The former called this syndrome "autistic disturbance of affective contact" and the latter, "autistic psychopathy." Although both Kanner and Asperger had described high-functioning children, the syndrome described by Kanner, consisting of severe impairments of social and communicative behavior, became known as autism and the syndrome described by Asperger, with a wider range of severity and better cognitive and communicative function, became known as Asperger's syndrome.

The American Psychiatric Association, recognizing that autism was a heterogeneous disorder affecting many, if not most, domains of a child's functioning, introduced the term "pervasive developmental disorder" in DSM-III as a generic term to include all shades and degrees of autism (22). In 1994, the DSM-IV incorporated five diagnoses under pervasive developmental disorders: autism, Rett disorder, childhood disintegrative disorder (CDD), Asperger disorder (ASP), and pervasive developmental disorder–not otherwise specified (PDD-NOS) (26). Not everyone agrees with the term "pervasive developmental disorder." According to Bernard Rimland, this term is meaningless because autism may not be pervasive in all children and other disorders such as mental retardation may cause more pervasive damage to a child's function. Other objections have been raised about the DSM-IV/ICD-10 classification of pervasive developmental disorders. DSM-IV does not differentiate autistic disorder clearly from other pervasive developmental disorders, especially Asperger's syndrome (58,59). DSM-IV criteria for Asperger's syndrome ignore the abnormal use of language by individuals with Asperger's syndrome (60,61). DSM-IV/ICD-10 system does not recognize the heterogeneity of presentation, functioning, response to treatment, and natural history within each group. While the symptoms of autism differ qualitatively and quantitatively at different ages, DSM-IV offers a common yardstick for all ages and developmental stages, increasing the possibility of diagnostic errors (62).

Because there are many shades of autism depending on which behavior is predominant and how severe it is, the term "autistic spectrum disorder" has been proposed as an umbrella term to include the whole range of autistic symptoms from mild to severe (63–65). Contributors to this volume prefer this term because it reflects the unifying social deficit more poignantly than the term 'pervasive developmental disorders,' and it mirrors the clinically common scenario of cases that do not meet the DSM-IV/ICD-10 criteria strictly but have significant impairments in social skills, pragmatic communication, or sensorimotor behavior. Another term, "broad autism phenotype," has gained currency among medical geneticists to include the relatives of children with autism who have subtle deficits in social and communicative domains, but do not meet the criteria of pervasive developmental disorders (66,67).

The National Center for Clinical Infant Programs/Zero to Three proposed the term "multisystem developmental disorder" (MSDD) for children who have dysfunction in many domains, such as communication, sensory processing, and motor planning, but have some capacity for engaging in an emotional and social relationship with the primary caregiver. The authors of the term emphasize that deficits in relating are not the defining characteristic of this condition in contrast to the pervasive developmental disorders of DSM-IV/ICD-10, but may be secondary to abnormalities of sensory processing and motor planning and, therefore, can improve with intervention. This term has not gained popularity, because the DSM-IV category of PDD-NOS includes atypical and subthreshold cases of autism (68).

Another term, multiple complex developmental disorder, has been proposed both as a separate category or as a subtype of pervasive developmental disorders. The defining characteristic of this disorder is deficit in affect regulation with secondary deficits in relatedness and thought. The symptoms of this condition include disturbed attachments, idiosyncratic anxiety reactions, episodes of behavioral disorganization, and wide emotional variability (69–71). Although both multiplex complex disorder and multisystem disorder have not become popular, they highlight abnormalities of affect regulation and sensory processing as part of the litany of problems in pervasive developmental disorder. The differential connotations of the terms used to describe pervasive developmental disorders are given in Table 2.

VI. TAXONOMY

Some of the foregoing difficulties may be resolved if autism is considered a heterogeneous disorder with many subtypes, but attempts to identify separate entities within autism have not fared well. Both categorical and dimensional approaches have been tried. The concept of autistic spectrum disorder is a popular dimensional approach but is vague with no clear-cut end points. It does not state clearly when normal variation ends and disorder begins. It does not address the issue of discordance among the three key domains of autistic symptoms—a child may have minimal abnormality in the communicative domain while having significant limitations in social reciprocity, making distinction from Asperger's syndrome impossible. Similarly, a child with a limited range of repetitive behaviors but few problems in the communicative and social domains may resemble a child with obsessive compulsive disorder. A vast range of permutations and combinations will be possible along the spectrum of the three key domains (Fig. 2). Both false positives and false negatives are likely to be high in this dimensional scheme. Lack of clear-cut diagnostic criteria in such a scheme can create doubt leading to conflicts in obtaining necessary services and cash benefits for some children. Neither does such an approach have any heuristic value. Thus instead of defining subtypes, this dimensional approach lumps different shades of the disorder under one rubric (Fig. 2).

Categorical subtyping of autism has been attempted on the basis of social behavior and intelligence quotient (IQ)/developmental level. Among the social typologies, Wing's (1997) "triad of subtypes" based on social interaction, communication, imagination, and behavior is the most accepted (72,73). The most severely autistic or aloof type avoid social contact except to fulfill a need, show poor attachment behaviors, have severe impairments in verbal and

Table 2 Various Terms in Vogue for Pervasive Developmental Disorders

	Social deficit	Communication		Stereotypies	Sensory disintegration	Affective dysregulation	Low nonverbal IQ
		Qualitative	Quantitative				
Autism							
High functioning	++	+	±	+	±	±	−
Low functioning	++	+	+	+	±	±	+
Asperger's syndrome	++	+	−	+	±	−	−
Multisystem disorder	±	±	±	±	++	±	±
Multiplex complex disorder	±	±	±	±	±	++	±
PDD-NOS	+	+	±	+	±	±	±
Language disorder	−	+	±	−	−	−	−

Affective dysregulation, lack of or inappropriate facial expression; +, mild; ++, severe; −, absent.

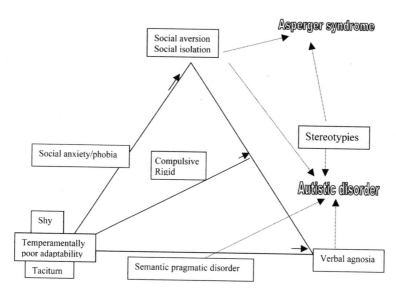

Figure 2 Autistic spectrum.

nonverbal communication, do not engage in pretend play or joint attention, have stereotypic behaviors and motor abnormalities such as toe-walking, and have low IQ. The passive type do not seek contact but are more accepting of social advances by others, imitate others in play or otherwise, have repetitive speech, and intermediate IQ. The active-but-odd type seek interactions but in odd and eccentric ways, talk but do not take turns in conversation, have poor eye contact, are motorically clumsy, and have higher IQ. Although there is some empirical support for aloof and active-but-odd subtypes (74,75), support for the third group (passive) is not so strong (76). Moreover, most of the variance in the groups is explained by IQ, aloof children having low IQ and active-but-odd having higher IQ (77).

Several studies have supported a two-type, low and high functioning, classification of autism, based on nonverbal IQ and adaptive behavior (78,79). Two groups emerged in the Autism and Language Disorders Nosology Project, a higher-functioning group that resembled Wing's active-but-odd group and a lower-functioning group that resembled Wing's aloof group. The former received the diagnosis of PDD-NOS and the latter, autistic disorder. The natural course of the first group was improvement, while the latter group remained stable (75). Cluster analyses have generally confirmed the two-type solution with a few overlapping intermediate subtypes (80–82).

Intellectual level has emerged as a strong predictor of outcome in most studies, high-functioning children with nonverbal IQ above 65 having better

Table 3 Two-Type Model of Pervasive Developmental Disorders

	High-functioning	Low-functioning
Onset	Later	Early
Nonverbal IQ (performance IQ)	Above 65	Below 65
Head circumference	Normal to large	Normal to small
Dysmorphic features	Attractive appearance with few dsysmorphic features	None to present
Seizures	Infrequent	Frequent
Neurological examination	Normal	Normal to abnormal
Development	Deviant	Delayed and deviant
Social behavior	"Active but odd"	"Aloof"
Identifiable cause	Unlikely	Likely
Prognosis	Better	Poor

outcome at school age than low-functioning children with nonverbal IQ of less than 65 (83,84). The two-type model has some heuristic value as well. DeLong has proposed that the low-functioning type is caused by bilateral brain damage in early life and the high-functioning type is idiopathic without evidence of brain damage and may be related to familial affective psychopathology (85). The differences between these two types are given in the Table 3.

Although the purpose of classification is to identify homogeneous subtypes that suggest a particular etiology, natural history, treatment approach, and outcome, such clear subtypes have not emerged in pervasive developmental disorders (86). This may never happen because autism, perhaps, represents several discrete disorders with a common overlapping phenotype. Until this happens a descriptive approach listing each child's behavior in the three DSM-IV/ICD domains of social behavior, communication skills, and stereotypic behaviors may be preferable to a diagnostic label. Additionally, severity of the condition may be judged by assessing the delay/deviance in relation to the child's nonverbal IQ, frequency of symptoms, and level of adaptive dysfunction (62).

REFERENCES

1. Bleuler E. Dementia Praecox Order Gruppe der Schizophrenien (1911). Translated by Zinkin J. New York: International Universities Press, 1950.
2. Kanner L. Autistic disturbances of affective contact. Nervous Child 1943; 2:217–250.
3. www.ama.org.br/kannereng12.htm, accessed on 9.12.02.

4. Eisenberg L, Kanner L. Childhood schizophrenia. Am J Orthopsychiatry. 1956; 26:556–566.
5. Asperger H. Die "Autistichen Psychopathen" Kindesalter. Arch Psychiatr Nervenkr 1944; 117:76–136.
6. Frith U. Autism—Explaining the Enigma. London: Blackwell Publishers, 1992.
7. Bender L. Schizophrenia in childhood. Nervous Child 1942; 27:138–140.
8. Anthony EJ. An experimental approach to the psychopathology of childhood. Br J Med Psychol 1958; 31:211–213.
9. Creak M, Cameron K, Cowie V, et al. Schizophrenic syndrome in childhood. Br Med J 1961; 2:889–890.
10. Werry JA. Childhood psychosis. In: Quay HC, Werry JI, eds. Psychopathological Disorders of Childhood. New York: Wiley, 1972.
11. Kolvin I, Ounsted C, Humphrey M, Mcnay A. Studies in the childhood psychoses. II. The phenomenology of childhood psychoses. Br J Psychiatry 1971; 118:385–395.
12. Eisenberg L. The classification of childhood psychosis reconsidered. J Autism Child Schiz 1972; 2:338–342.
13. American Psychiatric Association. The Diagnostic and Statistical Manual of Mental Disorders. 1st ed. Washington, DC: American Psychiatric Association, 1952.
14. American Psychiatric Association. The Diagnostic and Statistical Manual of Mental Disorders. 2nd ed. Washington, DC: American Psychiatric Association, 1968.
15. Ornitz EM, Ritvo ER. Perceptual inconstancy in early infantile autism. Arch Gen Psychiatry 1968; 18:79–98.
16. Makita K. Contemporary concept of autism and autismus infantum. Acta Paedopsychiatry 1975; 41:162–169.
17. Rutter M. Childhood schizophrenia reconsidered. J Autism Child Schiz 1972; 2:315–337.
18. Kolvin I. Infantile autism or infantile psychoses. Br Med J 1972; 23; 3(829):753–755.
19. Green WH, Campbell M, Hardesty AS, Grega DM, Padron-Gayol M, Shell J, Erlenmeyer-Kimling L. A comparison of schizophrenic and autistic children. J Am Acad Child Psychiatry 1984; 23:390–409.
20. Rutter M. Diagnosis and definition. In: Rutter M, Schopler E, eds. Autism: A Reappraisal of Concepts and Treatment. New York: Plenum, 1978:1–25.
21. Ritvo ER, Freeman BJ. Current research in the syndrome of autism: introduction— the National Society of Autistic Society's definition of the syndrome of autism. J Am Acad Child Adolesc Psychiatry 1978; 17:565–575.
22. American Psychiatric Association. The Diagnostic and Statistical Manual of Mental Disorders. 3rd ed. Washington, DC: American Psychiatric Publishing, Inc., 1980.
23. Volkmar FR, Stier DM, Cohen DJ. Age of recognition of pervasive developmental disorder. Am J Psychiatry 1985; 142:1450–1452.
24. American Psychiatric Association. The Diagnostic and Statistical Manual of Mental Disorders. 3rd ed. Revised. Washington, DC: American Psychiatric Publishing, Inc., 1987.
25. Factor DC, Freeman NL, Kardash A. A comparison of DSM-III and DSM-IIIR criteria for autism. J Autism Dev Discord 1989; 19:637–640.

26. American Psychiatric Association. The Diagnostic and Statistical Manual of Mental Disorders. 4th ed. Washington, DC: American Psychiatric Publishing, Inc., 1994.
27. International Statistical Classification of Diseases and Related Health Problems. 10th ed. Geneva, Switzerland: World Health Organization, 1994.
28. Volkmar FR, Klin A, Siegel B, et al. Field trial for autistic disorders in DSM-IV. Am J Psychriatry 1994; 151:1361.
29. Little WJ. On the influence of abnormal parturition, difficult labours, premature birth, and asphyxia neonatorum on the mental and physical condition of the child, especially in relation to deformities. Trans Obstet Soc Lond 1861; 3:293.
30. Kanner L. Problems of nosology and psychodynamics of early infantile autism. Am J Orthopsychiatry. 1949; 19:416–426.
31. Kanner L, Eisenberg L. Early infantile autism: 1943–1955. Am J Orthopsychiat 1956; 26:55–65.
32. Chess S. A remembrance. J Autism Dev Disord 1981; 11:259–263.
33. Bettelheim B. The Empty Fortress: Infantile Autism and the Birth of the Self. New York: Free Press, 1967.
34. Bakwin H. Loneliness in infants. Am J Dis Child 1942; 63:30–40.
35. Spitz RA. Hospitalism. In: Fenichel O, ed. The Psychoanalytic Study of the Child. New York: International Universities Press, 1945:53–74.
36. Bowlby J. Maternal Care and Mental Health. Geneva: World Health Organization, 1951.
37. Schopler E. New developments in the definition and diagnosis of autism. In: Lahey BB, Kazdin AE, eds. Advances in Clinical Child Psychology 1983; 6:93–127.
38. Favazza AR. Feral and isolated children. Br J Med Psychol 1977; 50:105–111.
39. Simon N. Kasper Hauser's recovery and autopsy: a perspective on neurological and sociological requirements for language development. J Autism Child Schizo 1978; 8:209–217.
40. Rutter M, Andersen-Wood L, Beckett C, Bredenkamp D, Castle J, Groothues C, Kreppner J, Keaveney L, Lord C, O'Connor TG. Quasi-autistic patterns following severe early global privation. English and Romanian Adoptees (ERA) Study Team. J Child Psychol Psychiatry 1999; 40:537–49.
41. Rogers SJ, Pennington BF. A theoretical approach to the deficits in infantile autism. Dev Psychopathol 1991; 3:137–162.
42. Rimland B. Infantile Autism: The Syndrome and Its Implications for a Neural Theory of Behavior. New York: Appleton-Century Crofts, 1964.
43. Crawley CA. Infantile autism—an hypothesis. J Ir Med Assoc 1971; 64:335–45.
44. Maudsley H. The Physiology and Pathology of Mind. London: Macmillan, 1867.
45. De Sanctis S. On some varities of dementia praecox. Riv Sper Freniatria 1906; 32:141–165. Translated and reprinted in Howells JG, ed. Modern Perspectives in International Child Psychiatry. Edinburgh: Oliver & Boyd, 1969:509–609.
46. Mouridsen SE, Rich B, Isager T. A comparative study of genetic and neurobiological findings in disintegrative psychosis and infantile autism. Psychiatry Clin Neurosci 2000; 54:441–446.
47. Witmer L. Orthogenic cases. XIV. Don: a curable case of arrested development due to a fear psychosis the result of shock in a three-year-old infant. Am Assoc Adv Sci 1920; 401:97–111.

48. Ssucharewa GE, Wolff S. The first account of the syndrome Asperger described? (Die shizolden Psychopathien lm Kindersalter). Eur Child Adolesc Psychiatry 1996; 5-119-32.
49. Demorsier G. Wild children and wolf children. Psychol Ekon Praxi (Charles University, Czechoslovakia) 1965; 24:148-155.
50. Lane Harlan. Wild Boy of Averon. Boston: Harvard University Press, 1976.
51. "Autistic psychopathy" in childhood. Translated by Uta Frith. In: Frith U, ed. Autism and Asperger Syndrome. Cambridge: Cambridge University Press, 1991.
52. Gayral L, Chabbert P, Baillaud-Citeau H. The first observations on the wild-boy of Lacaune (called "Victor" or "the wild-boy of Aveyron"): new documents. Ann Med-Psychol (Editions Elsevier, France) 1972; 2:465-490.
53. Stumpfe KD. The case of Kasper Hauser. Prax Kinderpsychol Kinderpsychiatr 1969; 18:292-299.
54. Oliver Sacks. Henry Cavendish: an early case of Asperger's syndrome? Neurology 2001; 57:1347.
55. Ledgin N, Temple Gardin. Diagnosing Jefferson. Arlington, TX: Future Horizons, Inc., 2002.
56. Houston Rab A, Houston RA, Frith U. Autism in History: The Case of Hugh Blair of Borgue. London: Blackwell Publishers, 2000.
57. Diagnosis and Detection: The Medical Iconography of Sherlock Holmes. Rutherford, NJ: Farleigh Dickinson University Press, 1987.
58. Eisenmajer R, Prior M, Leekam M, Wing L, Gould J, Welham M, et al. Comparison of clinical symptoms in autism and Asperger syndrome. J Am Acad Child Adolesc Psychiatry 1996; 35:1523-1531.
59. Volkmar F. Can you explain the difference between autism and Asperger syndrome? J Autism Dev Disord 1999; 29:185-186.
60. Mayes SD, Calhoun SL, Crites DL. Does DSM-IV Asperger's disorder exist? J Abnorm Child Psychol 2001; 29:263-271.
61. Ghaziuddin M, Gerstein L. Pedantic speaking style differentiates Asperger syndrome from high-functioning autism. J Autism Dev Disord 1996; 26:585-595.
62. Byrna Siegel. Toward DSM-IV: a developmental approach to autistic disorder. Psychiatry Clin North Am 1991; 14:53-68.
63. Wing L. The autistic spectrum. Lancet 1997; 350:1761-1766.
64. Filipek PA, Accardo PJ, Baranek GT. The screening and diagnosis of autistic spectrum disorders. J Autism Dev Disord 1999; 29:439-484.
65. Rapin I. The autistic-spectrum disorders. N Engl J Med 2002; 347:302-303.
66. Piven J, Palmer P, Jacobi D, Childress D, Arndt S. Broader autism phenotype: evidence from a family history study of multiple-incidence autism families. Am J Psychiatry 1997; 154:185-190.
67. Bolton P, MacDonald H, Pickles A, et al. A case-control family history study of autism. J Child Psychol Psychiatry 1994; 35:877-900.
68. Diagnostic Classification: 0-3. Diagnostic Classification of Mental Health and Developmental Disorders of Infancy and Childhood. Arlington, VA: ZERO TO THREE/National Center for Clinical Infant Programs, 1994.

69. Demb H B, Noskin O. The use of the term multiple complex developmental disorder in a diagnostic clinic serving young children with developmental disabilities: a report of 15 cases. Mental Health Aspects Dev Disabil 2001; 4:49–60.

70. Zalsman G, Cohen DJ. Multiplex developmental disorder. Isr J Psychiatry Relat Sci 1998; 35:300–306.

71. Van der Gaag RJ, Buitelaar J, Van den Ban E, Bezemer M, Njio L, Van Engeland H. A controlled multivariate chart review of multiple complex developmental disorder. J Am Acad Child Adolesc Psychiatry 1995; 34:1096–1106.

72. Wing L, Gould J. Severe impairments of social interaction and associated abnormalities in children: epidemiology and classification. J Autism Dev Disord 1979; 9:11–29.

73. Wing L. The autistic spectrum. Lancet 1997; 350:1761–1766.

74. Castelloe P, Dawson G. Subclassification of children with autism and pervasive developmental disorder: a questionnaire based on Wing's subgrouping scheme. J Autism Dev Disord 1993; 23:229–241.

75. Waterhouse L, Morris R, Allen D, Dunn M, Fein D, Feinstein C, Rapin I, Wing L. Diagnosis and classification in autism. J Autism Dev Disord 1996; 26:59–86.

76. Borden MC, Ollendick TH. An examination of the validity of social subtypes in autism. J Autism Dev Disord 1994; 24:23–37.

77. Volkmar FR, Cohen DJ, Bregman JD, Hooks MY, Stevenson JM. An examination of social typologies in autism. J Am Acad Child Adolesc Psychiatry 1989; 28:82–86.

78. Fein D, Stevens M, Dunn M, Waterhouse L, Allen D, Rapin I, Feinstein C. Subtypes of pervasive developmental disorders: clinical characteristics. Child Neuropsychol 1999; 5:1–23.

79. Stevens MC, Fein DA, Dunn M, Allen D, Waterhouse LH, Feinstein C, Rapin I. Subgroups of children with autism by cluster analysis: a longitudinal examination. J Am Acad Child Adolesc Psychiatry. 2000; 39:346–352.

80. Prior M, Eisenmajer R, Leekam S, Wing L, Gould J, Ong B, Dowe D. Are there subgroups within the autistic spectrum? A cluster analysis of a group of children with autistic spectrum disorders. J Child Psychol Psychiatry Allied Disc 1998; 39:893–902.

81. Eaves LC, Ho HH, Eaves DM. Subtypes of autism by cluster analysis. J Autism Dev Disord 1994; 24:3–22.

82. Siegel B, Anders TF, Ciaranello RD, Bienenstock B, Kraemer HC. Empirically derived subclassification of the autistic syndrome. J Autism Dev Disord 1986; 16:275–293.

83. Stevens MC, Fein DA, Dunn M, Allen D, Waterhouse LH, Feinstein C, Rapin I. Subgroups of children with autism by cluster analysis: a longitudinal examination. J Am Acad Child Adolesc Psychiatry 2000; 39:346–352.

84. Waterhouse L, Morris R, Allen D, Dunn M, Fein D, Feinstein C, Rapin I, Wing L. Diagnosis and classification in autism. J Autism Dev Disord 1996; 26:59–86.

85. DeLong GR. Autism: new data suggest a new hypothesis. Neurology 1999; 52(23):911–916.

86. Rutter M, Schopler E. Classification of pervasive developmental disorders: some concepts and practical considerations. J Autism Dev Disord 1992; 22:459–482.

2

The Epidemiology of Autism and Autism Spectrum Disorders

Tanya Karapurkar
Battelle Memorial Institute and Centers for Disease Control and Prevention, Atlanta, Georgia, U.S.A.

Nora L. Lee, Laura Kresch Curran, and Craig J. Newschaffer
Johns Hopkins Bloomberg School of Public Health, Baltimore, Maryland, U.S.A.

Marshalyn Yeargin-Allsopp
National Center on Birth Defects and Developmental Disabilities, Centers for Disease Control and Prevention, Atlanta, Georgia, U.S.A.

I. INTRODUCTION

In the 1940s, Dr. Leo Kanner described 11 children with "autistic disturbances of affective contact," and even today, that characterization continues to form the basis of the diagnostic criteria for autistic disorder (1). Epidemiological studies describing the prevalence and risk factors for autistic disorder and autism spectrum disorders (ASDs) did not appear in the scientific literature until the late 1960s and early 1970s (2–4). Since these earlier investigations, several population-based prevalence studies have been conducted. However, these vary in terms of their methods, case definitions, and population size; hence, comparisons of estimates from these studies are difficult. Other factors contributing to the lack of epidemiological understanding of autism stem from the paucity of well-designed studies that are able to examine trends over time, as well as a range of risk factors, both biological and sociodemographic, for autism.

For instance, there have been few studies that reflect racially heterogeneous populations, such as from the United States.

To examine the current prevalence of autism and trends in prevalence over time, we conducted a MEDLINE literature search for prevalence studies that have been published between 1966 and the present (January 2003). The criteria used for inclusion in the review included: peer-reviewed articles in the English language, book chapters, and summaries of articles published in other languages (1) that describe studies with temporally and geographically defined population-based cohorts; inclusion of case definitions that used clinical examinations or review by expert clinicians' assessment and diagnosis; and (2) that used the accepted clinical diagnostic criteria for autism/ASDs as a basis for case definition. This chapter will describe these studies according to (1) diagnostic criteria; (2) time period; (3) size of population; and (4) methods of ascertainment. We will also present what is currently known about autism risk factors and discuss challenges to conducting epidemiological studies of autism. In this chapter, we will use the term ASD to refer to the *Diagnostic and Statistical Manual of Mental Disorders*, 4th Edition (5) diagnosis of autistic disorder, Asperger disorder, and pervasive developmental disorder–not otherwise specified (PDD-NOS). Where possible, we will indicate those studies that attempted to differentiate between autistic disorder and the broader spectrum of ASDs.

II. EPIDEMIOLOGICAL CONCEPTS IN THE MEASUREMENT OF DISEASE OCCURRENCE

Two basic statistics are used to measure disease occurrence in a population: incidence and prevalence. In general, prevalence is a proportion with numerators that reflect the number of individuals with the disease and denominators that include the number of individuals in the study population at a particular point in time. Persons counted in the numerator must also be counted in the denominator. Point prevalence, involving an estimate taken at a particular point in time, is the most intuitive. Prevalence is typically described as a snapshot of the extent of disease in a population. It can be described either as a percentage or, more commonly, as the number of cases found per some unit of individuals in the population, the unit being dependent on how common the disease. Most of the published estimates of autistic disorder and ASD frequency are point prevalence estimates and are often described using a unit of 10,000 individuals.

On the other hand, incidence reflects the number of newly occurring cases emerging in a population over a defined period of time. Incidence differs from prevalence in that it counts *only* new cases in its numerator, limits its denominator to those who have *not yet but still may* develop the disease (excluding those in the numerator), and always incorporates an explicit time element. For example, the incidence rate is the number of new (or "incident") cases per 10,000 individuals per years of follow-up. Because of its emphasis on new cases, incidence reflects closely the underlying risk of disease occurrence, while prevalence, which counts both new and existing cases, reflects most closely the burden of disease in a population that is a function of both the risk and duration of a condition. Given its close relationship with risk, examination of time trends in disease incidence, not prevalence, is typically emphasized in classical epidemiology as a means of assessing whether the etiology of a disease (e.g., the risk factors contributing to disease causation and/or the population susceptibility) is changing over time. However, for autism and other developmental disabilities, there have been few attempts to directly estimate incidence. Instead, trends in prevalence have been more commonly used to make etiological inferences. The reasons for this are twofold. First, it is generally more difficult to develop studies that measure the true incidence of autism because of inherent difficulties defining newly occurring cases. The at-risk population consists of children typically diagnosed between 2 and 5 years of age although it is still not uncommon for older children and even adults to receive an initial first ASD diagnosis (6). Further, the clinical diagnosis of ASD may have more to do with the ability and willingness to make an ASD diagnosis than with the true onset of pathology. In fact, much neuropathological evidence supports a prenatal origin (7). The second reason why autism prevalence trends are often used to infer trends in incidence is that when the average duration of a disease is unchanging, trends in prevalence will approximate trends in incidence. For a lifelong condition with no cure that is not strongly associated with premature mortality, like autism, the average duration of disease is not expected to change drastically with time.

Unfortunately, *both* prevalence and incidence trends will be influenced by changes in the manner in which cases of disease are defined and detected. If available data are based on a diagnostic or ascertainment approach(s) that misses true cases, both the prevalence and incidence will be underestimated. For example, if education records are used to capture cases, young children who have not come to the attention of education authorities will be underascertained. In general, young children are more likely to be underascertained because they have not come to the attention of school officials. Furthermore, many clinicians or evaluators, including those at educational facilities, do not make it their practice to "label" children so young in age, particularly those children whose condition is less severe. Therefore, studies primarily using younger children or those that include younger children in their prevalence estimate might underestimate the true prevalence of the disorder. In addition, if the approach used to define and detect disease changes with time, this change will impact the trend for the estimation of prevalence or incidence—a trend not in any way attributable to a change in the real risk of disease occurrence. Considering this, the evolution of autism diagnostic criteria and the impact it has had on the prevalence of autism and ASDs will be described in this chapter.

III. INCIDENCE STUDIES

For the reasons described above, only four studies have attempted to report the *incidence* of autism (8–11). The investigators in all of these studies used the year of diagnosis as the year of onset of autism. However, the age of diagnosis in most studies is much later than the age of recognition of the behaviors that are characteristic of autism. In fact, although the current diagnostic criteria for autism require that the onset of behaviors that define the condition occur prior to 3 years of age, the mean age of recognition of the condition was closer to 4 years of age (12) in one study and was as late as 6 years of age in an earlier study (13). In addition to not having a precise time of onset, the diagnosis was not confirmed in any of these studies and the investigators did not take into account that the diagnostic criteria for autism that were used changed during the periods of study. Nevertheless, all of these studies, covering birth cohorts from the 1980s and 1990s, report increases over time. However, only carefully designed prospective studies after there was more certainty over how to detect the true biological onset of ASDs would allow us to determine precisely the onset of autism in the population, and thus, the true incidence of the disorder in a given population.

IV. TIME TRENDS IN DEFINED POPULATIONS

From our literature review, we were able to identify only three studies that described trends in autism prevalence *or* incidence within a defined population. In one study, the prevalence was estimated for two French birth cohorts (1972 and 1976) from the same region; no change in prevalence (5.1 and 4.9/10,000 children) occurred over that short period of time (14). In Göteborg, Sweden, the prevalence of autism was estimated for two time periods, 1962–1976 and 1975–1984 (15). Over the 1975–1984 time period, the prevalence increased from 4.0 to 11.6/10,000 children. The Swedish investigators offered a possible explanation for the increase. Rates of autism in children with mild mental retardation remained relatively stable, while the rates increased in children with severe mental retardation (IQ < 50) and in children with normal intelligence (IQ > 70). The investigators postulated that changes in the overall prevalence were influenced by the ability to better identify children with autism with very low as well as normal to high functioning. A third study that examined trends in autism occurrence measured incidence between 1991 and 1996 in preschool children in two areas on the west Midlands, UK, and found that although the rates for classical autism increased by 18% per year, there was a much larger increase for the other ASDs, i.e., 55% per year (8). The investigators attributed this increase in incidence to increased awareness among clinicians rather than to true changes in disease occurrence.

V. PREVALENCE STUDIES

We identified 35 studies that met inclusion criteria in our evaluation of autism point prevalence studies (Table 1). However, only 31 of the studies will be used in our evaluation of the trends in prevalence based on the criteria indicated earlier. The four studies that were excluded are: Hoshino et al., 1982; Fombonne and du Mazaubrun, 1992; Fombonne et al., 2001; and Yeargin-Allsopp et al., 2003. The Hoshino et al. and the Fombonne and du Mazaubrun studies were excluded because only an average prevalence rate was provided, without giving the sample sizes or the prevalence estimates used to derive that average rate. The Fombonne et al. and Yeargin-Allsopp et al. studies were excluded because separate rates for autism and other pervasive developmental disorders (PDDs) were not reported for those studies.

The trends in the prevalence estimates will be discussed in terms of weighted prevalence rates and mean prevalence rates. While the mean rate simply describes the prevalence in terms of the sum of the observed cases divided by the total sample size, the weighted prevalence estimate is derived by pooling the estimates of the individual prevalence studies and then weighting the estimates by the inverse of the variance. In contrast to the mean prevalence rate, the weighted prevalence estimate takes into account the variance heterogeneity that exists among the pooled studies. With the weighting approach, more weight is placed on those studies with larger sample sizes. This approach provides a more accurate portrayal of trends in the prevalence of autism as compared to using the mean rate, which may exaggerate the trends seen in certain populations owing to their size. Because other factors, such as the intensity of follow-up, play a role in the prevalence estimates, both the mean and weighted prevalence rates are described below.

VI. THE EFFECT OF DIAGNOSTIC CRITERIA
ON MEAN PREVALENCE RATES

To discuss the effect of changing diagnostic criteria on the classification of autism and ASDs over time, the evolution of the diagnostic criteria are provided here.

Table 1 Summary of Autism Prevalence Studies

Author	Year published	Country	Time period studied	Age range studied	Number of children in population	Criteria used	Methodology used	Prevalence rate (PR) for autism/other ASD per 10,000	IQ < 70 (%)
Lotter	1966	England	1964	8–10	78,000	Kanner	Case enumeration and direct exam	4.5/—	84
Brask	1970	Denmark	1962	2–14	46,500	Kanner	Case enumeration	4.3/—	NR
Treffert	1970	U.S.A.	1962–1967	3–12	899,750	Kanner	Case enumeration	0.7/2.4	70
Wing and Gould	1979	England	1970	0–14	35,000	Kanner	Case enumeration and direct exam	4.6/15.7	NR
Hoshino et al.[a]	1982	Japan	1977	0–17	234,039	Kanner	Case enumeration and direct exam	5.0/—	NR
Ishii and Takahashi	1983	Japan	1981	6–12	35,000	Rutter	Case enumeration and direct exam	16.0/—	NR
Bohman et al.	1983	Sweden	1979	0–20	69,000	Rutter	Case enumeration and direct exam	3.0/2.6	NR
McCarthy et al.	1984	Ireland	1978	8–10	65,000	Kanner	Case enumeration and direct exam	4.3/—	NR
Gillberg	1984	Sweden	1980	4–18	128,584	DSM-III	Case enumeration and direct exam	2.0/1.9	80,77
Steinhausen et al.	1986	Germany	1982	0–14	279,616	Rutter	Case enumeration and direct exam	1.9/—	44
Steffenberg and Gillberg	1986	Sweden	1984	<10	78,413	DSM-III	Case enumeration and direct exam	4.5/2.2	88
Matsuishi et al.	1987	Japan	1983	4–12	32,834	DSM-III	Case enumeration and direct exam	15.5/—	NR
Burd et al.	1987	U.S.A.	1985	2–18	180,986	DSM-III	Case enumeration and direct exam	1.2/2.1	NR

Bryson et al.	1988	Canada	1985	6–14	20,800	DSM-III	Case enumeration and direct exam	10.1/—	76
Tanoue et al.	1988	Japan	1977–1985	3–7	95,394	DSM-III	Case enumeration	13.8/—	NR
Cialdella and Mamelle	1989	France	1986	3–9	135,180	DSM-III	Case enumeration	5.1/5.2	NR
Sugiyama and Abe	1989	Japan	1979–1984	2–5	12,263	DSM-III	Population screen and direct exam	13.0/—	38
Ritvo et al.	1989	U.S.A.	1984–1988	8–12	184,822	DSM-III	Case enumeration and direct exam	4.0/—	NR
Gillberg et al.	1991	Sweden	1988	4–13	78,106	DSM-III-R	Case enumeration and direct exam	7.0/2.4	82,80
Fombonne and Mazaubrun[a]	1992	France	1985	9–13	274,816	ICD-10	Case enumeration and direct exam	4.9/—	87
Honda et al.	1996	Japan	1994	1.5–6	8,537	ICD-10	Population screen and direct exam	21.1/—	50
Fombonne et al.	1997	France	1992–1993	16–Aug	325,347	ICD-10	Case enumeration and direct exam	5.4/10.9	88
Arvidsson et al.	1997	Sweden	1994	3–6	1,941	ICD-10	Population screen and direct exam	31.0/15.0	100
Webb et al.	1997	Wales	1992	3–15	73,300	DSM-III-R	Case enumeration and direct exam	7.2/—	NR
Sponheim and Skjeldae	1998	Norway	1992	3–14	65,688	ICD-10	Case enumeration and direct exam	3.8/1.4	64
Kadesjo et al.	1999	Sweden	1992	6.7–7.7	826	ICD-10	Case enumeration and direct exam	60.0/60.0	60
Baird et al.	2000	England	1998	1.5–8	16,235	ICD-10	Population screen and direct exam	30.8/27.1	40
Powell et al.	2000	England	1995	1–4	29,200	DSM-III-R or DSM-IV	Case enumeration	9.6/10.6	NR
Kielinen et al.	2000	Finland	1996	18–Mar	152,732	DSM-IV	Case enumeration	12.2/1.2	73

Table 1 Continued

Author	Year published	Country	Time period studied	Age range studied	Number of children in population	Criteria used	Methodology used	Prevalence rate (PR) for autism/other ASD per 10,000	IQ < 70 (%)
Magnusson and Saemundsen	2000	Iceland	1997	5–14	43,153	ICD-10	Population screen and direct exam	8.6/4.6	95/65
Chakrabarti and Fombonne	2001	England	1998	2.5–6.5	15,500	DSM-IV	Population screen and direct exam	16.8/45.8	24,70
Fombonne et al.[b]	2001	UK	1999	5–15	12,529	DSM-IV	Population screen and direct exam	26.1	44
Bertrand et al.	2001	USA	1998	3–10	8,996	DSM-IV	Case enumeration and direct exam	40.0/67.0	49,58
Croen et al.	2001	USA	1987–1999	0–21	4.6 million	DSM-III-R or DSM-IV	Case enumeration	11.0/—	NR
Yeargin-Allsopp et al.[b]	2003	USA	1996	3–10	290,000	DSM-IV	Case enumeration	34	64,68[c]

NR, not reported; MR, mental retardation.
[a]The prevalence rate that is provided represents an average prevalence rate.
[b]The prevalence study provided overall rate only.
[c]64% had MR-based IQ data and 68% had cognitive impairment based on IQ and developmental tests.

Although Kanner recorded brilliant descriptions of the clinical features of autism, it was not until 1956 that he and Eisenberg published the Kanner diagnostic criteria for early infantile autism, which included (16):

1. a profound lack of affective contact with other people;
2. an anxiously obsessive desire for the preservation of sameness in the child's routines and environment;
3. a fascination for objects that are handled with skill in fine motor movements;
4. mutism or a kind of language that does not seem intended for interpersonal communication; and
5. good cognitive potential shown in feats of memory or skills on performance tests, especially the Séguin form board.

Kanner emphasized that the onset had to be from birth and before 30 months of age. In the same paper that listed these criteria, Kanner and Eisenberg modified the criteria by emphasizing that two features were essential for the diagnosis: a profound lack of affective contact and repetitive, ritualistic behaviors, which must be of an elaborate kind.

In 1978 Rutter published his criteria for childhood autism, which included (17):

1. early onset, by 30 months of age;
2. impaired and distinctive social development, i.e., social development that has a number of special characteristics out of keeping with the child's intellectual level;
3. delayed and deviant language development that also has certain defined features and is out of keeping with the child's intellectual level;
4. unusual behaviors, similar to the Kanner concept of "insistence on sameness," as shown by idiosyncratic responses to the environment, stereotyped play patterns, motor mannerisms, abnormal preoccupations, or resistance to change.

The Rutter criteria emphasized that the social and communication difficulties were not just a manifestation of any associated mental retardation.

With the publication of the American Psychiatric Association's third edition of the *Diagnostic and Statistical Manual of Mental Disorders* (DSM-III) in 1980 (18), autism and schizophrenia were differentiated. For the first time, autism was categorized as a developmental disorder, rather than a psychiatric one. Autism was listed under the more general term of PDD and a subgroup under PDD was infantile autism, which had as its features:

1. lack of responsiveness to others;
2. absence or abnormality of language;
3. resistance to change or attachment to objects;

4. absence of schizophrenic features; and
5. onset before 30 months of age.

DSM-III also included childhood-onset PDD (onset after 30 months of age and before 12 years of age) and described a subthreshold condition, atypical PDD.

In 1987 the DSM-III criteria were revised and led to the broadening of the concept of PDD. The concept of autism as a spectrum of disorders was first described by Wing and Gould in 1979 (19) and was likely influenced by the work of Hans Asperger, whose writings describing related behaviors did not become well known in the English literature until the 1980s (20). These writings introduced the concept of Asperger disorder, which represents behaviors that vary widely in their presentation as well as severity. These descriptions may have contributed to the changes seen with the revision of the DSM-III (21), which is referred to as the DSM-III-R. In this revision, the PDD category was retained but the subgroups were divided into autistic disorder and PDD-NOS and the age requirement was dropped. The DSM-III-R diagnostic criteria for autistic disorder were (21):

1. impairment in reciprocal social interaction (at least two from a list of five items);
2. impairment in verbal and nonverbal communication (at least one item from a list of six items);
3. markedly restricted repertoire of activities and interests (at least one from a list of five items);
4. a total of at least eight from among a list of 16 items.

The term PDD-NOS was used to refer to a qualitative impairment in the development of reciprocal social interaction and of verbal and nonverbal communication skills, but when criteria for autistic disorder, schizophrenia, or schizotypal or schizoid personality disorder were not met. It was also noted that some individuals with PDD-NOS will exhibit a markedly restricted repertoire of activities and interests (21).

With the fourth revision of the DSM, additional subgroups of PDD were described: autistic disorder, childhood disintegrative disorder, Rett disorder, Asperger disorder, and PDD-NOS (22). The diagnostic criteria for autistic disorder were revised and included:

A total of at least six items from (1), (2), and (3), with at least two from (1), and one each from (2) and (3):

1. qualitative impairments in social interaction;
2. qualitative impairments in communication;
3. restricted repetitive and stereotyped patterns of behavior, interests and activities.

In addition, there must be delays or abnormal functioning in at least one of these areas: (1) social interaction; (2) language; or (3) symbolic or imaginative play, and the behaviors cannot be due to Rett's disorder or childhood disintegrative disorder. DSM-IV also described research criteria for the subgroups.

The *International Classification of Diseases, Tenth Revision* (ICD-10), which was introduced in 1992 (23), has diagnostic and research criteria for autism overall and for the subgroups that are very similar to the PDD subgroups in DSM-IV. The umbrella term in ICD-10 is pervasive developmental disorders and the subgroups are childhood autism, which has diagnostic criteria similar to autistic disorder; atypical autism, which has criteria similar to PDD-NOS; and Rett's syndrome and other childhood disintegrative disorder, both of which have criteria similar to the criteria for these disorders in DSM-IV.

An examination of the 31 prevalence studies from 1966 to 2003 showed that the five studies that used the Kanner diagnostic criteria yielded a weighted prevalence rate of 0.9/10,000 and a mean prevalence of 3.9/10,000 (2–4,19,24). The three studies that used the Rutter criteria showed a slight increase in prevalence, with a weighted prevalence of 2.2/10,000 and a mean prevalence of 7.0/10,000 (25–27). The prevalence of autism increased further after the introduction of the DSM-III and, particularly, the DSM-III-R criteria as seen by the weighted (2.7 and 7.1/10,000) and mean prevalence rates (8.3 and 7.1/10,000), respectively (28–38). While the weighted prevalence rate decreased slightly to 5.5/10,000 with the introduction of the ICD-10 criteria, the weighted prevalence rate increased substantially with the introduction of the DSM-IV criteria, 13/10,000. The trend using the mean rates shows a very large increase in the mean prevalence reported from the 10 studies that used the ICD-10 and DSM-IV criteria, 21 and 23/10,000, respectively, as compared to previous investigations that used other diagnostic criteria (39–48). Two studies that used other criteria had a weighted prevalence of 10.9/10,000 and a mean prevalence of 10.3/10,000 (Fig. 1) (8,49). In summary, while there is a large difference in the

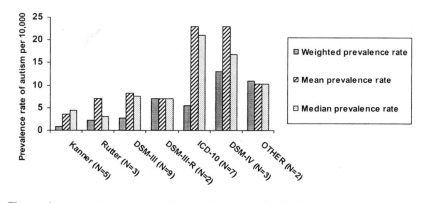

Figure 1   Trend in prevalence of autism by diagnostic criteria.

mean prevalence rates of studies that used DSM-IV or ICD-10 diagnostic criteria as compared with Kanner, Rutter, DSM-III, or DSM-III-R diagnostic criteria, the weighted prevalence shows a less exaggerated difference in the prevalence by diagnostic criteria, but more accurately shows the rise in prevalence based on the criteria that have been used over time. Further, these data support the notion that the broadening of the case definition at the time that the DSM-III or DSM-III-R was introduced may have contributed to the rise in prevalence seen in more recent investigations.

VII. THE RELATIONSHIP OF TIME PERIOD STUDIED TO PREVALENCE RATE

We examined trends in the weighted and mean prevalence rates of the 31 studies by time period studied. For the studies that reported period or birth prevalence rates over a specific range of time, we took the midpoint of that range of time to represent the year studied. For the studies that did not provide such information, we identified the study year as 2 years prior to the year of publication (31,44).

If we examine the weighted and mean prevalence rates of the 31 studies by year studied, there is an increasing trend over the four decades of published reports, with an exception in the weighted prevalence rate for those investigations that took place from 1980 to 1989 (Fig. 2). The weighted prevalence was 0.9/ 10,000 for the three studies published between 1960 and 1969 (2–4); 3.8/10,000 for the three investigations that were studied between 1970 and 1979 (19,24,26); 2.6/10,000 for the 12 studies that were conducted between 1980 and 1989 (25,27–37); and 10.1/10,000 for the 13 studies that were conducted between

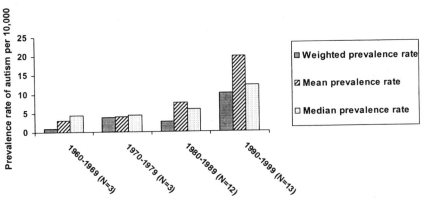

Figure 2   Trend in prevalence of autism by time period studied.

1990 and 1999 (8,38–49). The mean rates that were established for each decade that the studies were conducted show a similar pattern as the trend seen with the weighted prevalence estimates; however, larger differences are seen in the mean rates from one decade to the next. The mean prevalence rate ranges from 3.1 in the 1960s to 19.8 in the 1990s (Fig. 2). These data, showing the rise in prevalence by time period of study, may be reflective of the changing diagnostic criteria used over these four decades, but may also be reflective of other factors such as increased awareness and diagnosis of the disorder.

VIII. THE EFFECT OF POPULATION SIZE ON PREVALENCE RATE

As has been noted by Fombonne (50), when we examine the mean prevalence rates of the 31 studies by size of population (denominator), there is a trend toward higher prevalence rates in smaller populations. The weighted prevalence for studies with a population size of 100,000 or more children was 3.3/10,000, while the mean rate was 5.5/10,000 (4,27,28,31,34,36,40,45,49); for the one study with a population in the range of 80,000–99,999 (33), both the weighted and mean prevalence rate was 13.8/10,000. The lowest weighted and mean prevalence rates are seen in populations of 40,000–59,999 (weighted prevalence, 5.7/10,000 and mean prevalence, 6.4/10,000) (3,46) and 60,000–79,999 (weighted prevalence, 4.6/10,000 and mean prevalence, 4.9/10,000) (2,24,26,29,37,38,42). The weighted and mean prevalence starts to increase as the population becomes smaller, with a weighted prevalence of 9.2/10,000 and a mean prevalence of 11.2/10,000 for studies with a population of 20,000–39,999 (8,19,25,30,32). The prevalence is highest in the seven studies that had a population size of 0–19,999 children, with a weighted prevalence of 20.8 and a mean prevalence

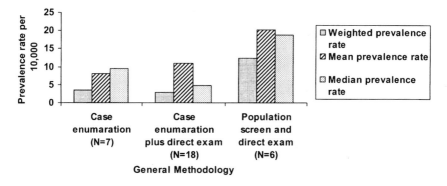

Figure 3   Trend in prevalence rate by case ascertainment methodology used.

of 30.4/10,000 (Fig. 3) (35,39,41,43,44,47,48). Based on these rates, we found that both the weighted and mean prevalence rates of studies using a population size of less than 20,000 individuals as the denominator were higher than those with a population of 100,000 or more. This finding supports the argument that more intensive surveillance for autism and its spectrum of disorders is possible in smaller populations and, therefore, may lead to greater identification of children; hence, the higher prevalence of the disorder in these study areas.

IX. THE EFFECT OF METHOD OF CASE ASCERTAINMENT ON PREVALENCE RATES

Of the 31 studies that were included in the review, over half (58%) of the investigators identified the cases using case enumeration, based on record review or surveys of a given population, followed by clinical examination of the children. For studies that used this methodology, a weighted prevalence of 2.9/10,000 and a mean prevalence of 10.9/10,000 was found (2,19,24–32,36–38,40,42,43,48). However, although the number of studies using case enumeration only ($N = 7$) (3,4,8,33,34,45,49) was almost the same as the number of studies using population screening followed by clinical examination ($N = 6$) (35,39,41,44,46,47), the weighted and mean prevalence rate of the studies using population screening and direct examination was higher than those using case enumeration only (Fig. 4). The weighted and mean prevalence estimates among the studies that used population screening and direct

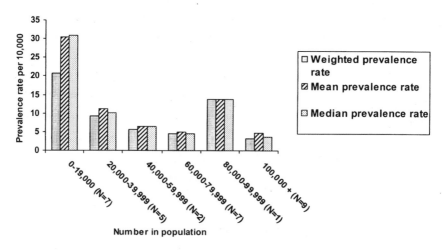

Figure 4   Trend in prevalence rate for autism by number in population.

examination were 12.4 and 20.2/10,000, respectively, while the weighted and mean rates for the studies that used case enumeration were only 3.6 and 8.1/10,000, respectively. It is worth noting that studies that used the method of population screening and direct examination were also those that had smaller study populations. Therefore, this method may have been more plausible in such populations and, again, reinforces the notion that perhaps, it is possible to do a more intensive and comprehensive survey in these populations, leading to a greater number of individuals identified with autism or ASD.

X. RISK FACTORS FOR AUTISM

The vast majority of autism cases are idiopathic, and no specific causal factor has been identified for ASDs. It is clear from twin (51–54) and family studies (55–58) that there is a substantive heritable component to ASDs. Although there is some consistent indication that suceptability genes may reside on chromosomes 7q (59–63) and 15q (64–67), no putative autism gene has been identified. At the same time, few nonheritable factors have been implicated in autism etiology. However, as much of the existing research on nonheritable factors are small studies with case groups defined under older, more restrictive diagnostic criteria, the evidence base ruling out particular factors of theoretical appeal is also quite weak. Nonheritable risk factors have increasingly become of concern in recent years owing to the apparent rise in autism prevalence. Should the prevalence increase prove to be attributable in part to a real increase in risk, this short-term fluctuation suggests the influence of a nonheritable as opposed to a heritable risk factor or factors. The remainder of this section discusses each class of potential nonheritable risk factors.

XI. OCCUPATIONAL EXPOSURES

Parental occupational exposures prior to conception have been reported to be associated with autism in two small, retrospective studies completed in the 1970s and 1980s. The parents self-reported exposures to chemicals and both studies found statistically significant associations with ASDs in the offspring (68,69). In the 1990s, a larger study was initiated in Leominster, Massachusetts, when ASDs appeared to be clustered among parents who resided near plastic manufacturing plants in the past, before conception of the affected child (70). The Massachusetts Department of Public Health followed up on this initial report by attempting to locate additional cases and reviewing a chromosomal study of the initial cases. They issued a report with the conclusion that further investigations were not warranted since their estimated prevalence of children with ASDs among former and current residents of Leominster was 7.6/10,000 (71). This estimated prevalence was lower than the generally accepted population prevalence of that time, which was 10–15/10,000.

XII. ENVIRONMENTAL EXPOSURES

Another cluster of ASD cases was investigated in the 1990s in the New Jersey community of Brick Township, but the concern was prenatal and postnatal exposure to environmental chemicals. Unlike Leominster, however, the prevalence of autistic disorder in Brick Township was higher than expected, 4/1000. After examining potential exposures such as swimming in the river, the local landfill, and drinking water, the Agency for Toxic Substances and Disease Registry reported "no apparent public health hazard" from these sources (72,73). Levels of chemicals in the river were not sufficient to cause adverse health effects. Trihalomethanes, tetrachloroethylene, and trichloroethylene were measured in the drinking water, but the sites and times of high measurements did not correspond with the residences of the cases during the study period.

XIII. XENOBIOTICS

A. Thalidomide

The discovery of a high prevalence of autism among a thalidomide-exposed cohort and subsequent follow-up of the autism subjects has established that prenatal xenobiotic exposure, defined as chemicals foreign to the body, can cause autism (74). In the mid-1990s a small, retrospective study of thalidomide embryopathy (75) first reported a higher-than-expected number of autism cases among a cohort prenatally exposed to the drug. The autism cases were all exposed between days 20 and 24 of gestation, the period when the neural tube is formed (76). Although today thalidomide exposure is not an important autism etiological factor since the drug is only approved for use in extremely limited circumstances, other in utero exposures during this critical window of embryonic development may play a role in autism etiology.

B. Other Pharmaceuticals

Other prenatal and intrapartum pharmaceutical agents have not shown such a strong correlation with autism as thalidomide, but the epidemiological evidence is limited. A few case reports point to prenatal use of valproic acid and other anticonvulsants as a possible cause of autism (77–79), but published epidemiological studies on this suggested link were not found. Interestingly, up to 30% of ASDs cases have comorbid epilepsy (80–82), and anticonvulsants appear to ameliorate ASD symptoms among nonepileptic children (83–85).

Two relatively large case-control studies, each with at least 50 cases, examined any prenatal medication use. One study, based on self-reporting, showed a slight increase in use among the ASDs group (86), but the other study, based on obstetrical records review, did not find any association (87). Epidemiological evidence on use of labor-inducing drugs and risk for autism is just as mixed. A 10-year birth cohort from four hospitals in Japan had twice the prevalence of autistic disorder from one hospital that routinely used labor-inducing drugs as well as more frequent use of general anesthesia, sedatives, and analgesics compared to the three other hospitals. In contrast, a case-control study of 180 children with ASDs that used two control groups—language impaired and cognitively impaired—found similar prevalences of labor induction (about 20%) among all groups. Two other relatively large case-control studies had conflicting results—one finding a significant difference in labor induction rates between the autism group and the general population (29% vs. 16%, respectively) (88) and the other finding no association with labor induction in 17% of both the autistic probands and their nonautistic siblings (87).

C. Vaccines

Beginning in the late 1990s, exposures via childhood vaccination, particularly the measles-mumps-rubella (MMR) vaccine and the ethylmercury-containing vaccine preservative thimerosal, have received considerable attention in both the scientific and lay media as potential autism risk factors. The epidemiological evidence that has since accumulated with respect to MMR has been consistent in showing no association with ASD risk (9–11,89–92). Fewer epidemiological studies have been able to assess thimerosal exposure. One unpublished analysis, based on CDC's Vaccine Safety Datalink, found no significant association (93). Reports on mercury-poisoned populations and populations with long-term low-dose methylmercury exposure have been reviewed and no unusual observations were found with regard to more frequent occurrence of autism (7). Further, the characteristic pathological features of brains of individuals with methylmercury poisoning do not appear to match those of the brains of persons with autism (7) and the toxicokinetics of ethyl- and methylmercury may differ with indications being that ethylmercury could be more efficiently eliminated (94).

XIV. INFECTIONS

A. Maternal

One of the earliest published reports of prenatal maternal infection possibly being associated with ASDs was a 1971 study of 243 preschool children with congenital rubella, 18 of whom had ASDs (95). In a follow-up report, however, six of the 18 ASD cases were reclassified so that only 12 of the 243 children had ASDs. A few other case reports of ASDs following prenatal maternal infection with herpes simplex, rubeola, syphilis, and varicella-zoster have been published (96).

Using a broader definition of infection exposure status, which includes documented fever in medical records to self-report of an ill person in the home, Deykin and MacMahon (97) analyzed maternal infection during pregnancy and found significantly increased risk of having a child with ASD following exposure to measles, mumps, rubella, and influenza. Other studies with broadly defined infection measures have not reported statistically significant associations, although risks were elevated in infection-exposed groups (86–88).

B. Child

Several published case studies describe sudden onset of autistic symptoms, or regressive autism, in older children after contracting herpes encephalitis (98–100). Secondary hydrocephalus (e.g., from bacterial meningitis) as a precursor to late-onset autism has also been reported in a few cases (98,100,101). Others have implicated the viral or bacterial infection, rather than the secondary hydrocephalus, as the pathogenic factor in autism (97,102,103). Deykin and MacMahon (97), using the broad definition of exposure as being in a household with another person who is infected during the first 18 months of the subject's life, found more autism cases exposed to mumps, chickenpox, herpes, and fever of unknown origin than their control siblings. The relative risks for autism when there was actual clinical illness during the first 18 months of life, after adjustment for sibship size, were even higher. These illnesses included measles, mumps, rubella, chickenpox, CNS infections, influenza, ear infections, and fever of unknown origin.

XV. PERINATAL COMPLICATIONS

No individual perinatal complication has emerged as a clear autism risk factor. Given the small sample sizes of many autism studies, another approach to studying perinatal risk factors is to consider combinations of perinatal events and factors as representing a pathophysiological cascade having a common source. This approach has been borrowed from other areas of perinatal research, producing a composite "optimality" score for pregnancy and delivery. Perinatal complications, or suboptimal conditions, may include maternal diabetes, neonatal respiratory distress (104), placental insufficiency (105), and frequency of intercourse during pregnancy (106). Optimality scores are generally heterogeneous, a combination of antepartum, intrapartum, and even postpartum factors into a single measure. While this approach may be valid as an indicator of perinatal mortality risk, it may not be appropriate for inferring autism risk. Some published studies using this approach, however, have found lower optimality scores among autism cases than controls (32,104,107,108), while others have not found any association between obstetric optimality and autism risk (109–111).

XVI. SUMMARY

Epidemiology is a tool that is useful for describing the occurrence of and risk factors for a disease or condition in human populations. In this chapter, we have described the epidemiology, specifically measures of occurrence, trends over time, and risk factors for autism and ASDs.

The most commonly used measure of disease frequency for most developmental disabilities, including autism, is prevalence, which has been used to approximate incidence because measurement of the true incidence of autism is problematic. Since the 1960s, with the conduct of the first prevalence studies of autism, a solid body of literature examining the prevalence of autism from population-based studies has been accumulating. We conducted a literature review and identified 35 population-based prevalence studies of autism/ASD, which we organized by diagnostic criteria, time period, size of population, and method of ascertainment in an attempt to better understand trends in autism prevalence over time; however, only 31 of the studies met our criteria for inclusion in the examination of possible trends.

When we examined trends in prevalence by diagnostic criteria used over time, we found that while there is a large difference in the mean prevalence rates of studies that used DSM-IV or ICD-10 diagnostic criteria as compared with other criteria, this trend toward increased prevalence rates based on use of these diagnostic criteria persisted, although the pattern was attenuated when weighted prevalence rates were used. When the 31 studies were examined by the year of study, overall, we found that the prevalence rates increased over time; however, the exact influences on such apparent trends cannot be easily elucidated. As noted previously, there seems to be a trend toward higher prevalence rates associated with smaller study populations. We were able to confirm this observation; i.e., we found that both the weighted and mean prevalence rates of studies with denominators of 20,000 or less yielded higher prevalence rates than study populations of 100,000 or more. The type of case ascertainment method is also believed to influence prevalence rates. Examining the 31 studies, we found that studies that used population screening followed by direct examination yielded higher rates than those using case enumeration only.

At this point there is no strong body of evidence supporting any specific nonheritable autism risk factor. However, it may be premature to interpret the lack of evidence in support of environmental and other nonheritable risk factors as being equivalent to strong evidence against their existence. Studies of autism risk factors completed to date have, for the most part, been conducted on small, select populations of cases and have often involved quite flawed exposure assessment approaches. Further, the fact that research attempting to fit models of inheritance to family data have not yet been able to characterize the familiality of autism suggests strongly that the etiological mechanism behind the disorder is quite complex. It is known from these studies, as well as others of chromosomal abnormalities and genetic conditions associated with autism, that there is undoubtedly a major genetic component to autism. One explanation consistent with this and the fact that no inheritance model appears to fit the family data is that genetic and nongenetic factors may interact—with certain nongenetic factors increasing risk only when key predisposing genes are present. If this is the case, not only will future epidemiological studies investigating nonheritable autism risk factors need to be of larger size and stronger design, they will also need to be able to look for these factors within strata defined by level of genetic susceptibility. This may require knowing the actual susceptibility genes but it may be possible to categorize by phenotypic markers for these genotypes before they are actually known. Either way, the challenges facing autism risk factor epidemiology are substantial but not insurmountable as genetic research proceeds apace and new efforts are now underway to conduct large, population-based studies of autism.

Our understanding of the prevalence of autism, trends in prevalence over time, and identification of specific genetic and environmental risk factors will be enhanced by our efforts to assemble large numbers of cases using the same case definitions and study methods over time and our ability to accurately classify these cases into relatively homogeneous grouping for further study of a range of pre-, peri-, and postnatal factors. Only by using the most rigorous scientific study methods will we be able to make significant progress in our understanding of this complex disorder.

REFERENCES

1. Kanner L. Autistic disturbances of affective contact. Nervous Child 1943; 2: 217–250.
2. Lotter V. Epidemiology of autistic conditions in young children: some characteristics of the parents and children. Soc Psychiatry 1966; 1:124–137.

3. Brask B. In: Nordic Symposium on the Comprehensive Care of Psychotic Children. Oslo, Norway: Barnepsykiatrisk, 1972:145–153.
4. Treffert D. Epidemiology of infantile autism. Arch Gen Psychiatry 1970; 22:431–438.
5. American Psychiatric Association. 1994. Diagnostic and Statistical Manual of Mental Disorders. 4th ed. Washington, DC: APA:65–78.
6. De Giacomo A, Fombonne E. Parental recognition of developmental abnormalities in autism. Eur Child Adolesc Psychiatry J 1998; 7:131–136.
7. Nelson K, Bauman M. Thimerosal and autism. Pediatrics 2003; 11:674–679.
8. Powell JE, Edwards A, Edwards M, Pandit BS, Sungum-Paliwal SR, Whitehouse W. Changes in the incidence of childhood autism and other autistic spectrum disorders in preschool children from two areas of the West Midlands, UK. Dev Med Child Neurol 2000; 42:624–628.
9. Taylor B, Miller E, Farrington CP, et al. Autism and measles, mumps, and rubella vaccine: no epidemiological evidence for a causal association. Lancet 1999; 353:2026–2029.
10. Kaye JA, del Mar Melero-Montes M, Jick H. Mumps, measles, and rubella vaccine and the incidence of autism recorded by general practitioners: a time trend analysis. Br Med J 2001; 322:460–463.
11. Dales L, Hammer SJ, Smith NJ. Time trends in autism and in MMR immunization coverage in California. JAMA 2001; 285:1183–1185.
12. Yeargin-Allsopp M, Rice C, Karapurkar T, Doernberg N, Boyle C, Murphy C. The prevalence of autism in a US metropolitan area. JAMA 2003.
13. Howlin P, Moore A. Diagnosis of autism: a survey of over 1200 patients in the UK. Autism 1997; 1:135–162.
14. Fombonne E, du Mazaubrun C. Prevalence of infantile autism in four French regions. Social Psychiatry Psychiatr Epidemiol 1992; 27:203–210.
15. Gillberg C, Wing L. Autism: not an extremely rare disorder. Acta Psychiatr Scand 1999; 99:399–406.
16. Kanner L, Eisenberg L. Early infantile autism 1943–1955. Am J Orthopsychiatry 1956; 26:55–65.
17. Rutter M. Diagnosis and definition. In: Rutter M, Schopler E, eds. Autism: A Reappraisal of Concepts and Treatment. New York: Plenum Press, 1978:1–25.
18. American Psychiatric Association. Diagnostic and Statistical Manual of Mental Disorders. 3rd ed. Washington, DC: APA, 1980:87–92.
19. Wing L, Gould J. Severe impairments of social interaction and associated abnormalities in children: epidemiology and classification. J Autism Dev Disord 1979; 9:11–29.
20. Asperger H. "Autistic psychopathy" in childhood. Translated and annotated by U. Frith. In: Frith U, ed. Autism and Asperger Syndrome. Cambridge: Cambridge University Press. 1944/1991:37–92.
21. American Psychiatric Association. Diagnostic and Statistical Manual of Mental Disorders, 3rd ed. Revised. Washington, DC: APA, 1987.
22. American Psychiatric Association. Diagnostic and Statistical Manual of Mental Disorders, 4th ed. Washington, DC: APA; 1994.

23. World Health Organization. International Statistical Classification of Diseases and Related Health Problems. 10th revision, Clinical Modification, ICD-10. Geneva, Switzerland: World Health Organization, 1992.

24. McCarthy P, Fitzgerald M, Smith M. Prevalence of childhood autism in Ireland. Irish Med J 1984; 77:129–130.

25. Ishi T, Takahashi O. The epidemiology of autistic children in Toyota, Japan: Prevalence. Jpn J Child Adolesc Psychiatry 1983; 24:311–321.

26. Bohman M, Bohman I, Bjorck P, et al. Childhood psychosis in a northern Swedish county: some preliminary findings from an epidemiological survey. In: Schmidt M, Remschmidt H, eds. Epidemiological Approaches in Child Psychiatry: II. New York: Thieme-Stratton, 1983:164–173.

27. Steinhausen H, Gobel D, Breinlinger M, et al. A community survey of infantile autism. J Am Acad Child Psychiatry 1986; 25:189–189.

28. Gillberg C. Infantile autism and other childhood psychoses in a Swedish urban region: epidemiological aspects. J Child Psychol Psychiatry 1984; 25:45–43.

29. Steffenburg S, Gillberg C. Autism and autistic-like conditions in Swedish rural and urban areas: a population study. Br J Psychiatry 1986; 149:81–87.

30. Matsuishi T, Shiotsuki Y, Yoshimura K, et al. High prevalence of infantile autism in Kurume City, Japan. J Child Neurol 1987; 2:268–271.

31. Burd L, Fisher W, Kerbeshian J. A prevalence study of pervasive developmental disorders in North Dakota. J Am Acad Child Adolesc Psychiatry 1987; 26:704–710.

32. Bryson S, Clark B, Smith IM. First report of a Canadian epidemiological study of autistic syndromes. J Child Psychol Psychiatry 1988; 29:433–446.

33. Tanoue Y, Oda S, Asano F, et al. Epidemiology of infantile autism in the Southern Ibaraki, Japan. J Autism Dev Disord 1988; 18:155–167.

34. Cialdella P, Mamelle N. An epidemiological study of infantile autism in a French Department Rhone: a research note. J Child Psychol Psychiatry 1989; 30:165–176.

35. Sugiyama T, Abe T. The prevalence of autism in Nagoya, Japan: a total population study. J Autism Dev Disord 1989; 19:87–96.

36. Ritvo E, Freeman B, Pingree C, et al. The UCLA–University of Utah epidemiological study of autism: prevalence. Am J Psychiatry 1989; 146:194–245.

37. Gillberg C. Outcome in autism and autistic-like conditions. J Am Acad Child Adolesc Psychiatry 1991; 30:375–382.

38. Webb E, Thompson W, Morey J, et al. A prevalence study of Asperger syndrome and high functioning autism. J Intellect Disabil Res 2000; 44:513.

39. Honda H, Shimizu Y, Misumi K, et al. Cumulative incidence and prevalence of childhood autism in children in Japan. Br J Psychiatry 1996; 169:228–235.

40. Fombonne E, du Mazaubrun C, Cans C, et al. Autism and associated medical disorders in a French epidemiological survey. J Am Acad Child Adolesc Psychiatry 1997; 36:1561–1569.

41. Arvidsson T, Danielsson B, Forsberg P, et al. Autism in 3–6 year-old children in a suburb of Goteborg, Sweden. Autism 1997; 1:163–171.

42. Sponheim E, Skjeldal O. Autism and related disorders: epidemiological findings in a Norwegian study using ICD-10 diagnostic criteria. J Autism Dev Disord 1998; 28:217–228.

43. Kadesjö B, Gillberg C, Hagberg B. Brief report. Autism and Asperger syndrome in seven-year-old children. J Autism Dev Disord 1999; 29:327–332.
44. Baird G, Charman T, Baron-Cohen S, et al. A screening instrument for autism at 18 months of age: a 6 year follow-up study. J Am Acad Child Adolesc Psychiatry 2000; 39:694–702.
45. Kielinen M, Linna S, Moilanen I. Austism Northern Finland. Eur Child Adolesc Psychiatry 2000; 9:162–167.
46. Mágnússon P, Sæmundsen E. Prevalence of autism in Iceland. J Autism Dev Disord 2001; 31:153–163.
47. Chakrabarti S, Fombonne E. Pervasive developmental disorder in preschool children. JAMA 2001; 285:3093–3099.
48. Bertrand J, Mars A, Boyle C, et al. Prevalence of autism in a United States population: the Brick Township, New Jersey, investigation. Pediatrics 2001; 108:1155–1161.
49. Croen L, Grether J, Hoogstrate J, et al. The changing prevalence of autism in California. J Autism Dev Disord 2001; 32:207–215.
50. Fombonne E. The epidemiology of autism: a review. Psychol Med 1999; 29:769–786.
51. Folstein S, Rutter M. Infantile autism: a genetic study of 21 twin pairs. J Child Psychol Psychiatry 1977; 18(4):297–321.
52. Ritvo ER, Freeman BJ, Mason-Brothers A, Mo A, Ritvo AM. Concordance for the syndrome of autism in 40 pairs of afflicted twins. Am J Psychiatry 1985; 142(1):74–77.
53. Steffenburg S, Gillberg C, Hellgren L, Andersson L, Gillberg IC, Jakobsson G, et al. A twin study of autism in Denmark, Finland, Iceland, Norway and Sweden. J Child Psychol Psychiatry 1989; 30(3):405–416.
54. Bailey A, Le Couteur A, Gottesman I, Bolton P, Simonoff E, Yuzda E, et al. Autism as a strongly genetic disorder: evidence from a British twin study. Psychol Med 1995; 25(1):63–77.
55. Smalley SL, Asarnow RF, Spence MA. Autism and genetics: a decade of research. Arch Gen Psychiatry 1988; 45(10):953–961.
56. Jorde LB, Hasstedt SJ, Ritvo ER, Mason-Brothers A, Freeman BJ, Pingree C, et al. Complex segregation analysis of autism. Am J Hum Genet 1991; 49(5):932–938.
57. Ritvo ER, Jorde LB, Mason-Brothers A, Freeman BJ, Pingree C, Jones MB, et al. The UCLA–University of Utah epidemiologic survey of autism: recurrence risk estimates and genetic counseling. Am J Psychiatry 1989; 146(8):1032–1036.
58. Jorde LB, Mason-Brothers A, Waldmann R, Ritvo ER, Freeman BJ, Pingree C, et al. The UCLA–University of Utah epidemiologic survey of autism: genealogical analysis of familial aggregation. Am J Med Genet 1990; 36(1):85–88.
59. Philippe A, Martinez M, Guilloud-Bataille M, Gillberg C, Rastam M, Sponheim E, et al. Genome-wide scan for autism susceptibility genes. Paris Autism Research International Sibpair Study. Hum Mol Genet 1999; 8(5):805–812.
60. A genomewide screen for autism: strong evidence for linkage to chromosomes 2q, 7q, and 16p. International Molecular Genetic Study of Autism Consortium. Am J Hum Genet 2001; 69(3):570–581.

61. Risch N, Spiker D, Lotspeich L, Nouri N, Hinds D, Hallmayer J, et al. A genomic screen of autism: evidence for a multilocus etiology. Am J Hum Genet 1999; 65(2):493–507.
62. Further characterization of the autism susceptibility locus AUTS1 on chromosome 7q. Hum Mol Genet 2001; 10(9):973–982.
63. An autosomal genomic screen for autism. Am J Med Genet 2001; 105(8):609–615.
64. Martinsson T, Johannesson T, Vujic M, Sjostedt A, Steffenburg S, Gillberg C, et al. Maternal origin of inv dup(15) chromosomes in infantile autism. Eur Child Adolesc Psychiatry 1996; 5(4):185–192.
65. Cook EH Jr, Lindgren V, Leventhal BL, Courchesne R, Lincoln A, Shulman C, et al. Autism or atypical autism in maternally but not paternally derived proximal 15q duplication. Am J Hum Genet 1997; 60(4):928–934.
66. Schroer RJ, Phelan MC, Michaelis RC, Crawford EC, Skinner SA, Cuccaro M, et al. Autism and maternally derived aberration of chromosome 15q. Am J Med Genet 1998; 76(4):327–333.
67. Wassink TH, Piven J, Patil SR. Chromosomal abnormalities in a clinic sample of individuals with autistic disorder. Psychiatr Genet 2001; 11(2):57–63.
68. The Autistic Syndromes. New York: American Elsevier Publishing Company, 1976.
69. Felicetti T. Parents of autistic children: some notes on a chemical connection. Milieu Ther 1981; 1(1):13–16.
70. Spiker D, Lotspeich L, Hallmayer J, Kraemer H, Ciaranello RD. Failure to find cytogenetic abnormalities in autistic children whose parents grew up near plastics manufacturing sites. J Autism Dev Disord 1993; 23(4):681–682.
71. Massachusetts Department of Public Health. Leominster Environment and Health Investigation. Boston, MA: Environmental Epidemiology Program, Bureau of Environmental Health Assessment, Massachusetts Department of Public Health. 6-12-0002, 1997.
72. Agency for Toxic Substances and Disease Registry. Chemical specific consultation: hazardous substance exposures and autism. Atlanta, GA, Agency for Toxic Substances and Disease Registry, Division of Toxicology, Emergency Response and Scientific Assessment Branch. 2-18-0002, 1999.
73. Agency for Toxic Substances and Disease Registry. Public health assessment: Brick Township investigation, Brick Township, Ocean County, New Jersey. 11-29-2000. Atlanta, GA, Agency for Toxic Substances and Disease Registry, Division of Health Assessment and Consultation, Superfund Site Assessment Branch. 6-13-2000.
74. London E, Etzel RA. The environment as an etiologic factor in autism: a new direction for research. Environ Health Perspect 2000; 108(suppl 3):401–404.
75. Stromland K, Nordin V, Miller M, Akerstrom B, Gillberg C. Autism in thalidomide embryopathy: a population study. Dev Med Child Neurol 1994; 36(4):351–356.
76. Rodier PM, Ingram JL, Tisdale B, Nelson S, Romano J. Embryological origin for autism: developmental anomalies of the cranial nerve motor nuclei. J Comp Neurol 1996; 370(2):247–261.

77. Moore SJ, Turnpenny P, Quinn A, Glover S, Lloyd DJ, Montgomery T, et al. A clinical study of 57 children with fetal anticonvulsant syndromes. J Med Genet 2000; 37:489–497.
78. Williams G, King J, Cunningham M, Stephan M, Kern B, Hersh JH. Fetal valproate syndrome and autism: additional evidence of an association. Dev Med Child Neurol 2001; 43:202–206.
79. Bescoby-Chambers N, Forster P, Bates G. Foetal valproate syndrome and autism: additional evidence of an association. Dev Med Child Neurol 2001; 43:847–848.
80. Deykin EY, MacMahon B. The incidence of seizures among children with autistic symptoms. Am J Psychiatry 1979; 136(10):1310–1312.
81. Bryson SE, Smith IE. Epidemiology of autism: prevalence, associated characteristics, and implications for research and service delivery. Ment Retard Dev Disabil Res Rev 1998; 4:97–103.
82. Berney TP. Autism-an evolving concept. Br J Psychiatry 2000; 176:20–25.
83. DiMartino A, Tuchman RF. Antiepileptic drugs: affective use in autism spectrum disorders. Pediatr Neurol 2001; 25(3):199–207.
84. Hollander E, Dolgoff-Kaspar R, Cartwright C, Rawitt R, Novotny S. An open trial of divalproex sodium in autism spectrum disorders. J Clin Psychiatry 2001; 62(7):530–534.
85. Plioplys AV. Autism: electroencephalogram abnormalities and clinical improvement with valproic acid. Arch Pediatr Adolesc Med 1994; 148(2):220–222.
86. Deykin EY, MacMahon B. Pregnancy, delivery, and neonatal complications among autistic children. Am J Dis Child 1980; 134:860–864.
87. Mason-Brothers A, Ritvo ER, Pingree C, Petersen PB, Jenson WR, McMahon WM, et al. The UCLA-University of Utah epidemiologic survey of autism: prenatal, perinatal, and postnatal factors. Pediatrics 1990; 86(4):514–519.
88. Juul-Dam N, Townsend J, Courchesne E. Prenatal, perinatal, and neonatal factors in autism, pervasive developmental disorder-not otherwise specified, and the general population. Pediatrics 2001; 107(4):E63.
89. Madsen KM, Hvid A, Vestergaard M, Schendel D, Wohlfahrt J, Thorsen P, et al. A population-based study of measles, mumps, and rubella vaccination and autism. N Engl J Med 2002; 347(19):1477–1482.
90. Fombonne E, Chakrabarti. No evidence for a new variant of measles-mumps-rubella-induced autism. Pediatrics 2001; 108(4):URL: http://www.pediatrics.org/cgi/content/full/108/4/e58
91. Gillberg C, Heijbel H. MMR and autism. Autism 1998; 2(4):423–424.
92. Farrington CP, Miller E, Taylor B. MMR and autism: further evidence against a causal association. Vaccine 2001; 19:3632–3635.
93. Institute of Medicine, Board on Health Promotion and Disease Prevention, Immunization Safety Review Committee. Immunization Safety Review: Thimerosal-Containing Vaccines and Neurodevelopmental Disorders. Washington, DC: National Academy Press, 2001.
94. Pichichero ME, Cernichiari E, Lopreiato J, Treanor J. Mercury concentrations and metabolism in infants receiving vaccines containing thiomersal: a descriptive study. Lancet 2002; 360(9347):1737–1741.

95. Chess S. Autism in children with congenital rubella. J Autism Child Schizophr 1971; 1(1):33–47.
96. Gillberg C, Coleman M. Infectious Diseases. The Biology of the Autistic Syndromes. London: Mac Keith Press, 1992:218–225.
97. Deykin EY, MacMahon B. Viral exposure and autism. Am J Epidemiol 1979; 109(6):628–638.
98. Delong GR, Bean SC, Brown FR. Acquired reversible autistic syndrome in acute encephalopathic illness in children. Arch Neurol 1981; 38(3):191–194.
99. Gillberg C. Onset at age 14 of a typical autistic syndrome. a case report of a girl with herpes simplex encephalitis. J Autism Dev Disord 1986; 16(3):369–375.
100. Gillberg IC. Autistic syndrome with onset at age 31 years: herpes encephalitis as a possible model for childhood autism. Dev Med Child Neurol 1991; 33(10):920–924.
101. Knobloch H, Pasamanick B. Some etiologic and prognostic factors in early infantile autism and psychosis. Pediatrics 1975; 55(2):182–191.
102. Ritvo ER, Mason-Brothers A, Freeman BJ, Pingree C, Jenson WR, McMahon WM, et al. The UCLA–University of Utah epidemiologic survey of autism: the etiologic role of rare disease. Am J Psychiatry 1990; 147(12):1614–1621.
103. Matarazzo EB. Treatment of late onset autism as a consequence of probable autoimmune processes related to chronic bacterial infection. World J Biol Psychiatry 2002; 3(3):162–166.
104. Gillberg C, Gillberg IC. Infantile autism: a total population study of reduced optimality in the pre-, peri-, and neonatal period. J Autism Dev Disord 1983; 13(2):153–166.
105. Eaton WW, Mortensen PB, Thomsen PH, Frydenberg M. Obstetric complications and risk for severe psychopathology in childhood. J Autism Dev Disord 2001; 31(3):279–285.
106. Torrey EF, Hersh SP, McCabe KD. Early childhood psychosis and bleeding during pregnancy. J Autism Child Schizophr 1975; 5(4):287–297.
107. Finegan J, Quarrington B. Pre, peri, and neonatal factors and infantile autism. J Child Psychol Psychiatry 1979; 20:119–128.
108. Bolton PF, Murphy M, Macdonald H, Whitlock B, Pickles A, Rutter M. Obstetric complications in autism: consequences or causes of the condition? J Am Acad Child Adolesc Psychiatry 1997; 36(2):272–281.
109. Lord C, Mulloy C, Wendelboe M, Schopler E. Pre- and perinatal factors in high-functioning females and males with autism. J Autism Dev Disord 1991; 21(2):197–209.
110. Piven J, Simon J, Chase GA, Wzorek M, Landa R, Gayle, J, et al. The etiology of autism: pre-, peri-, and neonatal factors. J Am Acad Child Adolesc Psychiatry 1993; 32(6):1256–1263.
111. Cryan E, Byrne M, O'Donovan A, O'Callaghan E. Brief report: a case-control study of obstetric complications and later autistic disorder. J Autism Dev Disord 1996; 26(4):453–460.

3

Etiology of Autism

Vidya Bhushan Gupta
*New York Medical College and Columbia University, New York,
New York, U.S.A.*

I. INTRODUCTION

Etiologically, autism can be divided into idiopathic (without an identifiable risk factor) and secondary (with an identifiable risk factor). About 80–85% of cases of autism are idiopathic and 15–20% are secondary (1). In a meta-analysis of 23 surveys of autism published between 1966 and 1998, "a medical condition of potential causal significance" was found in only 6% of cases (2). Although many causes of autism have been proposed for the idiopathic group, few meet the essential criteria of causation. According to Hill, to be causal, an association should be strong, consistent, sufficient, and necessary, and should precede the condition. There should be a dose relationship between the cause and the condition, a plausible and coherent biological explanation, and an experimental model (3). No single factor meets all these criteria, suggesting that autism is not due to a single cause. Most likely it is a heterogeneous disorder caused by many factors that work either independently, or in tandem, or in concert to cause neurological dysfunction, that, in turn, manifests as the syndrome of autism (Fig. 1). The foremost among these factors is genetic susceptibility.

II. GENETIC FACTORS

Kanner, in his seminal paper, noted that the parents of children in his case series were "highly intelligent, preoccupied with abstractions of a scientific, literary,

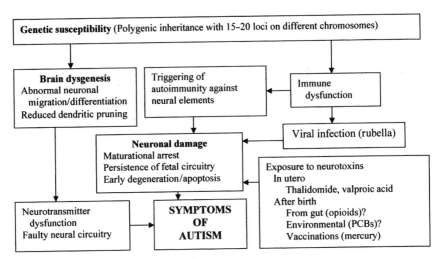

Figure 1   Etiological cascade in autism.

and artistic nature, limited in genuine interest in people, obsessive and lacking warm-heartedness" (4,5). Although he wrongly attributed autism to this lack of warmth in the parents, his observation was not without merit. Like Kanner, Piven et al. have also reported that the parents of autistic subjects have higher rates of aloof, rigid, hypersensitive, and anxious personality traits and of speech and language deficits (6). Family studies suggest that there is an increased prevalence of both autism and autistic-like behaviors in the first-degree relatives of persons with autism (7–9). The prevalence of autism in siblings is 3–9% (10,11), while the prevalence of a broad autism phenotype, comprising of subtle communication and social impairments, is 12.4–20.4% (7). Many families with multiple cases of autism (multiplex families) have been described. Relatives of multiple-incidence families have even higher rates of social and communication deficits and stereotypic behaviors (8). The recurrence rate for autism after the birth of one child is 8.6% and the relative risk of a sibling having autism is 50–175 (12,13). These data suggest that genetic factors cause subtle and obvious social, communication, and sensorimotor deficits among family members of the probands and influence the development of autism.

   A genetic basis of autism is also suggested by twin studies, because monozygotic twins have a higher concordance rate for autism than dizygotic twins (14–16). However, the concordance for typical autistic disorder in monozygotic twins is only 50%, and the symptoms of autism are often different in monozygotic twin pairs (17,18). Concordance for a broad autism phenotype consisting of social and language deficits, on the other hand, is much higher (92%) (17). This suggests that either a broad autism phenotype or a susceptibility to autism is inherited but the full manifestation of autism requires additional environmental factors.

Linkage studies suggest that the inheritance of autism is likely to be polygenic with involvement of three to seven or perhaps as many as 20 genes located on a number of chromosomes (19). The International Molecular Genetic Study of Autism Consortium (IMGSA, 1998) narrowed the search for susceptibility loci for autism to chromosome 7q and 16p, and to a lesser degree to chromosomes 4, 10, 19, and 22 (20), but Shao et al. identified candidate regions on chromosomes 2, 7, 15, 19, and X (21). Abnormalities of the long arm fifteenth chromosome, region 15q11–13, such as intrachromosomal and supernumerary [(isodicentric chromosome 15, or idic (15))] inverted duplications and deletions, have been reported frequently (22,23). The intrachromosomal inverted duplication is more likely to be associated with developmental delay and pervasive developmental disorder if it is maternally derived (24). The higher prevalence of autism in Prader Willi and Angelman syndromes and linkage disequilibrium at the Angelman syndrome gene UBE3A in autism families suggest that Prader-Willi/Angelman syndrome critical region (PWACR) may be an important locus for autism susceptibility genes (25).

Linkage with 7q has been found to be associated with severe developmental delay and delayed expressive language (21). Various genes on chromosome 7 seem to be promising candidates for autistic spectrum disorder. Autism-related gene (ARG-1), a new gene identified in a concordant twin pair with autism at 7q11.2 breakpoint in a translocation involving chromosomes 7 and 20, is highly expressed in adult and fetal brain (26). A gene has been identified at 7q22 that regulates the production of Reelin, a secretory glycoprotein responsible for cell lamination in cerebellun, and Bcl-2, a regulatory protein responsible for control of programmed cell death in the brain. This gene may be responsible for the observed Purkinje cell abnormalities. The risk of autism is increased 3.5 times if this gene is present (27). Deletion of a subtelomeric region of chromosome 2 is being reported with increasing frequency in autism (28,29).

No major genes on the X chromosome have been linked to autism (30). Although 2–5% of persons with fragile X have symptoms of autism, no specific abnormalities have been discovered in the FMR gene or in the fragile X region in individuals with autism (31,32).

About 3–5% of children with autism have a chromosomal anomaly (33,34). Although chromosomal abnormality of every chromosome has been described to be associated with autism in one or two individuals, Down syndrome and fragile X are the predominant chromosomal disorders among individuals with autistic disorder (35). Autistic disorder may occur in as many as 7% of individuals with Down syndrome. The likelihood of autistic disorder in children with Down syndrome is increased if there is history of autism or other pervasive developmental disorders in first- or second-degree relatives, infantile spasms, early hypothyroidism, and brain injury following heart surgery (36).

Between 2.5 and 6% of individuals with autism have fragile X syndrome (37,38) and 15–25% of persons with fragile X syndrome have symptoms of autism (39). The wide variation in the prevalence of autism in children with fragile X syndrome and of fragile X syndrome in autistic individuals is due to differences in methodology and diagnostic criteria in different studies. Some recent studies suggest that the usual behavioral phenotype of the fragile X anomaly is distinct from autism as usually defined and the two conditions are unrelated (40,41) Although 50–90% of children with fragile X syndrome have social anxiety that causes gaze aversion and difficulties in pragmatic use of language, ability to identify the emotional states of others and to understand the perspective of others in the theory of mind tasks is not impaired in fragile X syndrome (42,43). Among other sex chromosome aberrations, children with XYY syndrome seem to have a high prevalence of autism, especially those with perinatal brain damage (44).

Among the single-gene disorders, tuberous sclerosis and untreated phenylketonuria (PKU) seem to be the most important associations of autism. Autistic spectrum disorder has been reported in approximately 40% of persons with tuberous sclerosis (45,46), an autosomal dominant disorder that occurs due to mutation of the tuberous sclerosis complex 1 (TSC1) or TSC2 genes. Among autistic populations, the frequency of TSC is 1–4% and perhaps as high as 8–14% among those with mental retardation (MR) and seizures, particularly infantile spasms (2,46). Although the number of tubers seen on magnetic resonance imaging (MRI), especially in the temporal lobes, is correlated with severity of MR and autism (47), autism in tuberous sclerosis is not secondary to seizures or MR. According to Smalley, autism occurs due to effect of TSC gene mutation on brain development at a stage critical in the development of autism (46).

Untreated PKU was perhaps an important cause of autism before newborn screening became routine in the United States (48). Pearl S. Buck, in *The Child Who Never Grew*, describes the autistic features of a child with untreated PKU: "At three years she did not talk yet. The child's span of attention was very short indeed. Much of her fleet light running had no purpose—it was merely motion. Her eyes, so pure in their blue were blank when one gazed into their depths. They did not hold or respond. They were changeless" (49).

The behavioral phenotype of Smith-Lemli-Opitz syndrome, an inborn error of cholesterol biosynthesis, includes autism spectrum behaviors in as many as 46% cases. These children also demonstrate sleep cycle disturbance, sensory hyperreactivity, irritability, language impairment, self-injurious behavior, cognitive abilities from borderline intellectual functioning to profound mental retardation, and a characteristic movement disorder. This disorder should be considered in an autistic child who throws his upper body backward ("opisthokinesis") or stretches the upper body and flicks his hands (50).

The prevalence of autism is increased in neurofibromatosis (NF), a common single-gene disorder. In the French epidemiological study, 0.6% of children with autism had NF (51). Although the prevalence of neurofibromatosis type 1 (NF1) is increased about 150-fold in autistic patients, NF1 region is not a major susceptibility locus for autism (52).

The list of genetic syndromes occasionally associated with autism is too large to be mentioned, but some important associations are given in Table 1.

In summary, no single genetic abnormality has been proven to be a necessary or sufficient cause of autism. It seems that as many as 15–20 loci on different chromosomes may independently or additively play a minor role in increasing susceptibility to a broad autism phenotype consisting of abnormalities in social and communicative behavior, the typical syndrome occurring when a threshold or epistasis is reached by the combination of both genetic and exogenous causes (35,68).

From a practical point of view, a definitive cause, genetic or otherwise, is identified in about 15–20% of individuals with autism or PDD (69,70). Others have reported identifying an etiology in even fewer cases of autism (2,71). An etiology is more likely to be identified in low-functioning children with mental retardation, epilepsy, or dysmorphic features. Therefore, search for the etiology of autism should be individualized according to the clinical presentation of each case. Genetic counseling, too, should be individualized. If an obvious cause is identified, the recurrence rate depends on the recurrence risk of the identified condition. In idiopathic cases, if no other case is identified in the family,

Table 1 Syndromes Associated with Autism

Down syndrome (7%) (53,54)
Fragile X syndrome (3–6%) (31–39)
Prader Willi syndrome (5%) (55,56)
Angelman syndrome (57–59)
Hypomelanosis of Ito (10%) (60)
Williams syndrome (61,62)
XYY syndrome (35)
Duchenne muscular dystrophy (63)
Cornelia de Lange syndrome (67)
Tuberous sclerosis (45,46)
Neurofibromatosis (52)
Möbius syndrome (64,65)
Joubert syndrome (66)

the prevalence of autism in siblings is 3–9% (10,11) while the broad autism phenotype, comprising more subtle communication/social impairments or stereotypic behaviors, can occur in as many as 12.4–20.4% of siblings (7). The risk of autism is particularly high if one of the parents has autism or Asperger's syndrome (72).

III. IMMUNOLOGICAL FACTORS

The immune system and brain communicate with each other through neurotransmitters, hormones, and cytokines. The cytokines and immune cells can activate neuronal pathways and release tropic hormones such as ACTH. The latter, in turn, can influence immunological function by stimulating the release of end-organ hormones, such as corticosteroids. The immune, nervous, and endocrine systems are, therefore, tightly interwoven to regulate homeostasis and changes in one can affect the other, and it is biologically plausible that immune dysfunction can cause neurological dysfunction. Two broad categories of immunological abnormalities have been described in autism—qualitative or quantitative abnormalities of immune cells, and autoantibodies against neural elements. However, it is difficult to make meaningful generalizations from the available studies because of small and heterogeneous samples, selection bias, and lack of uniform diagnostic criteria across studies. The findings are often inconsistent and contradictory. While decreased lymphocyte proliferation in response to mitogens, such as phytohemagglutinin (PHA), concanavalin A, and pokeweed mitogen, was reported in a few studies (73,74), other studies found normal (75), and both high and low rates of T-cell proliferation in response to mitogens (76). Decreased number of T cells, proportional to the severity of symptoms, was reported by one group (74,77), but another group reported normal numbers of T and B cells (75). Changes in the distribution of T-cell subtypes have also been described in autism. The T lymphocytes are characterized by cluster of differentiation (CD) surface molecules. CD4+ T cells, also called helper cells, stimulate the differentiation of B lymphocytes into plasma and memory cells and induce suppressor/cytotoxic cells, thus helping both the cellular and humoral components of immune response. CD8+ cells, also called T suppressor cells, kill the infected cells and suppress autoimmune response. The lack of T helper cells can impair cell-mediated and humoral immune response, while the lack of suppressor cells can set the stage for autoimmune mechanisms to occur. Warren et al. reported reduced numbers of CD4+ cells, in particular of the CD4 + CD45RA + lymphocytes that induce suppressor/cytotoxic cells (77). A reversal of T helper/suppressor ratio due to a selective decrease in CD4 helper cells has also been reported (78,79). Plioplys et al., on the contrary, have reported normal CD4:CD8 ratios for the whole group, with increased ratio in some and decreased ratio in others (75). Gupta et al. reported lower proportions of (Th1) T cells and increased proportions of (Th2) T cells in autistic children as compared to healthy controls (80). T helper-1 cells promote the expansion of active T cells by producing cytokines IL-2 and IFN-γ. Decreased numbers of Th1 cells can affect cell-mediated immunity and NK cell activity, making an individual more susceptible to infection, particularly by viruses.

Other studies have focused on the activity of natural killer (NK) cells in autistic patients. These cells have the ability to function without prior exposure to a particular antigen and are involved in the removal of viral-infected cells as well as tumor cells. It is believed that these cells may have a regulatory role in the immune system, preventing autoimmunity, because their activity has been demonstrated to be reduced in several autoimmune disorders, such as systemic lupus erythematosus, rheumatoid arthritis, and multiple sclerosis. Warren et al. reported significantly reduced killing activity by NK cells in 40% of autistic subjects (81). Reduced NK cell activity can presumably place an individual, or fetus, at an increased risk for the development of neurological damage by viruses.

The second hypothesis linking the etiology of autism to the immune system involves the breakdown of self-recognition mechanisms, or autoimmunity. Autoimmunity is characterized by cellular and humoral immunological reactions against components of the self. Production of autoantibodies to neuron-specific antigens in autistic children has been described in several studies. Singh et al. reported antibodies to neuron-axon filament proteins (NAFP) and myelin basic proteins in children with autism (82,83), while Plioplys et al. reported antibodies against cerebellar neurofilaments (84). Vojdani et al. measured autoantibodies against nine different neuron-specific antigens, including myelin basic protein, neurofilament proteins, and tubulin, and three cross-reactive peptides from *Chlamydia* pneumonia, *Streptococcus* group A, and milk. In this study, autistic children showed the highest levels of IgG, IgM, and IgA antibodies against all neurological antigens as well as the three cross-reactive peptides compared to controls (85).

Several studies have reported antibodies against neurotransmitter receptors such as serotonin (5-HT) receptors (86,87), α2-adrenergic receptors (88), and brain endothelia cell proteins (89) in children with autism. However, the autoantibodies reported in the above studies are not specific to patients with autism and are seen in demyelinating neuropathies such as multiple sclerosis and Guillain-Barré syndrome as well. Antibodies reactive to CNS proteins are not seen in the sera of most patients with autism. Unlike myasthenia gravis, in which a clear antibody-receptor interaction has been identified, no consistent antibody receptor interaction has been found in autism. There are few pathological findings suggestive of immune reaction or autoimmunity such as inflammation or demyelination in patients with autism. Clustering of autoimmune disease in families who have children with autism also suggests the role of autoimmune factors in some individuals with autism (90). Forty-six percent of families with autism had two or more family members with an autoimmune disorder, compared to only 26% of controls. Although the risk of autism showed a positive correlation with the number of affected family members with an autoimmune disorder, patients with autism themselves did not exhibit an increase in autoimmune disorders. Unlike autoimmune disorders, which have a progressive or remitting-relapsing time course, the neurobehavioral symptoms of autism tend to remain stationary or get better rather than intensify with time. Moreover, the neuronal injury in autism is postulated to occur so early during gestation, at or before 5–6 weeks of pregnancy, that immunological dysfunction is unlikely to be the primary cause of autism.

It is unclear if immune dysfunction is the cause or effect of autism. Is it primary or secondary to a genetic abnormality or an infection? Reduced expression of C4B gene, a major histocompatibility complex gene that regulates the immune system and is involved in eliminating viruses and bacteria from the body, has been described in autism (91). A viral infection in utero can damage the developing immune system of the fetus. Congenital rubella infection is associated with immune dysfunction, autoimmune diseases, and autism. Other prenatal infections, such as rubella, cytomegalovirus, herpes simplex, syphilis, and toxoplasmosis, have been implicated in the causation of autism. Infections can alter antigenic determinants on cell surface, activate immune cells, and influence the nervous system through cytokine release. Over 60 different microbial peptides have been reported to cross-react with human brain tissue and myelin basic protein and are potentially capable of triggering autoimmune encephalomyelitis. But the association between congenital infections and autism is not strong as originally reported, with less than 1% of patients with autism having histories of congenital rubella or other congenital infections. An attempt to find viral genomes or proteins in blood and CSF of patients with autism has also produced inconsistent results.

The support for immune hypothesis of autism from trials of immunomodulant therapies, such as intravenous gamma globulin, has been weak and inconsistent. While a few open-label trials have suggested clinical improvement with intravenous gammaglobulins in a small group of autistic children (91,92), others reported transient or no improvement (93,94). Although immune dysfunction may be involved in the causal pathway of autism in a few individuals, the evidence for a major role of immune dysfunction in the etiology of autism is meager at present and further research is needed to elucidate the nexus between immune system and autism (Fig. 2).

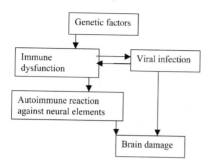

Figure 2   The immune system and autism.

IV. GASTROINTESTINAL FACTORS

During the last two decades there has been a growing interest in the "central nervous system and gut nexus." The enteric nervous system develops from the cells of neural crest (95) and shares neurotransmitters, such as serotonin, vasoactive intestinal peptide (VIP), and secretin, with the main nervous system. There is some evidence that VIP regulates immune response by microglia and secretin affects GABA transmission in the Purkinje cells of the cerebellum (96,97). Thus it is theoretically conceivable that the gut and brain can influence each other.

The main premise of the "gut" theory of autism is that the gastrointestinal (GI) tract is unable to adequately metabolize opioids derived from dietary sources, in particular foods that contain gluten and casein, and permits them to be absorbed via an abnormally permeable intestinal membrane (98–102). These peptides cross the blood-brain barrier and bind to the opioid receptors producing symptoms of autism, such as inattention, inability to learn, and poor social interaction (103,104). Children with autism have been reported to have increased urinary excretion of low-molecular-weight peptides (99,105,106) and increased opioid levels in cerebrospinal fluid (98,99).

The proponents of this theory cite increased rate of the gastrointestinal symptoms, such as bulky, malodorous, loose stools or intermittent diarrhea, in children with autistic spectrum disorder (103). A variety of gastrointestinal abnormalities, such as lymphoid nodular hyperplasia of the terminal ileum, enterocolitis with infiltration of T, plasma, and Paneth cells, mild duodenitis, disaccharide malabsorption, and esophageal reflux, have been described in children with autistic spectrum disorders (ASD) referred to the GI clinics (103,107,108). The now largely discounted (109) association between MMR vaccination and autism was allegedly mediated by vaccine-induced enterocolits resulting in absorption of toxic peptides (101).

A variety of other GI problems have been reported in small case series. Colonization of the gut by neurotoxin-producing bacteria such as *Clostridium* species was reported in a small group of children with regressive autism (110). A poorly absorbed oral antibiotic, vancomycin, led to significant improvement in a few children who developed regressive autism and persistent diarrhea following treatment with antibiotics, but the improvement was not sustained when the antibiotic was discontinued, suggesting that the association may have been fortuitous (111). Horvath et al. reported an increase in the volume of pancreatobiliary fluid after an intravenous injection of secretin in autistic children as an evidence of altered secretin receptor sensitivity in autism. Because secretin reactive receptors have been identified in the cerebellum, they argued that the anecdotal reports of the benefits of secretin in autism are biologically plausible (102). Megson has proposed that symptoms of autistic spectrum disorder are caused by increased intestinal permeability and malabsorption of vitamin A and other nutrients due to an inherited defect in G-alpha subunit proteins, but there is no clinical or laboratory evidence for this hypothesis (112).

Most studies reporting an association between gastrointestinal symptoms and autism have been clinic-based. Population-based studies of autism, on the contrary, do not suggest an association between autism and inflammatory bowel disease (IBD) or gastrointestinal symptoms. In a French population-based study, no children with autism were diagnosed with IBD. The onset of IBD in children is after the age of 5 years while the onset of ASD symptoms usually occurs at the age of 1–2 years (113,114). Except for food refusal and food fads gastrointestinal symptoms are unusual in children with ASD. Many intervention studies based on the gut theory, although initially promising, could not be replicated. Lucarelli et al. noticed a marked improvement in the behavioral symptoms of patients after a period of 8 weeks on a gluten- and/or casein-free diet (115), but a recent study found no significant difference in the behavior pattern between the diet and control groups of autistic children (116). In 1999, Horvath et al. (102) reported increased expressive language and eye contact in three autistic children with chronic diarrhea who received a single dose of hormone secretin during endoscopy, but follow-up studies showed no effect of intravenous secretin on the language or behavior of children with autism (117,118). Pharmacological trials with the opiate antagonist naltrexone have produced mixed results and direct measurement of blood or spinal fluid levels of endorphins do not suggest a link between opiate excess and the core symptoms of ASD (119).

In summary, although a few clinic-based studies have shown increased prevalence of GI symptoms in children with autism, population-based studies have failed to show an association of GI disorders, including IBD, with autism. The available evidence does not justify GI evaluation of every child with autism. However, a child with autism who presents with GI symptomatology may be worked up according to the "gut theory" of autism. The work-up for such patients may include: stool studies for malabsorption and *Clostridium*, urine for opioid and peptide levels, serum levels of IgG and IgM antibodies for casein, lactalbumin, and β-lactoglobulin, and upper and lower endoscopic studies to evaluate for lymphoid nodular hyperplasia and other signs of gut epithelial dysfunction. Moreover, well-designed population-based studies are needed to evaluate the prevalence of abnormalities of the GI tract and to test the hypothesis that gut dysfunction can cause autism through the gut-brain nexus.

V. TERATOGENIC FACTORS

Because many studies point toward a prenatal onset of autism, it is conceivable that a teratogen damages the fetal brain directly or makes it vulnerable to injury by another factor. Time of neural tube closure seems critical for the development of autism, because cases of thalidomide embryopathy with symptoms of autism were exposed to thalidomide at the time of neural tube closure (120,121). Rodier et al. have produced an animal model of autism using valproic acid, an inhibitor of neural tube closure (122). Moore et al. reported autistic symptoms in 60% of children exposed to anticonvulsants including valproic acid in utero (123).

Other substances that have been suspected to be associated with autism are alcohol, cocaine, polychlorinated polyphenyls (PCBs), retinoids, and methylmercury. Although a few cases of fetal alcohol syndrome have been reported to have symptoms of autism, autism is uncommon in fetal alcohol syndrome (124). One case series reported high prevalence of autism in children exposed to cocaine in utero (125), but this has not been replicated. A study that examined children exposed to both cocaine and alcohol in utero found that exposure to alcohol accounted for most of the effect (126). The neurotoxic theory of autism was examined by the Center for Disease Control (CDC) in Brick Township of New Jersey. This town is close to several Superfund sites and has three contaminants in drinking water, tetrachloroethylene, trichloroethylene, and trihalomethanes (THMs). Although the town was believed to have higher prevalence of autism, an epidemiological study by CDC did not find the prevalence of autism in Brick Township to be higher than in other small communities (127). Studies that have examined exposure to polychlorinated biphenyls (PCBs), dioxin, and methylmercury have not shown any association with autism (128). Thus the search for a chemical teratogen that is necessary or sufficient to cause autism has been elusive so far.

VI. MMR VACCINATION AND AUTISM

The saga of measles, mumps, and rubella (MMR) vaccination and autism started when Wakefield et al. reported a series of 12 cases that allegedly developed regressive autism after receiving MMR vaccination. The symptoms were apparently mediated by MMR vaccine-induced enterocolitis that, in turn, allowed neurotoxic metabolites to be absorbed from the gut (129,130). However, population-based studies of autism have not found any association between autism and MMR vaccination (131,132). In a retrospective cohort study involving 537,303 children, Madsen et al. found no association between the date of vaccination and the onset of autism. The relative risk of autism and autistic spectrum disorder in the vaccinated group was not higher than in the unvaccinated group (132). The prevalence of autism has increased in the 1990s, while the MMR vaccine has been used in the United States since 1963 and the rates of MMR vaccination have remained stable during the 1980s and 1990s. There is no correlation between MMR time trends and autism prevalence (133).

Similarly, it is not proven that MMR vaccination causes enterocolits (134). In a retrospective study that linked MMR vaccination with the hospital discharge data, none of the autistic children were hospitalized for inflammatory bowel disease (135). Even with the most sophisticated assays, measles viral material has not been demonstrated consistently in the intestines of children with inflammatory bowel disease (136,137). A detailed discussion of the GI theory of autism was presented earlier in this chapter.

Because intrauterine exposure to high doses of methylmercury, often from seafood contamination, is associated with neurobehavioral complications such as developmental delay, cognitive deficits, and seizures, it has been suggested that autism can occur due to intrauterine or postnatal exposure to mercury either from contaminated fish or from thimerosal, an ethylmercury-containing preservative used in infant vaccines (138). But, the symptoms of mercury poisoning include seizures, ataxia, photophobia, and dysarthria, symptoms not seen in autism. According to the Food and Drug Administration, if a child receives multiple thimerosal containing vaccinations, he may be exposed to mercury in excess of the federal safety guidelines (139). Although the association is not proven, most infant vaccines are now made without thiomerosal.

The U.S. Institute of Medicine and the American Academy of Pediatrics have both concluded that there is little evidence that MMR vaccination causes regressive autism (140,141). Similarly, multiple vaccinations, whether given as multiple injections or as tetra- or pentavaccines, do not increase the risk of autism.

VII. INFECTIOUS FACTORS

Cases of autism have been described in children who had intrauterine rubella (142,143) and cytomegalovirus infection (144). Autism has also been described after perinatal and postnatal herpes simplex encephalitis (145). Most of these cases have clear evidence of brain damage with additional manifestations such as mental retardation and seizures. Besides damaging the brain directly, viruses can damage the brain indirectly by triggering an autoimmune response against the neural elements of the host. Investigations are ongoing into the possibility of previously unrecognized viruses specifically causing the syndrome of autism without producing recognizable cytopathic effects. Hornig and Lipkin have produced symptoms suggestive of autism in newborn Lewis rats by infecting them with Borna virus (146). These rats have been noted to have abnormalities in cerebellum and hippocampus that resemble the lesions reported in autism. Thus it is biologically plausible for a viral infection occurring at a critical time of development to result in neurodevelopmental disability with no overt signs of encephalitis at the time of infection. Persistent viral infections can, theoretically, cause neurotransmitter dysfunction without causing inflammation, histological injury, or cytopathic effect and may not be detected by traditional neurological investigations (147). Thus a viral infection at a key time in early stages of neurological development can predispose an individual to autism, but no specific viral cause of autism has been confirmed so far.

VIII. PERINATAL FACTORS

Perinatal and obstetric factors have not emerged as important in the etiology of autism. Several case control studies have found no association between obstetric factors and autism. Others have reported weak associations between various obstetric factors and autism, but no single obstetric event has emerged as a preeminent antecedent of autism. Higher incidence of second- or third-trimester uterine bleeding and prolonged labor have been reported in several studies (148–151). Hyperbilirubinemia was noted more often in autistic children in three studies (148–151). Other complications that have been reported inconsistently include induction of labor, prolonged and precipitous labor, and oxygen requirement at birth. Data on vaginal infections during pregnancy are conflicting and may be confounded by socioeconomic status and number of sexual partners, factors not controlled for in the studies. Prematurity is not associated with autism. Overall the complications that have been reported have been mild and none have emerged as necessary or sufficient to cause autism (152).

Studies that have used the optimality approach to assess the obstetric factors in autism have also reported mixed to negative results. This approach looks at obstetric and neonatal risk as a composite score. Deb et al. found no significant difference in the scores of obstetric optimality between the overall group of autistic children and their siblings, but among children with severe autism there was a significant correlation between severity of autism and obstetric and neonatal complication scores. This observation supports the notion of two types of autism: low-functioning, which is secondary to some known obstetric and other etiological factor, and high-functioning, which is idiopathic (153). Cryan et al., on the other hand, did not find any association between autism and obstetric complications score (154). Because some of the variance in obstetric adversity may be due to birth order, Piven et al. studied the association between perinatal factors and autism, correcting for birth order. They did not find any association between perinatal factors and autism (155).

In summary, obstetric and perinatal complications do not, by themselves, cause autism but may occur because the fetus and pregnancy are compromised by the primary cause of autism. Alternatively, common risk factors may cause both autism and the obstetric complication (149,152).

IX. METABOLIC FACTORS

Features of autism have been described in a few children with metabolic conditions such as D-glyceric aciduria, phenylketonuria, histidinemia, adenylosuccinate lyase deficiency, dihydropyrimidine dehydrogenase deficiency, 5'-nucleotidase superactivity, and phosphoribosylpyrophosphate synthetase deficiency (156,157). Although hyperuricosuria has been described in a few children with autism, defects of purine metabolism such as adenylosuccinate lyase deficiency are infrequent (158). Metabolic defects of detoxification, such as a defect of sulfation, have also been suggested (159). Other metabolic disorders, such as mitochondrial respiratory complex defects, fatty acid oxidation defects, carnitine deficiency, and organic acidopathies, are being explored, but, at present, there is little evidence to support the notion that autism is a metabolic disorder or that metabolic defects are common in autism.

X. SUMMARY

It seems from the foregoing that the etiology of autism is still elusive. Many hypotheses have been proposed, some based on empirical observations, some by analogy, and some by deductive reasoning. Only the salient hypotheses have been presented in this chapter. Because autism is such a disheartening condition, there is a tendency to say "eureka" whenever any association is observed. Explosion in the prevalence of autism has made it a political disease. And the media smells for rats, ready to sensationalize any anecdote, any suggestion, and any insinuation as a potential cause. In this charged environment it is the responsibility of the professionals to be rational while keeping an open mind. Instead of rushing to judgment, the professionals should measure every association with Hill's criteria and plan and inform accordingly. Because of the fervor with which the scientific community and the society at large are responding to this apparent epidemic of autism, it is likely that we shall find the etiological factors associated with autism in the near future and be able to stall the tide of autism.

ACKNOWLEDGMENTS

I wish to acknowledge the help of Rohit Kohli, M.D., in the section on gastrointestinal factors and of Divya Aggarwal, M.D., in the section on teratogenic factors.

REFERENCES

1. DeLong GR. Autism: new data suggest a new hypothesis. Neurology 1999; 23;52:911–916.
2. Fombonne E. The epidemiology of autism: a review. Psychol Med 1999; 29:769–786.
3. Hill AB. The environment and disease: association or causation? Proc R Soc Med 1965; 58:295–300.
4. Kanner L. Autistic disturbances of affective contact. Nervous Child 1943; 2:217–250.
5. www.ama.org.br/kannereng12.htm, accessed on 9.12.02.
6. Piven J, Palmer P, Landa R, Santangelo S, Jacobi D, Childress D. Personality and language characteristics in parents from multiple-incidence autism families. Am J Med Genet 1997; 74:398–411.
7. Bolton P, MacDonald H, Pickles A, et al. A case-control family history study of autism. J Child Psychol Psychiatry 1994; 35:877–900.
8. Piven J, Palmer P, Jacobi D, Childress D, Arndt S. Broader autism phenotype: evidence from a family history study of multiple-incidence autism families. Am J Psychiatry 1997; 154:185–190.
9. Spiker D, Lotspeich L, Kraemer HC, et al. Genetics of autism: characteristics of affected and unaffected children from 37 multiplex families. Am J Med Genet 1994; 54:27–35.
10. Smalley SL, McCracken J, Tanguay P. Autism, affective disorders, and social phobia. Am J Med Genet 1995; 60:19–26.
11. Jones MB, Szatamari P. Stopagge rules and genetic studies of autism. Autism Dev Disord 1988; 18:31–40.
12. Ritvo ER, Jorde LB, Mason-Brothers A, Freeman BJ, Pingree C, Jones MB, McMahon WM, Petersen PB, Jenson WR, Mo A. The UCLA–University of Utah epidemiologic survey of autism: recurrence risk estimates and genetic counseling. Am J Psychiatry 1989; 146:1032–1036.
13. Silverman JM, Smith CJ, Schneidler J, et al. Symptom domains in autism and related conditions: evidence for familiarity. Am J Med Genet (Neuropsychiatry) 2002; 114:64–73.

14. Folstein S, Rutter M. Infantile autism: a genetic study of 21 twin pairs. J Child Psychol Psychiatry 1977; 18:297–321.
15. Ritvo ER, Freeman BJ, Mason-Brothers A, Mo A, Ritvo AM. Concordance of the syndrome of autism in 40 pairs of afflicted twins. Am J Psychiatry 1985; 142:74–77.
16. Steffenburg S, Gillberg C, Hellgren L, et al. A twin study of autism in Denmark, Finland, Iceland, Norway and Sweden. J Child Psychol Psychiatry 1989; 30:405–416.
17. Bailey A, Le Couteur A, Gottesman I, et al. Autism as a strongly genetic disorder: evidence from a British twin study. Psychol Med 1995; 25:63–77.
18. Le Couteur A, Bailey A, Goode S, Pickles A, Robertson S, Gottesman I, Rutter M. A broader phenotype of autism: the clinical spectrum in twins. J Child Psychol Psychiatry. 1996; 37:785–801.
19. Risch N, Spiker D, Lotspeich L, Nouri N, Hinds D. A genomic screen of autism: evidence for a multilocus etiology. Am J Hum Genet 1999; 65:493–497.
20. International Molecular Genetic Study of Autism Consortium. A full genome screen for autism with evidence for linkage to a region on chromosome 7q. Hum Mol Genet 1998; 7:571–578.
21. Shao Y, Wolpert CM, Raiford KL, Menold MM, Donnelly SL, Ravan SA, Bass MP, McClain C, von Wendt L, Vance JM, Abramson RH, Wright HH, Ashley-Koch A, Gilbert JR, DeLong RG, Cuccaro ML, Pericak-Vance MA. Genomic screen and follow-up analysis for autistic disorder. Am J Med Genet. 2002; 114:99–105.
22. Wolpert CM, Menold MM, Bass MP, Qumsiyeh MB, Donnelly SL, Ravan SA, Vance JM, Gilbert JR, Abramson RK, Wright HH, Cuccaro ML, Pericak-Vance MA. Three probands with autistic disorder and isodicentric chromosome 15. Am J Med Genet. 2000; 96:365–372.
23. Cook EH Jr. Genetics of autism. Ment Retard Dev Disabil Res Rev 1998; 4:113–120.
24. Cook EH Jr, Lindgren V, Leventhal BL, Courchesne R, Lincoln A, Shulman C, Lord C, Courchesne E. Autism or atypical autism in maternally but not paternally derived proximal 15q duplication. Am J Hum Genet 1997; 60:928–34
25. Nurmi EL, Bradford Y, Chen Y, Hall J, Arnone B, Gardiner MB, Hutcheson HB, Gilbert IR, Pericak-Vance MA, Copeland-Yates SA, Michaelis RC, Wassink TH, Santangelo SL, Sheffield VC, Piven J, Folstein SE, Haines JL, Sutcliffe JS. Linkage disequilibrium at the Angelman syndrome gene UBE3A in autism families. Genomics 2001; 77:105–113.
26. Sultana R, Yu J, Raskind W, Disteche C. Cloning of a candidate gene (ARG1) from the breakpoint of t(7;20) in an autistic twin pair. In: Abstracts of the Annual Meeting of the American Society for Human Genetics, program no. 230. Bethesda, Maryland, 1999.
27. Fatemi SH. Dysregulation of reelin and Bcl-2 proteins in autistic cerebellum. J Autism Dev Disord 2001; 31:529–535.
28. Wolff DJ, Clifton K, Karr C, Charles J. Pilot assessment of the subtelomeric regions of children with autism: detection of a 2q deletion. Genet Med 2002; 4:10–14.
29. Ghaziuddin M, Burmeister M. Deletion of chromosome 2q37 and autism: a distinct subtype? J Autism Dev Disord 1999; 29:259–263.
30. Hallmayer J, Hebert JM, Spiker D et al. Autism and the X chromosome: multipoint sib-pair analysis. Arch Gen Psychiatry 1996; 53:985–989.

31. Gurling HM, Bolton PF, Vincent J, Melmer G, Rutter M. Molecular and cytogenetic investigations of the fragile X region including the Frax A and Frax ECGG trinucleotide repeat sequences in families multiplex for autism and related phenotypes. Hum Hered 1997; 47:254–262.

32. Vincent JB, Konecki DS, Munstermaun E, et al. Point mutation analysis of the FMR-1 gene in autism. Mol Psychiatry 1996; 1:227–231.

33. Ritvo ER, Mason-Brothers A, Freeman BJ, Pingree C, Jenson WR, McMahon WM, Peterson PB, Jorde LB, Mo A, Ritvo A. The UCLA–University of Utah epidemiologic survey of autism: the etiologic role of rare diseases. Am J Psychiatry 1990; 147:1614–1621.

34. Weidmer-Mikhail E, Sheldon S, Ghaziuddin M. Chromosomes in autism and related pervasive developmental disorders: a cytogenetic study. J Intellect Disabil Res 1998; 42 (Pt 1):8–12.

35. Gillberg C, Coleman M. The Biology of the Autistic Syndromes. Clinics in Developmental Medicine No. 126. 2nd ed. London: MacKeith Press, 1992.

36. Rasmussen P, Borjesson O, Wentz E, Gillberg C. Autistic disorders in Down syndrome: background factors and clinical correlates. Dev Med Child Neurol 2001; 43:750–754.

37. Bailey A, Bolton P, Butler L, LeCouteur A, Murphy M, Scott S, Webb T, Rutter M. Prevalence of the fragile X anomaly amongst autistic twins and singletons. J Child Psychol Psychiatry 1993; 34:673–688.

38. Brown WT, Jenkins EC, Cohen IL, Fisch GS, Wolf-Schein EG, Gross A, Waterhouse L, Fein D, Mason-Brothers A, Ritvo E, et al. Fragile X and autism: a multicenter survey. Am J Med Genet 1986; 23:341–352.

39. Reiss AL, Freund L. Behavioral phenotype of fragile X syndrome: DSM-III-R autistic behavior in male children. Am J Med Genet 1991; 43:35–46.

40. Einfeld S, Molony H, Hall W. Autism is not associated with the fragile X syndrome. Am J Med Genet 1989; 34:187–193.

41. Rapin I. Legitimacy of comparing fragile X with autism questioned. J Autism Dev Disord 2002; 32:60–61.

42. Sudhalter V, Cohen IL, Silverman W, Wolf-Schein EG. Conversational analyses of males with fragile X, Down syndrome, and autism: comparison of the emergence of deviant language. Am J Ment Retard 1990; 94:431–441.

43. Cohen IL, Vietze PM, Sudhalter V, Jenkins EC, Brown WT. Parent–child dyadic gaze patterns in fragile X males and in non-fragile X males with autistic disorder. J Child Psychol Psychiatry 1989; 30:845–856.

44. Gillberg C, Wahlstrom J. Chromosome abnormalities in infantile autism and other childhood psychoses: a population study of 66 cases. Dev Med Child Neurol 1985; 27:293–304.

45. Gutierrez GC, Smalley SL, Tanguay PE. Autism in tuberous sclerosis complex. J Autism Dev Disord 1998; 28:97–103.

46. Smalley SL. Autism and tuberous sclerosis. J Autism Dev Disord 1998; 28:407–414.

47. Bolton PF, Griffiths PD. Association of tuberous sclerosis of temporal lobes with autism and atypical autism. Lancet 1997; 349:392–395.

48. Kratter FE. The physiognomic, psychometric, behavioral and neurological aspects of phenyketonuria. J Pediatr 1959; 55:182–191.

49. Buck PS, Michener JA. The Child Who Never Grew. Bethesda, MD: Woodbine House, 1992.

50. Tierney E, Nwokoro NA, Kelley RI. Behavioral phenotype of RSH/Smith-Lemli-Opitz syndrome. Ment Retard Dev Disabil Res Rev 2000; 6:131–134.

51. Fombonne E, Du Mazaubrun C, Cans C, Grandjean H. Autism and associated medical disorders in a French epidemiological survey. J Am Acad Child Adolesc Psychiatry 1997; 36:1561–1569.

52. Mbarek O, Marouillat S, Martineau J, Barthelemy C, Muh JP, Andres C. Association study of the NF1 gene and autistic disorder. Am J Med Genet 1999; 88:729–732.

53. Kent L, Evans J, Paul M, Sharp M. Comorbidity of autistic spectrum disorders in children with Down syndrome. Dev Med Child Neurol 1999; 41:153–158.

54. Rasmussen P, Borjesson O, Wentz E, Gillberg C. Autistic disorders in Down syndrome: background factors and clinical correlates. Dev Med Child Neurol 2001; 43:750–754.

55. Demb HB, Papola P. PDD and Prader-Willi syndrome. J Am Acad Child Adolesc Psychiatry 1995; 34:539–540.

56. Dykens EM, Cassidy SB, King BH. Maladaptive behavior differences in Prader-Willi syndrome due to paternal deletion versus maternal uniparental disomy. Am J Ment Retard 1999; 104:67–77.

57. Steffenburg S, Gillberg CL, Steffenburg U, Kyllerman M. Autism in Angelman syndrome: a population-based study. Pediatr Neurol 1996; 14:131–136.

58. Penner KA, Johnston J, Faircloth BH, Irish P, Williams CA. Communication, cognition, and social interaction in the Angelman syndrome. Am J Med Genet 1993; 46:34–39.

59. Summers JA, Allison DB, Lynch PS, Sandler L. Behaviour problems in Angelman syndrome. J Intellect Disabil Res 1995; 39(Pt 2):97–106.

60. Pascal-Castroviejo I, Roche C, Martinez-Bermejo A, Arcas J, Lopez-Martin V, Tendero A, Equiroz JL, Pascal-Pascal SI. Hypomelanosis of Ito: a study of 76 infantile cases. Brain Dev 1998; 20:36–43.

61. Gosch A, Pankau R. "Autistic" behavior in two children with Williams-Beuren syndrome. Am J Med Genet 1994; 15;53:83–84.

62. Gillberg C, Rasmussen P. Brief report: four case histories and a literature review of Williams syndrome and autistic behavior. J Autism Dev Disord. 1994; 24:381–93.

63. Komoto J, Usui S, Otsuki S. Infantile autism and Duchenne muscular dystrophy. J Autism Dev Disord 1984; 14:191–195.

64. Gillberg C, Steffenburg S. Autistic behaviour in Moebius syndrome. Acta Paediatr Scand 1989; 78:314–316.

65. Stromland K, Sjogreen L, Miller M, Gillberg C, Wentz E, Johansson M, Nylen O, Danielsson A, Jacobsson C, Andersson J, Fernell E. Mobius sequence—a Swedish multidiscipline study. Eur J Paediatr Neurol 2002; 6:35–45.

66. Holroyd S, Reiss AL, Bryan RN. Autistic features in Joubert syndrome: a genetic disorder with agenesis of the cerebellar vermis. Biol Psychiatry 1993; 33:854–855.

67. Berney TP, Ireland M, Burn J. Behavioral phenotype of Cornelia de Lange syndrome. Arch Dis Child 1999; 81:333–336.
68. Jones MB, Szatmari P. A risk-factor model of epistatic interaction, focusing on autism. Am J Med Genet 2000; 114:558–565.
69. Chudley AE, Gutierrez E, Jocelyn LJ, Chodirker BN. Outcomes of genetic evaluation in children with pervasive developmental disorder. J Dev Behav Pediatr 1998; 19:321–325.
70. Steffenburg S. Neuropsychiatric assessment of children with autism: a population-based study. Dev Med Child Neurol 1991; 33:495–511.
71. Chakraborti S, Fombone E. Pervasive developmental disorders in preschool children. JAMA 2001; 285:3093–3099.
72. Gillberg C. Clinical and neurobiologicl aspects in six family studies of Asperger syndrome. In: Frith U, ed. Autism and Asperger Syndrome. Cambridge: Cambridge University Press, 1991:122–146.
73. Stubbs EG, Crawford ML. Depressed lymphocyte responsiveness in autistic children. J Autism Child Schizophr 1977; 7:49–55.
74. Warren RP, Margaratten NC, Pace NC, Foster A. Immune abnormailites in patients with autism. J Autism Dev Disord 1986; 16:189–197.
75. Plioplys AV, Greaves A, Kazemi K, Silverman E. Lymphocyte function in autism and Rett syndrome. Neuropsychobiology 1994; 29:12–16.
76. Singh VK, Fudenberg HH, Emerson D, Coleman M. Immunodiagnosis and immunotherapy in autistic children. Ann NY Acad Sci 1988; 540:602–604.
77. Warren RP, Yonk LJ, Burger RA, Cole P, Odell JD, Warren WL, White E, Singh VK. Deficiency of suppressor-inducer (CD4+CD45RA+) T cells in autism. Immunol Invest 1990; 19:245–251.
78. Yonk LJ, Warren RP, Burger RA, Cole P, Odell JD, Warren WL, White E, Singh VK. CD4+ helper T cell depression in autism. Immunol Lett 1990; 25:341–345.
79. Denney DR, Frei BW, Gaffhey GR. Lymphocyte subsets and interleukin-2 receptors in autistic children. J Autism Dev Disord 1996; 26:87–97.
80. Gupta S, Aggarwal S, Rashanravan B, Lee T. Th1- and Th2-like cytokines in CD4+ and CD8+ T cells in autism. J Neuroimmunol 1998; 85:106–109.
81. Warren RP, Foster A, Margaretten NC. Reduced natural killer cell activity in autism. J Am Acad Child Adoleso Psychiatry 1987; 26:333–335.
82. Singh VK, Warren RP, Averett R, Ghaziuddin M. Circulating autoantibodies to neuronal and glial filament proteins in autism. Pediatr Neurol 1997; 17:88–90.
83. Singh VK, Warren RP, Odell JD, Warren WL, Cole P. Antibodies to myelin basic protein in children with autistic behavior. Brain Behav Immun 1993; 7:97–103.
84. Plioplys AV, Greaves A, Yoshida W. Anti-CNS antibodies in childhood neurologic diseases. Neuropediatrics 1989; 20:93–103.
85. Vojdani A, Campbell AW, Anyanwu E, Kashanian A, Bock K, Vojdani E. Antibodies to neuron-specific antigens in children with autism: possible cross-reaction with encephalitogenic proteins from milk, *Chlamydia pneumoniae* and *Streptococcus* group A. J Neuroimmunol 2002; 129:168–177.
86. Singh VK, Singh EA, Warren RP. Hyperserotoninemia and serotonin receptor antibodies in children with autism but not mental retardation. Biol Psychiatry 1997; 41:753–755.

87. Todd RD, Ciaranello RD. Demonstration of inter- and intraspecies differences in serotonin binding sites by antibodies from an autistic child. Proc Natl Acad Sci USA 1985; 82:612–616.
88. Cook EH Jr., Perry BD, Dawson G, Wainwright MS, Leventhal BL. Receptor inhibition by immunoglobulins: specific inhibition by autistic children, their relatives, and control subjects. J Autism Dev Disord 1993; 23:67–78.
89. Connolly AM, Chez MG, Pestronk A, Arnold ST, Mehta, Deuel RK. Serum autoantibodies to brain in Landau-Kleffner variant, autism, and other neurologic disorders. J Pediatr 1999; 134:607–613.
90. Comi AM, Zimmerman AW, Frye VH, Law PA, Peeden JN. Familial clustering of autoimmune disorders and evaluation of medical risk factors in autism. J Child Neurol 1999; 14:388–394.
91. Warren RP, Yonk J, Burger RW, Odell D, Warren WL. DR-positive T cells in autism: association with decreased plasma levels of the complement C4B protein. Neuropsychobiology 1995; 31:53–57.
92. Gupta S. Treatment of children with autism with intravenous inimunoglobulin. J Child Neurol 1999; 14:203–205.
93. Plioplys AV. Intravenous immunoglobulin treatment in autism. J Autism Dev Disord 2000; 30:73–74.
94. DelGiudice-Asch G, Simon L, Schmeidler J, Cunningham-Rundles C, Hollander E. Brief report: a pilot open clinical trial of intravenous immunoglobulin in childhood autism. J Autism Dev Disord 1999; 29:157–160.
95. Gershon MD. The enteric nervous system: a second brain. Hosp Pract (Off Ed). 1999; 34:31–32, 35–38, 41–42.
96. Yung WH, Leung PS, Ng SS, Zhang J, Chan SC, Chow BK. Secretin facilitates GABA transmission in the cerebellum. J Neurosci 2001; 21:7063–7068.
97. Delgado M. Vasoactive intestinal peptide and pituitary adenylate cyclase-activating polypeptide inhibit CBP-NF-kappaB interaction in activated microglia. Biochem Biophys Res Commun 2002; 297:1181–1185.
98. Reichelt KL, Hole K, Hamberfer A, et al. Biologically active peptide containing fractions in schizophrenia and childhood autism. Adv Biochem Psychopharmacol 1981; 28:627–643.
99. Israngkun PP, Newman HAI, Patel ST, DuRuibe VA, Abou-Issa H. Potential biochemical markers for infantile autism. Neurochem Pathol 1986; 5:51–70.
100. D'Eufemia P, Celli M, Finocchiaro R, et al. Abnormal intestinal permeability in children with autism. Acta Paediatr 1996; 85:1076–1079.
101. Wakefield AJ, Murch SH, Anthony A. Ileal-lymphoid-nodular hyperplasia, non-specific colitis, and pervasive developmental disorder in children. Lancet 1998; 351(9103):637–641.
102. Horvath K, Papadimitriou JC, Rabsztyn A, Drachenberg C, Tildon JT. Gastrointestinal abnormalities in children with autistic disorder. J Pediatr 1999; 135:559–563.
103. Reichelt KL, Knivsberg A, Lind G, Nodland M. Probable etiology and possible treatment of childhood autism. Brain Disfunct 1991; 4:308–319.
104. Knivsberg A, Reichelt KL, Nodland M, et al. Autistic syndromes and diet: a follow-up study. Scand J Educ Res 1995; 39:222–236.

105. Reichelt KL, Saelid, G, Lindback T, et al. Childhood autism: a complex disorder. Biol Psychiatry 1986; 21:1279–1290.
106. Shattock P, Kennedy A, Rowell F, et al. The role of neuropeptides in autism and their relationship with classical neurotransmitters. Brain Dysfunct 1990; 3:328–345.
107. Furlano RI, Anthony A, Day R. Colonic CD8 and gammadelta T-cell infiltration with epithelial damage in children with autism. J Pediatr 2001; 138:366–372.
108. Goodwin MS, Cowen MA, Goodwin TC. Malabsorption and cerebral dysfunction: a multivariate and comparative study of autistic children. J Autism Child Schizophr 1971; 1:48–62.
109. Madsen KM, Hviid A, Vestergaard M, Schendel D, Wohlfahrt J, Thorsen P, Olsen J, Melbye M. A population-based study of measles, mumps, and rubella vaccination and autism. N Engl J Med 2002; 7(347):1477–1482.
110. Finegold SM, Molitoris D, Song Y, Liu C, Vaisanen ML, Bolte E, McTeague M, Sandler R, Wexler H, Marlowe EM, Collins MD, Lawson PA, Summanen P, Baysallar M, Tomzynski TJ, Read E, Johnson E, Rolfe R, Nasir P, Shah H, Haake DA, Manning P, Kaul A. Gastrointestinal microflora studies in late-onset autism. Clin Infect Dis 2002; 1(35)(suppl 1):S6–S16.
111. Sandler RH, Finegold SM, Bolte ER, Buchanan CP, Maxwell AP, Vaisanen ML, Nelson MN, Wexler HM. Short-term benefit from oral vancomycin treatment of regressive-onset autism. J Child Neurol 2000; 15:429–435.
112. Megson MN. Is autism a G-alpha protein defect reversible with natural vitamin A? Med Hypoth 2000; 54:979–983.
113. Fombonne E, Du Mazaubrun C, Cans C, Grandjean H. Autism and associated medical disorders in a French epidemiological survey. J Am Acad Child Adolesc Psychiatry 1997; 36:1561–1569.
114. Fombonne E. Inflammatory bowel disease and autism (letter). Lancet 1998; 351:955.
115. Lucarelli S, Frediani T, Zingoni AM, et al. Food allergy and infantile autism. Panminerva Med 1995; 37:137–141.
116. Cornish E. Gluten and casein free diets in autism: a study of the effects on food choice and nutrition. J Hum Nutr Diet 2002; 15:261–269.
117. Sandler AD, Sutton KA, DeWeese J, et al. Lack of benefit of a single dose of synthetic human secretin in the treatment of autism and pervasive developmental disorder. N Engl J Med 1999; 341:1801–1806.
118. Lightdale JR, Hayer C, Duer A. Effects of intravenous secretin on language and behavior of children with autism and gastrointestinal symptoms: a single-blinded, open-label pilot study. URL: http://www.pediatrics.org/cgi/content/full/108/5/e90.
119. Feldman HM, Kolmen BK, Gonzaga AM. Naltrexone and communication skills in young children with autism. J Am Acad Child Adolesc Psychiatry, 1999; 38:587–593.
120. Miller MT. Thalidomide embryopathy: an insight into autism? Teratology 1993; 47:387–388.
121. Stromland K, Nordin V, Miller M, Akerstrom B, Gilberg C. Autism in thalidomide embryopathy: a population study. Dev Med Child Neurol 1994; 36:351–356.

122. Rodier PM, Ingram JL, Tisdale B, Croog VJ. Linking etiologies in humans and animal models: studies of autism. Reprod Toxicol 1997; 11:417–422.

123. Moore SJ, Turnpenny P, Quinn A, Glover S, Llyod DJ, Montgomery T, Dean JC. A clinical study of 57 children with fetal anticonvulsant syndromes. J Med Genet 2000; 37:489–497.

124. Nanson JL. Autism in fetal alcohol syndrome: a report of five cases. Alcohol Clin Exp Res 1990; 14:322.

125. Davis E, Fennoy I, Laraque D, Kanem N, Brown G, Mitchell J. Autism and developmental abnormalities in children with perinatal cocaine exposure. J Natl Med Assoc 1992; 84:315–319.

126. Delaney-Black V, Covington C, Templin T, Compton S, Sokol R, Ager J, Martier S. Influence of prenatal alcohol/cocaine exposure on the report of autistic-like behaviors among first grade students. Alcohol Clin Exp Res 1997; 21(3 suppl):117A.

127. Bertrand J, Mars A, Boyle C, Bove F, Yeargin-Allsopp M, Decoulfe P. Prevalence of autism in a United States population: the Brick Township, New Jersey, investigation. Pediatrics 2001; 108:1155–1161.

128. Trask CL, Kosofsky BE. Developmental considerations of neurotoxic exposures. Neurol Clin. 2000; 18:541–562.

129. Wakefield AJ, Anthony A, Murch SH, et al. Enterocolitis in children with developmental disorders. Am J Gastroenterol 2000; 95:2285–2295.

130. Wakefield AJ, Murch SH, Anthony A, et al. Ileal-lymphoid-nodular hyperplasia, nonspecific colitis, and pervasive developmental disorder in children. Lancet 1998; 351:637–641.

131. Taylor B, Miller E, Farrington CP, et al. Autism and measles, mumps, and rubella vaccine: no epidemiologic evidence for a causal association. Lancet 1999; 353:2026–2069.

132. Madsen KM, Hviid A, Vestergaard M, Schendel D, Wohlfahrt J, Thorsen P, Olsen J, Melbye M. Population-based study of measles, mumps, and rubella vaccination and autism. N Engl J Med. 2002; 347:1477–1482.

133. Dales L, Hammer SJ, Smith NJ. Time trends in autism and in MMR immunization coverage in California. JAMA 2001; 285:1183–1185.

134. Thjodleifsson B, Davidsdottir K, Agnarsson U, Sigthorsson G, Kjeld M, Bjarnason I. Effect of Pentavac and measles-mumps-rubella (MMR) vaccination on the intestine. Gut 2002; 51:816–817.

135. Makela A, Nuorti JP, Pelota H. Neurologic disorders after measles-mumps-rubella vaccination. Pediatrics 2002; 110:957–963.

136. Haga Y, Funakoshi O, Kuroe K, Kanazawa K, Nakajima H, Saito H, Murata Y, Munakata A, Yoshida Y. Absence of measles viral genomic sequence in intestinal tissues from Crohn's disease by nested polymerase chain reaction. Gut 1996; 38:211–215.

137. Afzal MA, Minor PD, Begley J, Bentley ML, Armitage E, Ghosh S, Ferguson A. Absence of measles-virus genome in inflammatory bowel disease. Lancet 1998; 351:646–647.

138. Bernard S, Enayati A, Redwood L, Roger H, Binstock T. Autism: a novel form of mercury poisoning. Med Hypoth 2001; 56:462–471.

139. Redwood L, Bernard S, Brown D. Predicted mercury concentrations in hair from infant immunizations: cause for concern. Neurotoxicology 2001; 22:691–697.
140. Institute of Medicine, and Immunization Safety Review Committee. Immunization Safety Review: Measles-Mumps-Rubella Vaccine and Autism. Washington, DC: National Academy Press, 2001.
141. Halsey NA, Hyman S. Members of the AAP-Autism Writing Panel. Measles-mumps-rubella vaccine and autism spectrum disorder: report from the new challenges in childhood immunizations conference. Pediatrics 2001; 107:E84.
142. Chess S. Autism in children with congenital rubella. J Autism Child Schizophr 1971; 1:33–47.
143. Chess S. Follow-up report on autism in congenital rubella. J Autism Child Schizophr 1977; 7:69–81.
144. Ivarsson SA, Bjerre I, Vegfors P, Ahlfors K. Autism as one of several disabilities in two children with congenital cytomegalovirus infection. Neuropediatrics 1990; 21:102–103.
145. Ghaziuddin M, Al-Khouri I, Ghaziuoddin N. Autistic symptoms following herpes encephalitis. Eur Child Adolesc Psychiatry 2002; 11:142–146.
146. Hornig M, Lipkin WI. Infectious and immune factors in the pathogenesis of neurodevelopmental disorders: epidemiology, hypotheses, and animal models. Ment Retard Dev Disabil Res Rev 2001; 7:200–210.
147. Lipkin WI, Battenberg ELF, Bloom FE, et al. Viral infections can depress neurotransmitter mRNA levels without histologic injury. Brain Res 451:333–339.
148. Juul-Dam N, Townsend J, Courchesne E. Prenatal, perinatal, and neonatal factors in autism, pervasive developmental disorder-not otherwise specified, and the general population. Pediatrics 2001; 107:E63.
149. Deykin EY, MacMahon B. Pregnancy, delivery, and neonatal complications among autistic children. Am J Dis Child 1980; 134:860–864.
150. Gilberg C, Gilberg IC. Infantile autism: a total population study of reduced optimality in the pre-, peri-, and neonatal period. J Autism Dev Disord 1983; 13:153–166.
151. Finegan JA, Quarrington B. Pre-, peri-, and neonatal factors and infantile autism. J Child Psychol Psychiatry 1979; 20:119–128.
152. Bolton PF, Murphy M, Macdonald H, Whitlock B, Pickles A, Rutter M. Obstetric complications in autism: consequences or causes of the condition? J Am Acad Child Adolesc Psychiatry 1997; 36:272–281.
153. Deb S, Prasad KB, Seth H, Eagles JM. A comparison of obstetric and neonatal complications between children with autistic disorder and their siblings. J Intellect Disabil Res 1997; 41(pt 1):81–86.
154. Cryan E, Byrne M, O'Donovan A, O'Callaghan E. A case-control study of obstetric complications and later autistic disorder. J Autism Dev Disord 1996; 26:453–460.
155. Piven J, Simon J, Chase GA, et al. The etiology of autism: pre-, peri- and neonatal factors. J Am Acad Child Adolesc Psychiatry 1993; 32:1256–1263.

156. Topcu M, Saatchi I, Haliloglu G, Keismer M, Coskun T. D-glyceric aciduria in a six-month-old boy presenting with West syndrome and autistic behaviour. Neuropediatrics 2002; 33:47–50.
157. Page T. Metabolic approaches to the treatment of autism spectrum disorders. J Autism Dev Disord 2000; 30:463–469.
158. Page T, Coleman M. Purine metabolism abnormalities in a hyperuricosuric subclass of autism. Biochim Biophys Acta 2000; 1500:291–296.
159. Alberti A, Pirrone P, Elia M, Waring RH, Romano C. Sulphation deficit in "low-functioning" autistic children: a pilot study. Biol Psychiatry 1999; 46:420–424.

4

Neurological Basis of Autism

Vidya Bhushan Gupta
New York Medical College and Columbia University, New York,
New York, U.S.A.

I. INTRODUCTION

Brain is the final pathway to which all the etiological factors discussed in the last chapter lead. There is sufficient evidence in the neuroscience literature that autistic symptoms occur because of functional or structural abnormalities of the brain. About 15–30% of children with autism have macrocephaly (1–5), due to larger brain volume (6,7), with increases in both gray and white matter (8). While autistic individuals continue to have a larger head circumference throughout their life, their brain volume decreases after increasing for a few years after birth (8–10), suggesting a neuropathological process that begins before birth but continues postnatally. Increased head circumference in autism is not correlated with IQ, verbal ability, seizure disorder, or autistic symptoms.

Despite a litany of studies pointing to the neurogenic origin of autistic symptoms, the core areas of the brain that are involved and the specifics of their dysfunction are unknown. The attempts to find a single source of autistic symptoms in the brain have been unsuccessful and it is likely that this syndrome is neurologically heterogeneous with different symptoms originating from different structures of the brain. Perhaps autism occurs due to an insult to the developing nervous system at an earlier stage when a localized insult branches off to other areas of the brain because of the "interdependent nature of early brain development" (11). Depending on sensory inputs and other factors during subsequent maturation, this "branching off" takes its unique course in every individual, giving rise to unique pathology in every individual. Reported abnormalities in the key brain structures that have been incriminated as the "home of autism in the brain" (12) are described below.

II. CEREBELLUM

Several neuropathological studies have found low Purkinje and granular cell count in the cerebellar hemispheres of individuals with autism (13–15). Smaller Purkinje cells have been reported. Fatemi et al. attributed small this reduction in the size of Purkinje cells to reduction in Reelin and Bcl-2 proteins in the cerebellum (16,17). Proton magnetic resonance studies have found lower concentration of N-acetyl aspartate (NAA) in the cerebellum, suggesting reduced activity of Purkinje cells (18,19).

Hypoplasia of cerebellar vermal lobules VI and VII was reported as the "eureka" of autism in 1988 by Courchesne et al. (20), but since then other findings, such as hypoplasia of vermal lobuli VIII–X (21,22), hypoplasia of vermal lobuli I–V (23), and a combination of vermal hypo- and hyperplasia, have been described (24). A report of pervasive developmental disorder in two children with Joubert's syndrome, a condition characterized by the agenesis of cerebellar vermis, provided some support to the cerebellar hypothesis of autism (25), but a later study refuted this association (26). Not all individuals with autism have vermal hypoplasia (27,28) and vermal hypoplasia has been described in individuals without autism, such as acute lymphoblastic leukemia survivors (29,30). According to Ciesielski and Knight, involvement of the cerebellum in such diverse conditions may be due to its prolonged course of maturation, making it vulnerable to injury (30).

Morphometric studies of cerebellum have also shown inconsistent and contradictory results. Both small (31) and large (32) cerebella have been described, and in studies that report large cerebella, increase in cerebellar size out of proportion to the overall brain size (32) as well as increase in cerebellar size proportional to the overall brain size has been reported (27,33).

Limited support for the cerebellar hypothesis of autism comes from an animal model in which exposure to valproic acid early during gestation damages the brainstem cranial nerve nuclei and reduces the number of neurons in the deep cerebellar nuclei, changes analogous to thalidomide embryopathy with autism (34).

Although it is difficult to conclude from the inconsistent and contradictory data presented above that cerebellar abnormalities are the source of autistic symptoms in every person with autism, they may be responsible for some symptoms of autism in a subset of patients. The cerebellum plays an important role in language, emotion, and motor-attentional systems through its connections with frontal lobe, thalamus, olivary nuclei, and other areas of the brain. It is plausible that abnormalities of the cerebellum or a disruption of its neural networks with the other areas of the brain contributes to symptoms pertaining to these domains (35,36).

III. LIMBIC SYSTEM

The limbic system includes subcallosal, cingulate, orbitofrontal and parahippocampal gyri, underlying hippocampal formation, dentate nucleus, amygdaloid complex, anterior thalamus, mamillary bodies, fornix, and septal nuclei. The limbic system is believed to be the socio-emotional brain, and is, thus, a plausible candidate for the source of social symptoms in autism (37). Citing a functional MRI (fMRI) study in which patients with autism or Asperger's syndrome did not activate their amygdala when judging what that other person might be thinking or feeling by looking at his face, Baron-Cohen et al. proposed an "amygdale theory of autism" (38). Howard et al. showed that people with high-functioning autism have a neuropsychological profile characteristic of amygdala damage, in particular impairment in recognizing faces and facial expressions. Using quantitative magnetic resonance (MR) images analysis techniques, they demonstrated bilateral enlargement of the amygdala in these individuals (39). Bitemporal ablation of the hippocampus and amygdala in monkeys was reported to produce behavioral effects suggestive of autism (40), but this finding has been recently refuted by Amaral and Corbett (41).

Limbic system involvement is suggested by the findings of smaller anterior cingulate gyrus (42) and area dentata in MRIs of brains of individuals with autism (43). Functional neuroimaging has shown reduced glucose metabolism in cingulate gyrus of individuals with autism (44). Autopsy studies have revealed small, sparsely branched, but tightly packed, neurons in hippocampus and amygdala of the brains of individuals with autism (45,46), suggesting arrested maturation of the limbic system. However, other studies have not confirmed these findings (13).

As in the case of cerebellum, the data on the involvement of limbic system in autism are inconsistent and contradictory (13,47). It seems that structural or functional abnormalities of the limbic system may be responsible for social-cognitive deficits (theory of mind deficits) in a subset of individuals with autism, but are by no means universal.

IV. BRAINSTEM

Association between autism and Möbius sequence suggests that brainstem may be involved in a few cases of autism (48,49). Möbius sequence is characterized by hypoplasia of cranial nerve nuclei resulting in congenital palsy of the sixth and seventh cranial nerves. Rodier et al. found cellular abnormalities of the facial and other brainstem nuclei in the brain of a woman with autism. The association between cranial nerve involvement and autism has also been seen in thalidomide embryopathy (50). Rodier et al. reproduced the lesion seen in thalidomide embryopathy in rats by exposing them to valproic acid at the time of neural tube closure (50). Autopsy studies have revealed smaller pons, midbrain, and medulla oblongata (51–53) and abnormalities of inferior olivary nucleus in the brains of individuals with autism (54). It has been suggested that autism occurs because of the persistence of a transitional zone (lamina desiccans) beneath the Purkinje cells where the climbing olivary fibres synapse until 24–30 weeks of gestation. The lesions in brainstem at an early stage of embryogenesis perhaps damage the cerebral-cerebellar connections that are necessary for the development of higher cognitive functions (55). Such brainstem-cerebellar dysfunction was suggested by the finding of abnormal oculomotor movements and brainstem potentials in children with autism in a study (56). However, the evidence for brainstem involvement in autism is far from conclusive. Studies of auditory brainstem responses of autistic probands and their relatives report contradictory results including prolongation, shortening (57,58), and no abnormalities of transmission latencies (59). Few children with autism have cranial nerve palsies.

The brainstem plays a role in arousal and shifting of attention, and modulates both general sensory input and motor response to it. Ornitz et al. found abnormal responses to vestibular stimulation in autistic children (60). Therefore, it is plausible that brainstem dysfunction can cause some symptoms of autism such as transitioning from one activity to another, vestibular dysfunction, and abnormal sensory processing.

V. BASAL GANGLIA

Basal ganglia include caudate nucleus, putamen, globus pallidus, nucleus accumbens, and substantia nigra. An increase in the volume of the caudate nuclei, proportional to the increased total brain volume, was found to be associated with compulsions and rituals, complex motor mannerisms, and resistance to change in autism in an MRI study of the brain (61). The caudate may be part of the abnormal neural networks that are responsible for the ritualistic-repetitive behaviors of the autism (61). Enhanced activity of basal ganglia cells has been incriminated in stereotyped movements of Rett's syndrome (62). A boy with right putamen infarct showed sterotypies similar to those seen in autism (63). Animal models have localized behavioral stereotypies and self-injurious behavior to basal ganglia (64). Although direct evidence of basal ganglia involvement in autism is meager, circumstantial evidence is compelling that structural or chemical abnormalities of the basal ganglia cause stereotypic and repetitive behavior in autism. According to Thong, stereotypic and ritualistic behavior in autism occurs due to injury to the more primitive striatal complex, mammalian counterpart of the brain of reptiles (65).

VI. CEREBRAL CORTEX

Cognitive and communication deficits in autism make cerebral cortex a plausible "home for autism." Findings in structural MRIs of the brains of individuals with autism have included changes in the size of anterior horns of lateral ventricles and right lenticular nucleus (66), smaller parietal lobes (67), and findings suggestive of abnormal neuronal migration, such as polymicrogyria, schizencephaly, and macrogyria (68).

Functional neuroimaging of the brain of autistic individuals suggests involvement of cerebral cortex but no particular region emerges as the preeminent source of autistic behaviors. Many studies have reported involvement of temporal lobes and auditory cortex in autism (69,70). Chugani et al. showed reduced bitemporal hypometabolism on positron emission tomography (69). George et al. reported reduction in total brain as well as frontal and right temporal lobe perfusion, but this finding was not confirmed in another study (70,71). Using functional MRI during a theory of mind task, Baron-Cohen et al. showed less activation of the superior temporal gyrus, an area that is usually activated in such tasks in normal individuals (72). The role of the temporal lobe in autism is suggested by the association between autistic symptoms and temporal tubers and temporal lobe epileptiform discharges in tuberous sclerosis (73), and focal EEG abnormalities in the temporal region in West syndrome (74). DeLong has proposed that low-functioning autism occurs due to bitemporal, especially mesial temporal, involvement, while higher-functioning autism occurs due to left hemispheric dysfunction with sparing and even better functioning of the right hemisphere (75). Reversed hemispheric dominance with decreased blood flow to the left cortical areas devoted to language and handedness in children has been reported by others as well (76,77).

Abnormalities of other cortical areas have also been reported in autism. Prefrontal dysfunction is suggested by abnormalities in voluntary suppression of oculomotor responses to visual targets (78). Delayed metabolic maturation of frontal lobes causing functional deficits in object permanence and theory of mind has been reported (79).

Electrophysiological studies, like electro- and magnetoencephalography, nonspecifically suggest that there is cortical dysfunction in autism but do not help in clinical diagnosis or explain the neurological source of autistic behaviors. Traditional EEG of individuals with autism shows paroxysmal activity in

20–70% of cases while magnetoencephalography shows epileptiform activity in as many as 82% of cases (80,81). Epileptiform activity is mostly focal or multifocal with centrotemporal spikes, with occipital spikes in a minority of patients (82). Although epileptiform activity is more common in children with regression, it is not certain if this activity causes regression and whether anticonvulsants can stall regression (83,84). The effects of the epileptiform discharge on cognitive functioning may be due to the extension of epileptic activity in temporal or parietal lobes, but this has not been confirmed.

Epilepsy has been reported in as many as 4–30% of children with autism and pervasive developmental disorders, providing additional support for the neurogenic basis of autism. Clinical seizures, usually partial, occur more often in infancy and adolescence (86–90).

In the absence of a core deficit area in autism, abnormality of neural networks has been proposed to be the primary problem in autism (35). Damage to the developing neural networks can result in secondary problems in the regions interconnected by these networks. Recent finding of small and less compact minicolumns in key frontal and temporal lobe gyri of the brains of individuals with autism supports this view (91). Because of environmental vulnerability and neural plasticity of the networks, each child may have a unique neurological and symptomatic profile. Other mechanisms that have been incriminated in autistic neuropathology are listed in Table 1.

It is likely that dysfunction of different areas of the brain contributes to different aspects of autistic symptomatology (Table 2). For example, attentional deficits and inflexibility may be caused by prefrontal dysfunction, communication abnormalities due to temporal lobe dysfunction, theory of mind deficits due to dysfunction of the orbitofrontal cortex and limbic system, and stereotypies due to dysfunction of the basal ganglia.

Table 1 Possible Neuropathological Processes in Autism

Delayed maturation
Maturational arrest with persistence of fetal circuitry
Abnormal development of neuropil (reduced dendritic pruning or abnormal proliferation)
Early damage to neural circuits/networks
Abnormal neuronal migration
Abnormal differentiation (microcolumnar changes)
Early degeneration (neurofibrillay tangles)
Abnormal apoptosis
Disconnect between various areas of the brain
Abnormalities of cerebral regional blood flow

Table 2 Possible Sources of Autistic Symptoms in the Brain

Symptom complex	Source in the brain	Reported associations
Impairment in social interaction	Limbic system	Enlargement of amygdala
Theory of mind tasks		Tightly packed small neurons
Impairments in communication	Temporal cortex	Bitemporal hypometabolism Temporal lobe epileptiform discharges
Cognitive impairment	Cerebral cortex	Abnormal neuronal migration
Inattention, hyperactivity, impulsivity, and inflexibility	Prefrontal cortex	Abnormalities in voluntary suppression of oculomotor responses to visual targets
Restricted and stereotyped behaviors	Basal ganglia	Larger caudate nuclei
Fine-tuning of communicative, emotional, attentional, and motor responses to the context	Cerebellum	Low Purkinje cell count Vermal hypoplasia
Difficulties in transitioning from one activity to another, vestibular and sensory dysfunction	Brainstem	Smaller brainstem structures Cranial nerve nuclear hypoplasia Abnormalities of inferior olivary nuclei
Inability to discriminate between competing sensory information	Frontal and temporal cortex	Small, less compact, numerous minicolumns

VII. NEUROCHEMICAL FACTORS

Because the symptoms of autism originate in multiple areas of the brain, abnormal chemical neurotransmission among these areas may be the root cause of autism. There is some evidence to support the neurochemical basis of autism, but like neuroimaging, neurochemical findings in autism are inconsistent and contradictory. While many studies have reported increased serotonin levels in whole blood and platelets in individuals with autism (92–94), a few have reported low whole-blood serotonin levels in children with autism (95). Based on the finding of autoantibodies to brain serotonin receptors (96), it has been suggested that serotonin-blocking antibodies inhibit the specific binding of serotonin to its receptor in autistic children, causing serotonergic dysfunction (97), but research support for this hypothesis is lacking (98,99).

The finding of increased serotonin in blood platelets generated interest in the role of serotonin transporter gene (5-HTT) in increasing 5-HT uptake in platelets, but the findings have been inconclusive. While some studies have suggested an association between the serotonin transporter gene and autistic disorder (100,101), others have not (102,103). Serotonin transporter promoter alleles have also been examined, because they can modify the severity of autistic behaviors in the social and communication domains, without increasing the risk for autism (104,105). Clinical pharmacological evidence about serotonergic dysfunction in autism is contradictory, because clinical improvement occurs with agents that enhance its transmission, such as clomipramine (106), fluoxetine, and paroxetine (107), and those that deplete serotonin, such as fenfluramine (108), or block its transmission, such as risperidone (109). Serotonin is involved in perception and sensory filtration of stimuli and in social attachment (110) and its dysfunction can plausibly cause autistic symptoms; the exact nature of serotonergic dysfunction in autism is still unknown despite a litany of studies.

Improvement in behavioral symptoms of autism by haloperidol, a dopamine antagonist, suggests that dopaminergic systems are involved in autism (111). Risperidone, an atypical neuroleptic and a potent antagonist of the postsynaptic dopamine D2 receptor, is effective in controlling some symptoms of autism, such as tantrums, aggression, and self-injurious behavior (109). Higher levels of homovanillic acid, a metabolite of dopamine, have been reported in low-functioning autistic children (112). The dopaminergic system influences selective attention and motor behavior (113). Dysfunction of dopaminergic transmission in the prefrontal cortex may cause symptoms of inattention and hyperactivity in autism, while in the basal ganglia it may cause motor stereotypies (114). The role of dopamine in autism is, however, inconclusive, because drugs that antagonize dopamine, such as risperidone, as well as those that enhance its transmission, such as methylphenidate, are helpful in children with autism.

Opioid overactivity in the brain has been proposed to be the cause of poor socialization, decreased sensitivity to pain, and self-injurious behaviour in autism (115). The limbic system, which is implicated in the causation of socio-emotional and theory of mind problems of autism, is rich in endogenous opioid receptors (116). But drug trials with the opiate antagonist naltrexone and direct measurement of blood or spinal fluid levels of endorphins have not demonstrated strong evidence of opiate excess being responsible for the core symptoms of autistic spectrum disorder (117–121).

An unsubstantiated theory about the role of exogenous opioids in autism is in vogue in the alternative medicine camp. According to this theory, an excess of opioids enter the bloodstream from the gut through a defective mucosal barrier. Opioids are produced in the gut from incompletely digested gluten and/or casein due to the failure of intestinal peptidases to convert opioids to innocuous metabolites (122,123). The results of two systematic trials of dietary exclusion of gluten and casein have been equivocal (124,125).

Dysfunction of other neurotransmitter systems, such as catecholamines, glutamate, γ-amino butyric acid (GABA), neuropeptides (126), and nicotine (127), has been proposed to cause symptoms of autism. Catecholamines are plausible candidates for involvement in autism because noradrenergic cells in the locus ceruleus regulate attention, behavioral flexibility, filtering of irrelevant stimuli, arousal, anxiety, and learning, which are impaired in autistic individuals (128). Plasma norepinephrine has been reported to be elevated in some children with autism (129). Increased levels of neuroexcitatory neurotransmitters, such as glutamate and upregulation of their receptors, can damage neural pathways, resulting in symptoms of autism. Reduced levels of gluatamic acid decarboxylase have been reported in the brains of autistic children. This can theoretically result in elevated levels of glutamate in blood and platelets (130). Evidence for both these neurotransmitters is weak and unreliable. Hormones such as oxytocin, insulin-like growth factor, and testosterone have also been suggested to have or affect neurotransmitter function (131).

It seems that no single neurotransmitter has a monopoly on the symptoms of autism, but they modulate one another's actions to cause a unique mix of symptoms in each patient. Because of the unique pattern of neurochemical dysfunction in each patient, no single drug works in all the patients. Various neurotransmitters putatively involved in autism are presented in Table 3.

Table 3 Neurotransmitters Involved in Autism

Neurotransmitter	Symptom	Evidence
Serotonin	Social orientation, attunement, and cognition	Increased serotonin levels in whole blood and platelets Autoantibodies to brain serotonin receptors
Dopamine In prefrontal cortex Basal ganglia	Inattention, hyperactivity, behavioral flexibility, stereotypies, mannerisms	Higher levels of homovanillic acid
Norepinephrine	Hyper- or hypoarousal Regulation of attention, anxiety	Elevated plasma norepinephrine
Others	Opioids, glutamate, γ-amino butyric acid (GABA), neuropeptides, and nicotine	

REFERENCES

1. Fombonne E, Roge B, Claverie J, Courty S, Fremolle J. Microcephaly and macrocephaly in autism. J Autism Dev Disord 2000; 30:365.
2. Bolton PF, Roobol M, Allsopp L, Pickles A. Association between idiopathic infantile macrocephaly and autism spectrum disorders. Lancet 2001; 358(9283): 726–727.
3. Fidler DJ, Bailey JN, Smalley SL. Macrocephaly in autism and other pervasive developmental disorders. Dev Med Child Neurol 2000; 42:737–740.
4. Parmeggiani A, Posar A, Giovanardi-Rossi P, Andermann F, Zifkin B. Autism, macrocrania and epilepsy: how are they linked? Brain Dev 2002; 24:296–299.
5. Davidovitch M, Patterson B, Gartside P. Head circumference measurements in children with autism. J Child Neurol 1996; 11:389–393.
6. Piven J, Arndt S, Bailey J, Andreasen N. Regional brain enlargement in autism: a magnetic resonance imaging study. J Am Acad Child Adolesc Psychiatry 1996; 35:530–536.
7. Piven J, Arndt S, Bailey J, Havercamp S, Andreasen NC, Palmer P. An MRI study of brain size in autism. Am J Psychiatry 1995; 152:1145–1149.
8. Courchesne E, et al. Unusual brain growth patterns in early life in patients with autism. Neurology 2001; 57:245–254.
9. Lainhart JE, Piven J, Wzorek M, et al. Macrocephaly in children and adults with autism. J Am Acad Child Adolesc Psychiatry 1997; 36:282–290.
10. Aylward EH, Minshew NJ, Field K, Sparks BF, Singh N. Effects of age on brain volume and head circumference in autism. Neurology 2002; 59:175–183.
11. Schultz RT, Klin A. Genetics of childhood disorders: XLIII. Autism, Part 2: Neural Foundations. J An Acad Child Adolesc Psychiatry 2002; 41:1259–1262.
12. Rapin I. Autism in search of a home in the brain. Neurology 1999; 52:902–904.
13. Kemper TL, Bauman M. Neuropathology of infantile autism. J Neuropathol Exp Neurol 1998; 57:645–652.
14. Bailey A, Luthert P, Dean A, Harding B, Janota I, Montogomery M, Rutter M, Lantos P. A clinicopathological study of autism. Brain 1998; 121 (Pt 5):889–905.
15. Ritvo ER, Freeman BJ, Scheibel AB, et al. Lower Purkinje cell counts in the cerebellum of four autistic subjects: initial findings of the UCLA-NSAC Autopsy Research Report. Am J Psychiatry 1986; 143:862–866.
16. Fatemi SH, Halt AR, Realmuto G, Earle J, Kist DA, Thuras P, Merz A. Purkinje cell size is reduced in cerebellum of patients with autism. Cell Mol Neurobiol 2002; 22:171–175.
17. Fatemi SH, Stary JM, Halt AR, Realmuto GR. Dysregulation of Reelin and Bcl-2 proteins in autistic cerebellum. J Autism Dev Disord 2001; 31:529–535.
18. Chugani DC, Sunderam BS, Behen M, et al. Evidence of altered energy metabolism in autistic children. Prog Neuropsychopharmacol Biol Psychiatry 1999; 23:635–641.
19. Otsuka H, Harda M, Mori K, et al. Brain metabolism in the hippocampus-amygdala region and cerebellum in autism: an iH-MR spectroscopy study. Neuroradiology 1999; 41:517–519.

20. Courchesne E, Yeung-Courchesne R, Press GA, Hesselink JR, Jernigan TL. Hypoplasia of cerebellar vermal lobules VI and VII in autism. N Engl J Med 1988 26; 318:1349–1354.
21. Levitt JG, Blanton R, Capetillo-Cunliffe L, Guthrie D, Toga A, McCracken JT. Cerebellar vermis lobules VIII–X in autism. Prog Neuropsychopharmacol Biol Psychiatry 1999; 23:625–633.
22. Hashimoto T, Tayama M, Miyazaki M, Murakawa K, Kuroda Y. Brainstem and cerebellar vermis involvement in autistic children. J Child Neurol 1993; 8:149–153.
23. Ciesielski KT, Harris RJ, Hart BL, Pabst HF. Cerebellar hypoplasia and frontal lobe cognitive deficits in disorders of early childhood. Neuropsychologia 1997; 35:643–655.
24. Saitoh O, Courchesne E. Magnetic resonance imaging study of the brain in autism. Psychiatry Clin Neurosci 1998; 52(suppl):S219–22.
25. Holroyd S, Reiss AL, Bryan RN. Autistic features in Joubert syndrome: a genetic disorder with agenesis of the cerebellar vermis. Biol Psychiatry 1993; 33:854–855.
26. Ozonoff S, Williams BJ, Gale S, Miller JN. Autism and autistic behavior in Joubert syndrome. J Child Neurol 1999; 14:636–641.
27. Garber HJ, Ritvo ER. Magnetic resonance imaging of the posterior fossa in autistic adults. Am J Psychiatry 1992; 149:245–247.
28. Piven J, Saliba K, Bailey J, Arndt S. An MRI study of autism: the cerebellum revisited. Neurology 1997; 49:546–551.
29. Schaefer GB, Thompson JN, Bordensteiner JB, McConnell JM, Kimberling WJ, Gay CT, Dutton WD, Hutchings DC, Gray SB. Hypoplasia of the cerebellar vermis in neurogenetic syndromes. Ann Neurol 1996; 39:382–385.
30. Ciesielski KT, Knight JE. Cerebellar abnormality in autism: a nonspecific effect of early brain damage? Acta Neurobiol Exp (Warsz) 1994; 54:151–154.
31. Courchesne E, Townsend J, Saitoh O. The brain in infantile autism: posterior fossa structures are abnormal. Neurology 1994; 44:214–223.
32. Hardan AY, Minshew NJ, Harenski K, Keshavan MS. Posterior fossa magnetic resonance imaging in autism. J Am Acad Child Adolesc Psychiatry 2001; 40:666–672.
33. Sparks BF, Friedman SD, Shaw DW, Aylward EH, Echelard D, Artru AA, Maravilla KR, Giedd JN, Munson J, Dawson G, Dager SR. Brain structural abnormalities in young children with autism spectrum disorder. Neurology 2002; 59:184–192.
34. Rodier PM. Animal model of autism based on developmental data. MRDD Res Rev 1996; 2:249–256.
35. Zimmerman AW and Gordon B. Neural mechanisms in autism. In: Accardo PJ, Magnusen C, Capute AJ, eds. Autism, Clinical and Research Issues. Baltimore: York Press, 2000.
36. Kern JK. The possible role of the cerebellum in autism/PDD: disruption of a multisensory feedback loop. Med Hypoth 2002; 59:255–260.
37. Brothers L. The social brain: a project for integrating primate behavior and neurophysiology in a new domain. Concepts Neurosci 1990; 1:27–51.

38. Baron-Cohen S, Ring HA, Bullmore ET, Wheelwright S, Ashwin C, Williams SC. The amygdala theory of autism. Neurosci Biobehav Rev 2000; 24:355–364.

39. Howard MA, Cowell PE, Boucher J, Broks P, Mayes A, Farrant A, Roberts N. Convergent neuroanatomical and behavioural evidence of an amygdala hypothesis of autism. Neuroreport 2000; 11:2931–2935.

40. Bachevalier J. Medial temporal lobe structures and autism: a review of clinical and experimental findings. Neuropsychologia 1994; 32:627–648.

41. Amaral DG, Corbett BA. The amygdale, autism, and anxiety. In: Autism: Neural Basis and Treatment Possibilities. Wiley, Chichester, England (Novartis Foundation Symposium 251), 2003:177–197.

42. Haznedar MM, Buchsbaum MS, Metzger M, Solimando A, Spiegel-Cohen J, Hollander E. Anterior cingulate gyrus volume and glucose metabolism in autistic disorder. Am J Psychiatry 1997, 154:1047–1050.

43. Saitoh O, Karns CM, Courchesne E. Development of the hippocampal formation from 2 to 42 years: MRI evidence of smaller area dentate in autism. Brain 2001; 124(Pt 7):1317–1324.

44. Hardenar MM, Buchsbaum MS, Wei TC, Hof PR, Cartwright C, Bienstock CA, Hollander E. Limbic circuitry in patients with autism spectrum disorders studied with positron emission tomography and magnetic resonance imaging. Am J Psychiatry 2000; 157:1994–2001.

45. Kemper TL, Bauman ML. The contribution of neuropathologic studies to the understanding of autism. Neurol Clin 1993; 11:175–187.

46. Raymond GV, Bauman ML, Kemper TL. Hippocampus in autism: a Golgi analysis. Acta Neuropathol (Berl) 1996; 91:117–119.

47. Piven J, Bailey J, Ranson BJ, Arndt S. No difference in hippocampus volume detected on magnetic resonance imaging in autistic individuals. J Autism Dev Disord 1998; 28:105–110.

48. Gillberg C, Steffenburg S. Autistic behaviour in Möbius syndrome. Acta Paediatr Scand 1989; 78:314–316.

49. Stromland K, Sjogreen L, Miller M, Gillberg C, Wentz E, Johansson M, Nylen O, Danielsson A, Jacobsson C, Andersson J, Fernell E. Mobius sequence—a Swedish multidiscipline study. Eur J Paediatr Neurol 2002; 6:35–45.

50. Rodier PM, Ingram JL, Tisdale B, Nelson S, Romano J. Embryological origin for autism: developmental anomalies of the cranial nerve motor nuclei. J Comp Neurol 1996 24; 370:247–261.

51. Hashimoto T, Tayama M, Miyazaki M, Murakawa K, Kuroda Y. Brainstem and cerebellar vermis involvement in autistic children. J Child Neurol 1993; 8:149–153.

52. Hashimoto T, Tayama M, Miyazaki M, et al. Brainstem involvement in high functioning autistic children. Acta Neurol Scand 1993; 88:123–128.

53. Hashimoto T, Tayama M, Murakawa K, et al. Development of the brainstem and cerebellum in autistic patients. J Autism Dev Disord 1995; 25:1–18.

54. Bauman M, Kemper TL, Histoanatomic observations of the brain in early infantile autism. Neurology 1985; 35:866–874.

55. Skoyles JR. Is autism due to cerebral-cerebellum disconnection? Med Hypoth 2002; 58:332–336.

56. Rosenhall U, Johansson E, Gillberg C. Oculomotor findings in autistic children. J Laryngol Otol 1988; 102:435–439.
57. Maziade M, Mérette C, Cayer M, Roy M, Szatmari P, Côté R, Thivierge J. Prolongation of brainstem auditory-evoked responses in autistic probands and their unaffected relatives. Arch Gen Psychiatry 2000; 57:1077–1083.
58. Sersen EA, Heaney G, Clausen J, Belser R, Rainbow S. Brainstem auditory-evoked responses with and without sedation in autism and Down's syndrome. Biol Psychiatry 1990; 27:834–840.
59. Klin A. Auditory brainstem responses in autism: brainstem dysfunction or peripheral hearing loss? J Autism Dev Disord 1993; 23:15–35.
60. Ornitz EM, Atwell CW, Kaplan AR, Westlake JR. Brain-stem dysfunction in autism: results of vestibular stimulation. Arch Gen Psychiatry 1985; 42:1018–1025.
61. Sears LL, Vest C, Mohamed S, Bailey J, Ranson BJ, Piven J. An MRI study of the basal ganglia in autism. Prog Neuropsychopharmacol Biol Psychiatry 1999; 23:613–624.
62. Leontovich TA; Mukhina JK; Fedorov AA; Belichenko PV. Morphological study of the entorhinal cortex, hippocampal formation, and basal ganglia in Rett syndrome patients. Neurobiol Dis 1999; 6:77–91.
63. Maraganore DM, Lees AJ, Marsden CD. Complex stereotypies after right putaminal infarction: a case report. Mov Disord 1991; 6:358–361.
64. Breese GR, Criswell HE, Duncan GE, Moy SS, Johnson KB, Wong DF, Mueller RA. Model for reduced dopamine in Lesch-Nyhan syndrome and the mentally retarded: neurobiology of neonatal-6-OH-dpamine-lesioned rats. MRDD Res Rev 1995; 1:111–119.
65. Thong YH. Reptilian behavioural patterns in childhood autism. Med Hypoth 1984; 13:399–405.
66. Gaffney GR, Kuperman S, Tsai L, Minchin S. Forbrain structure in infantile autism. J Am Acad Child Adolesc Psychiatry 1989; 28:534–537.
67. Courchesne E, Press GA, Yeung-Courchesne R. Parietal lobe abnormalities detected with MR in patients with infantile autism. Am J Roentgenol 1993; 160:387–393.
68. Piven J, Berthier ML, Starkstein SE, Nehme E, Pearlson G, Folstein S. Magnetic resonance imaging evidence for a defect of cerebral cortical development in autism. Am J Psychiatry 1990; 147:734–739.
69. Chugani HT, Da Silva E, Chugani DC. Infantile spasms. III. Prognostic implications of bitemporal hypometabolism on positron emission tomography. Ann Neurol 1996; 39:643–649.
70. George MS, Costa DC, Kouris K, Ring HA, Ell PJ. Cerebral blood flow abnormalities in adults with infantile autism. J Nerv Ment Dis 1992; 180:413–417.
71. Zilbovicius M, Garreau B, Tzourio N, Mazoyer B, Bruck B, Martinot J-L, Raymond C, Samson Y, Syrota A, Lelord G. Regional cerebral blood flow in childhood autism: a SPECT study. Am J Psychiatry 1992; 149:924–930.

72. Baron-Cohen S, Ring HA, Wheelwright S, Bullmore ET, Brammer MJ, Simmons A, Williams SC. Social intelligence in the normal and autistic brain: an fMRI study. Eur J Neurosci 1999; 11:1891–1898.

73. Bolton PF, Park RJ, Higgins JN, Griffiths PD, Pickles A. Neuro-epileptic determinants of autism spectrum disorders in tuberous sclerosis complex. Brain 2002; 125(Pt 6):1247–1255.

74. Riikonen R. Long-term outcome of patients with West syndrome. Brain Dev 2001; 23:683–687.

75. DeLong GR. Autism: new data suggest a new hypothesis. Neurology 1999; 52:911–916.

76. Muller RA, Behen ME, Rothermel RD, Chugani DC, Muzik O, Mangner TJ, Chugani HT. Brain mapping of language and auditory perception in high-functioning autistic adults: a PET study. J Autism Dev Disord 1999; 29:19–31.

77. Chiron C, Leboyer M, Leon F, Jambaque I, Nuttin C, Syrota A. SPECT of the brain in childhood autism: evidence for a lack of normal hemispheric asymmetry. Dev Med Child Neurol 1995; 37:849–860.

78. Minshew NJ, Luna B, Sweeney JA. Oculomotor evidence for neocortical systems but not cerebellar dysfunction in autism. Neurology 1999; 52:917–922.

79. Zilbovicius M, Garreau B, Samson Y, et al. Delayed maturation of the frontal cortex in childhood autism. Am J Psychiatry 1995; 152:248–252.

80. Rossi PG, Parmeggiani A, Bach V, Santucci M, Visconti P. EEG features and epilepsy in patients with autism. Brain Dev 1995; 17:169–174.

81. Lewine JD, Andrews R, Chez M, Patil AA, Devinsky O, Smith M, Kanner A, Davis JT, Funke M, Jones G, Chong B, Provencal S, Weisend M, Lee RR, Orrison WW Jr. Magnetoencephalographic patterns of epileptiform activity in children with regressive autism spectrum disorders. Pediatrics 1999; 104(3Pt 1):405–418.

82. Rossi PG, Parmeggiani A, Bach V, Santucci M, Visconti P. EEG features and epilepsy in patients with autism. Brain Dev 1995; 17:169–174.

83. Tuchman RF, Rapin I. Regression in pervasive developmental disorders: seizures and epileptiform electroencephalogram correlates. Pediatrics 1997; 99:560–566.

84. Rapin I. Autistic regression and disintegrative disorder: how important the role of epilepsy? Semin Pediatr Neurol 1995; 2:278–285.

85. Nass R, Gross A, Devinsky O. Autism and autistic epileptiform regression with occipital spikes. Dev Med Child Neurol 1998; 40:453–458.

86. Wong V. Epilepsy in children with autistic spectrum disorder. J Child Neurol 1993; 8:316–322.

87. Giovanardi RP, Posar A, Parmeggiani A. Epilepsy in adolescents and young adults with autistic disorder. Brain Dev 2000; 22:102–106.

88. Rossi PG, Parmeggiani A, Bach V, Santucci M, Visconti P. EEG features and epilepsy in patients with autism. Brain Dev 1995; 17:169–174.

89. Olsson I, Steffenburg S, Gillberg C. Epilepsy in autism and autisticlike conditions: a population-based study. Arch Neurol 1988; 45:666–668.

90. Tuchman RF, Rapin I, Shinnar S. Autistic and dysphasic children. II. Epilepsy. Pediatrics 1991; 88:1219–1225.

91. Casanova MF, Buxhoeveden DP, Switala AE, Roy E. Minicolumnar pathology in autism. Neurology 2002; 12;58:428–432.

92. Cook EH, Leventhal BL. The serotonin system in autism. Curr Opin Pediatr 1996; 8:348–354.

93. Cook EH. Autism: review of neurochemical investigation. Synapse 1990; 6:292–308.

94. Kuperman A, Beeghly JHL, Burns TL, Tsai LY. Association of serotonin concentration to behavior and IQ in autistic children. J Autism Dev Disord 1987; 17:133–140.

95. Herault J, Petit E, Martineau J, Perrot A, Lenoir P, Cherpi C, Barthelemy C, Sauvage D, Mallet J, Muh JP. Autism and genetics: clinical approach and association study with two markers of HRAS gene. Am J Med Genet 1995; 60:276–281.

96. Todd RD, Ciaranello RD. Demonstration of inter- and intraspecies differences in serotonin binding sites by antibodies from an autistic child. Proc Natl Acad Sci USA 1985; 82:612–616.

97. Singh VK, Singh EA, Warren RP. Hyperserotoninemia and serotonin receptor antibodies in children with autism but not mental retardation. Biol Psychiatry 1997; 41:753–755.

98. Cook EH Jr, Perry BD, Dawson G, Wainwright MS, Leventhal BL. Receptor inhibition by immunoglobulins: specific inhibition by autistic children, their relatives, and control subjects. J Autism Dev Disord 1993; 23:67–78.

99. Yuwiler A, Shih JC, Chen CH, Ritvo ER, Hanna G, Ellison GW, King BH. Hyperserotoninemia and antiserotonin antibodies in autism and other disorders. J Autism Dev Disord 1992; 22:33–45.

100. Kim SJ, Cox N, Courchesne R, Lord C, Corsello C, Akshoomoff N, Guter S, Leventhal BL, Courchesne E, Cook EH Jr. Transmission disequilibrium mapping at the serotonin transporter gene (SLC6A4) region in autistic disorder. Mol Psychiatry 2002; 7:278–288.

101. Yirmiya N, Pilowsky T, Nemanov L, Arbelle S, Feinsilver T, Fried I, Ebstein RP. Evidence for an association with the serotonin transporter promoter region polymorphism and autism. Am J Med Genet 2001; 105:381–386.

102. Klauck SM, Poustka F, Benner A, Lesch KP, Poustka A. Serotonin transporter (5-HTT) gene variants associated with autism? Hum Mol Genet 1997; 6:2233–2238.

103. Herault J, Petit E, Martineau J, Cherpi C, Perrot A, Barthelemy C, Lelord G, Muh JP. Serotonin and autism: biochemical and molecular biology features. Psychiatry Res 1996; 65:33–43.

104. Tordjman S, Gutknecht L, Carlier M, Spitz E, Antoine C, Slama F, Carsalade V, Cohen DJ, Ferrari P, Roubertoux PL, Anderson GM. Role of the serotonin transporter gene in the behavioral expression of autism. Mol Psychiatry 2001; 6:434–439.

105. Persico AM, Pascucci T, Puglisi-Allegra S, Militerni R, Bravaccio C, Schneider C, Melmed R, Trillo S, Montecchi F, Palermo M, Rabinowitz D, Reichelt KL,

Conciatori M, Marino R, Keller F. Serotonin transporter gene promoter variants do not explain the hyperserotoninemia in autistic children. Mol Psychiatry 2002; 7:795–800.

106. Gordon CT, State RC, Nelson JE, Hamburger SD, Rapoport JL. A double-blind comparison of clomipramine, desipramine, and placebo in the treatment of autistic disorder. Arch Gen Psychiatry 1993; 50:441–447.

107. Awad GA. The use of selective serotonin reuptake inhibitors in young children with pervasive developmental disorders: some clinical observations. Can J Psychiatry 1996; 41:361–366.

108. Aman MG, Kern RA. Review of fenfluramine in the treatment of the developmental disabilities. J Am Acad Child Adolesc Psychiatry 1989; 28:549–565.

109. McCracken JT, McGough J, Shah B, Cronin P, Hong D, Aman MG, Arnold LE, Lindsay R, Nash P, Hollway J, McDougle CJ, Posey D, Swiezy N, Kohn A, Scahill L, Matin A, Koenig K, Volkmar F, Carroll D, Lancor A, Tierney E, Ghuman J, Gonzalez NM, Grados M, Vitiello B, Ritz L, Davies M, Robinson J, McMahon D. Risperidone in children with autism and serious behavioral problems. N Engl J Med 2002; 347:314–321.

110. Chamberlain RS, Herman BH. A novel biochemical model linking dysfunctions in brain melatonin, proopiomelanocortin peptides, and serotonin in autism. Biol Psychiatry 1990; 28:773–793.

111. Anderson LT, Campbell M, Grega DM, Perry R, Small AM, Green WH. Haloperidol in the treatment of infantile autism: effects on learning and behavioral symptoms. Am J Psychiatry 1984; 141:1195–1202.

112. Cohen DJ, Caparulo BK, Shaywitz BA, et al. Dopamine and serotonin metabolism in neuropsychiatrically disturbed children: CSF homovanillic acid and 5-hydroxyindolacetic acid. Arch Gen Psychiatry 1977; 34:545–550.

113. Young JG, Kavanagh ME, Anderson GM, et al. Clinical neurochemistry of autism and associated disorders. J Autism Dev Disord 1982, 12:147–165.

114. Grados MA, McCarthy D. Stereotypies and repetitive behaviors in autism. In: Accardo PJ, Magnusen C, and Capute AJ, eds. Autism, Clinical and Research Issues. Baltimore: York Press, 2000.

115. Gillberg C, Terenius L, Lonnerholm G. Endorphin activity in childhood psychosis. Arch Gen Psychiatry 1985; 43:780–783.

116. Schwartz JC, Opiate Schwartz JC, Roques BP. Opioid peptides as intercellular messengers. Biomedicine 1980; 32:169–175.

117. Willemsen-Swinkels SH, Buitelaar JK, van Engeland H. The effects of chronic naltrexone treatment in young autistic children: a double-blind placebo-controlled crossover study. Biol Psychiatry 1996; 15;39:1023–1031.

118. Sher L. Autistic disorder and the endogenous opioid system. Med Hypoth 1997; 48:413–414.

119. Nagamitsu S, Matsuishi T, Kisa T, Komori H, Miyazaki M, Hashimoto T, Yamashita Y, Ohtaki Y, Kato H. CSF beta-endorphin levels in patients with infantile autism. J Autism Dev Disord 1997; 27:155–163.

120. Bouvard MP, Leboyer M, Launay JM, Recasens C, Plumet MH, Waller-Perotte D, Tabuteau F, Bondoux D, Dugas M, Lensing P, et al. Low-dose naltrexone effects on plasma chemistries and clinical symptoms in autism: a double-blind, placebo-controlled study. Psychiatry Res 1995; 16;58:191–201.

121. Feldman HM, Kolmen BK, Gonzaga AM. Naltrexone and communication skills in young children with autism. J Am Acad Child Adolesc Psychiatry 1999; 38(5):587–593.

122. Reichelt KL, Knivsberg AM, Lind G, et al. Probable etiology and possible treatment of childhood autism. Brain Dysfunct 1991; 4:308–319.

123. Sahley, TL, Panksepp, J. Brain opioids and autism: an updated analysis of possible linkages. J Autism Dev Disord 1987; 17, 201–216.

124. Knivsberg A, Reichelt K, Høien T, et al. Parents' observations after one year of dietary intervention for children with autistic syndromes. In: Shattock P, Linfoot G, eds. Psychobiology of Autism: Current Research and Practice. Sunderland: Autism Research Unit, University of Sunderland and Autism North, 1998:13–24.

125. Whiteley P, Rodgers J, Savery D, et al. A gluten-free diet as an intervention for autism and associated spectrum disorders: preliminary findings. Autism 1999; 3:45–65.

126. Tsai LY. Psychopharmacology in autism. Psychosom Med 1999; 61:651–665.

127. Lee M, Martin-Ruiz C, Graham A, Court J, Jaros E, Perry R, Iversen P, Bauman M, Perry E. Nicotinic receptor abnormalities in the cerebellar cortex in autism. Brain 2002; 125:1483–1495.

128. Aston-Jones G. Locus ceruleus and regulation of behavioral flexibility and attention. Prog Brain Res 2000; 126:165–82.

129. Cook EH. Autism: review of neurochemical investigation. Synapse 1990; 6:292–308.

130. Fatemi SH, Halt AR, Stary JM, Kanodia R, Schulz SC, Realmuto GR. Glutamic acid decarboxylase 65 and 67 kDa proteins are reduced in autistic parietal and cerebellar cortices. Biol Psychiatry 2002; 52:805–810.

131. Insel TR, O'Brien DJ, Leckman JF. Oxytocin, vasopressin, and autism: is there a connection? Biol Psychiatry 1999; 45:145–157.

5

Early Clinical Characteristics of Children with Autism

Chris Plauché Johnson
University of Texas Health Science Center at San Antonio, San Antonio, Texas, U.S.A.

I. INTRODUCTION

Most neurodevelopmental disorders are recognized either by their phenotype (physical appearance) and/or by their genotype (chromosomal and/or molecular appearance). Unfortunately, there is neither a specific phenotype nor a consistent genotype that reliably defines autism spectrum disorder (ASD). Relatively new to the field of neurodevelopmental disorders is the recognition of "behavioral" phenotypes. Although the characteristic behaviors of some "syndromes" have been recognized for quite some time, it has only been in the recent past that sophisticated genetic diagnostic techniques [e.g., fluorescent in situ hybridization (FISH)] have provided the corresponding genetic characteristics allowing the two to be reliably linked to one another. Examples of such behavioral phenotypes (and their corresponding genotype) include, but are not limited to: hand-wringing and hyperventilation characteristic of Rett's syndrome (MECP2), self-hugging in Smith-Magenis (17p11.2 deletion), excessive smiling and wide-based puppet-like gait in Angelman's syndrome (15 q11–13 deletion of maternal origin), extreme hyperphagia in Prader-Willi syndrome (15 q11–13 deletion of paternal origin), and self-biting and tissue destruction of lips and hands in Lesch-Nyhan (X q26–27).

In addition to the absence of a defining genotype or characteristic physical phenotype, ASD also does not have a specific behavioral phenotype. For many years ASD was conceptualized as primarily a communication disorder. In 1991,

Rogers and Pennington (1) proposed a novel developmental model, suggesting that an abnormal developmental cascade resulted in sequential deficits in joint attention, social referencing, communication, symbolic play, and repetitive restricted behaviors. The model accounted for deficits in all three main symptom areas: social relatedness, communication, and restricted, repetitive behaviors, and fostered recognition of children with ASD at much younger ages (2). Also contributing to the de-emphasis of communication skills as the defining characteristic of autism was the recent recognition of the full spectrum of autism in which some children with high-functioning autism, or Asperger's syndrome, have relatively minor language deficits during early development (but later demonstrate significant pragmatic deficits). Moreover, abnormalities in language development are not specific to ASD and, in fact, are more commonly seen in children with mental retardation, hearing loss, and communication disorders. Although delayed echolalia, advanced expressive language skills relative to receptive ones, and pragmatic deficits are somewhat unique to ASD, not all children demonstrate these abnormalities. Although stereotypies may be obvious and will readily alert the clinician to a problem, they often do not become apparent until after 3 years of age. These are also seen in children with severe or profound mental retardation or severe visual impairment. Thus, language deficits and stereotypies do not distinguish ASD from other childhood disorders. All children with ASD, however, do demonstrate unique deficits in social skills. Although not pathognomonic, a few of the early recognizable social deficits are very characteristic and considered by some to quite possibly be specific for ASD.

Currently, the DSM-IV (discussed in Chapter 6) is the gold standard in regard to diagnostic criteria (3–5). Unfortunately, DSM-IV criteria are not as reliable in children less than 3 years of age since, due to the natural evolution of developmental skills, many of the defining criteria may not be present in very young children later diagnosed with autism. For example, "failure to form age-appropriate peer relationships" is really not applicable in very young children. Additionally, in a preverbal child, it is difficult to demonstrate abnormal conversational skills and stereotypic language. Ritualistic behaviors, a need for routines, and stereotypies are often not found in children less than 3. Thus, even children appearing to have severe autism may not meet full criteria at very young ages. Instead, they usually receive the "threshold" provisional diagnosis of PDD-NOS. Later, if additional signs appear, full criteria may be met and the diagnosis of autistic disorder is then made. Realizing this diagnostic dilemma, especially now that earlier diagnosis is emphasized, modified DSM criteria have been suggested for children less than 3 years of age (6):

A1: Decreased use of nonverbal behavior (eye-to-eye gaze, facial expression, body posture, gestures)
A2: Lack of social and emotional reciprocity

A4: Lack of seeking to share enjoyment, interests, or achievements with other people (absent showing, bringing, or pointing to objects of interest)

B1: Delayed or absent language skills

The authors state that all four criteria should be present to make the provisional diagnosis of ASD in the very young child. It is important to note that three of the four are social skill criteria. Recognizing the importance of social skills in defining and detecting ASD in very young children, this chapter will focus on social skill deficits and how they impact later development of language and play skills. A short discussion of additional DSM criteria in the language and restricted, repetitive play domains, as well as brief discussions regarding physical characteristics, motor development, savant skills, and autism regression variant, will follow.

"Social skills" as discussed in this chapter are defined more loosely than in the DSM-IV. Indeed, behaviors described in this chapter overlap with some of the DSM-IV criteria listed in the language and repetitive/restricted play domains. Additionally, deficits in social skills negatively impact the later development of language and cognitive skills. Whereas very early social skills depend on facial and gestural interactions, later ones depend on the child's ability to verbalize. Social development parallels cognitive development in normal or globally delayed children; in children with ASD, the development of social skills is characteristically "out of sync" with the child's overall level of functioning. This discrepancy between social and general levels of functioning is one of the most important defining criteria of ASD. The discrepancy can be first noted in infants aged 8–12 months, but it becomes more evident as the child approaches 18–24 months. The purpose of this chapter is not to discuss the social skills as strictly defined by the DSM-IV, but rather to discuss a more inclusive set of social-emotional characteristics that impact not only social skill development but also language, cognitive, and play development. Ultimately, the goal is to help the clinician recognize the expanded range of social deficits to raise the index of suspicion for ASD at an earlier age than would occur if one focuses only on failure to achieve later-occurring language milestones. This is extremely important as recent literature has demonstrated that children with ASD, who are recognized *early* and referred to an appropriate and intensive intervention program, improve and demonstrate decreased symptomatology (7–9).

In the past, the definitive diagnosis of autistic disorder has usually not been made until after 3 years of age, more likely between 4 and 6 years of age. Howlin (10,11) demonstrated that parents usually become concerned by 18 months, but do not present to the child's primary care provider with these concerns until 6 months later. In one study published in 1997, over 50% of parents were reassured and told "not to worry." The usual interval between first parental concern and the final definitive diagnosis was approximately 4 years. Denial, lack of familiarity with the spectrum of distinguishing characteristics that define ASD, and scarce subspecialty resources, among other reasons, contributed to late diagnosis.

Parents usually first become concerned when they realize that their child's expressive language is delayed. Indeed, this has been the historical hallmark of the disorder and will likely continue to be so as these deficits are easily recognized. Although earlier social skill deficits are now better known in professional circles, they are not as easily recognized by parents. There is one exception. In families where there are two children with ASD, parents often recognize the early social signs in the younger child prior to any concerns about language. Indeed, now that experts in the field have begun to focus on these earlier social deficits, often by the use of screening (e.g., the CHAT) or diagnostic (e.g., the ADOS) tools that target such skills, the average age of diagnosis has decreased. These instruments have facilitated a "provisional," if not definitive, diagnosis of ASD much earlier. In Europe, it has been reported that these techniques have resulted in decreasing the average age of diagnosis from 4 years to 30 months (12). The recent emphasis on social skill deficits has also led to better ascertainment of children who are high functioning with few language deficits, i.e., children with Asperger's syndrome. Indeed, it is both the earlier recognition of ASD and the recognition of additional children with ASD who are high-functioning and/or more mildly affected that has been responsible, at least in part, for the apparent rise in prevalence.

The recognition of the importance of deficits in social skills as defining characteristics of ASD will *not* likely represent our final stage in the evolution of our understanding of this disorder (Table 1). Our understanding of autism has "come a long way," especially during the 1990s. It has moved away from the belief that most children with autism are nonverbal, make no eye contact, sit in the corner, and engage in bizarre stereotypies. It is now known that more subtle deficits in social skills, particularly in joint attention, may indicate a disorder somewhere "on the spectrum." But the journey is not yet over. At the time of this publication, a multicenter study designed to evaluate signs in even younger infants is in progress, but results are not available. The "Baby Sibs Project" has been expanded from its original study site in Canada under the leadership of Lonnie Zwaigenbaum to a multicenter project with international funding (13). The goal of this project is to identify ASD in siblings (between the ages of 3 and 6 months) of children with known ASD. Siblings have an increased incidence of ASD—3–9% when there is one older sibling with ASD (14) and up to 25% when there are two (15). The study infants will be prospectively observed for the above distinguishing early social deficits as well as for new, potentially unknown early behavioral signs of ASD.

II. DEFICITS IN SOCIAL SKILLS

As noted above, abnormalities in social relatedness are now the sine qua non of autism; however, these are rarely defined (16). Rogers and Benneto suggest that it is a kind of "interpersonal synchrony of bodies, voices, movements, expressions and... complementary feeling states. It is the interpersonal coordination that people feel, see and hear through the matching of their movements (face, body, voice) with those of their social partners." Infants with other disabilities, for example cerebral palsy or blindness, may have difficulties with this synchrony due to their respective motor and visual deficits; however, they do manage to maintain social connectedness by using compensatory strategies. Infants who are blind use voice, touch, and language through which emotions can be shared and connectedness experienced. Those with severe cerebral palsy establish social relatedness through eye contact, facial expressions, sounds, and conversations. With time both partners ignore the asynchronies and attend to whatever interpersonal coordinations are indeed present. Children with autism make no (or very few) such attempts to compensate.

A. Joint Attention

The single most distinguishing characteristic of very young children with ASD is a deficit in "joint attention." Currently it is thought to be associated with abnormalities in the amygdala. It is a core feature of the DSM-IV and includes a limited inclination to share enjoyment, interests, or achievements with other people. Joint attention is the triadic ability to coordinate one's own attention between an object and another person. It is dependent on four developmental components: 1) orienting and attending to a social partner, 2) coordinating attention between people and objects, 3) sharing affect or emotional states with people, and 4) ultimately being able to draw others' attention to objects or events for the purpose of indicating a need of sharing experiences. Children with autism may have difficulty with all of these components. Mastery of joint attention reflects a child's ability and motivation to share in mental states of others.

Joint attention serves both a communicative and a social function. In its purely communicative function, it may be used to regulate the behavior of others to get them to do something (request) or to stop doing something (protest). Although children with ASD may occasionally use gestures to accomplish this, they rarely alternate eye gaze between the object and the person's face. When they do happen to look at the adult's face, they neither follow his/her gaze nor use the adult's facial expressions to influence their own behavior (see "Social Orienting," below). Even more rare is the use of joint attention for the pure social function of drawing another's attention to an object or event out of mere interest (as in to comment or label).

Just like other developmental skills, joint attention appears to develop in graduated stages. Very early skills include true reciprocal smiling at the mere sight of a caregiver's smile. At approximately 8 months of age, a typically developing infant may demonstrate an early form of joint attention called "gaze monitoring." For example, an infant sitting on his mother's lap and facing her is engaged and making eye contact with her while she sings to him. At some point, something catches the mother's visual attention causing her to look away from the child and toward the object of interest. The child in turn will follow mother's gaze and also look in the same direction. It is the loss of mother's eye contact that stimulates the child to jointly look in the same direction . . . not the stimulus itself as it is visualized later in time. If the environmental stimulus catches the child's attention first (as in an auditory stimulus that is heard by both mother and baby simultaneously), then the spontaneous head turning is *not* an indication of joint attention, but instead marks the child's ability to "localize to sound" (a receptive language milestone, not a social one).

At about 10–12 months of age, the child will "follow a point." In this situation, the child is engaged in some activity without particular regard for the parent. The parent sees something of interest, points in its direction, and says, for example, "Oh look! The kitty cat has come inside." The child intuitively will look in the direction that the parent is pointing. Upon seeing the object of interest he may smile or look back at the parent to reassure himself. If he does not see the object, he may even look back quizzically at the parent. This joint attention milestone can easily be elicited during a clinic visit in a typically developing 10-month-old. However, a child with autism may appear oblivious to the examiner's request to look at the targeted object. If there is no response, one may need to increase the intensity of the stimulus by calling louder, adding the child's name, or touching his shoulder first to get his attention, and then pointing and exclaiming. Finally, if this still does not elicit a response, a familiar caregiver may be asked to repeat the maneuvers. Often, no degree of intensity is successful in getting the child to look at the desired stimulus.

Unlike these passive or reactive joint-attention milestones, the next ones to emerge are "active" where the child, not the caregiver, initiates the interaction. At approximately 12–14 months of age, the child begins to point. At first he may point to a desired object that is out of reach. Typically, a child will verbalize during the act of pointing. Depending on his language level, the verbalizations may not be recognizable words, but instead any vocalization used to solicit the caregiver's attention. The typically developing child will look back and forth from the object to the caregiver in an effort to make the caregiver understand that he desires the object. Here, pointing is used as a "command" and is often called "protoimperative" pointing. The object is the goal; the caregiver is the means by which the child can obtain that goal. Alternating eye contact between the object and the caregiver is critical in designating this as a joint-attention skill. A child with ASD rarely masters this skill at the usual time. Instead he is more likely to take the caregiver's hand and lead him to the object, for example, to the refrigerator if he is hungry or thirsty. At that point the caregiver must open the refrigerator door and guess what the child wants by offering him various items and asking, "Is this what you want?" The child will then grasp the desired object. Some children develop certain self-help skills (such as opening a refrigerator door, climbing onto cabinets) at an advanced rate to circumvent the need to solicit help. Another possibility might involve a more primitive pointing stage whereby the child opens and closes his hand in repetitive grasping motion in the direction of the refrigerator and cries or whines. There is little or no eye contact with the caregiver. Some consider this to be a transitional skill leading to later more mature protoimperative pointing.

At 14–16 months of age, in a typically developing child, pointing and accompanying verbalization may take on a new function. Instead of being used as a "command," pointing is used to "comment" or to point out an object/event of interest. This type of gesturing is more social in nature and is often called "protodeclarative pointing." The same triad exists (child, caregiver, object), but the goal is reversed. The child sees something of interest, perhaps a helicopter flying overhead. He points to the sky and may vocalize to some degree (depending on his language level) to get the caregiver's attention. He will then alternatively look at the object and the caregiver to make sure the caregiver has seen the object of interest. The reward is the caregiver's approval either by smiling at the child or through some type of verbalization that acknowledges the object of interest. Children with autism consistently fail to demonstrate protodeclarative pointing skills at age-appropriate times. If and when these skills finally emerge, there is often a qualitative difference in that the child is less likely to show positive affect during acts of joint attention. Also around 14–16 months, children should master the social skill of "showing." This occurs when the child has found something or made something (a scribble on a piece of paper) and holds it out to the parent as if to say, "Look at this!" This act is to be distinguished from bringing an item to the parent to get help, for example, bringing a bottle of bubbles to the parent and putting his/her hand on the lid to indicate that he wants it opened. Although this skill is also often delayed in children with ASD, it is not a pure joint-attention milestone. Instead, it is a "reenactment." Reenactments can be motor, as just described, or verbal (see discussion of echolalia, below). In reenactment attempts, the child repeats an event to make it happen again. It may serve as a building block and actually herald the emergence of joint-attention skills in some children (17).

The ability to communicate using gestural joint attention (showing or pointing to direct attention) emerges before words in typical development and appears to be a core deficit in autism that impedes later functional language development. Joint-attention skills (but not global social skills) appear to be

Table 1 Evolution of Clinical Characteristics of Autism Spectrum Disorder with Age

		Signs in infancy (<18 months)		
Motor	Perceptual	Socioemotional	Language	Mental representation

Inactive hypoactive
Flaccid muscle tone
Rarely cries
Decreased facial expression
Irritable
Hyperactive, restless
Only soothed when in constant motion
Rigid when held
Arches away from close physical contact
	Unusual mix of hyper- and hypo-sensitivities to sensory stimuli; i.e., sensory integration deficits
	Auditory
	Appears deaf to voice but jolts or panics to environmental sounds
	Tactile
	Tactile defensiveness
	Refuses food with rough texture
	Adverse reaction to wool fabrics and seams
	Prefers smooth or rough surfaces
	Visual
	Sensitive to light
	May panic at change in illumination
	Preoccupied with observing own hand and finger movements
		Temperament swings from good to inconsolable
		Crying and unpredictable mood
		Late, rare or absent social smile
		Decreased looking at faces
		Avoids eye contact when held
		Doesn't recognize parent's face
		Lack of anticipatory response to being picked up
		Fails to show stranger anxiety
		Lack of gaze monitoring
		Does not follow a point
		Seems to dislike being held
		Seems content to be left alone
		Fails to visually follow coming and going of parent
		Doesn't play peek-a-boo, patty cake, or wave bye-bye
		Delayed attachment in some
		Poor social referencing
		Decreased "showing" parents interesting objects
			Delayed or absent cooing and/or expressive vocalization
			Failure to respond to name
			Failure to imitate words, sounds
			Little communicative use of gestures
			Absent to-fro babbling in response to parent's voice
			Lack of usual progression from monotone babbling to immature jargoning with inflection/animation
			Decreased protoimperative pointing; instead leads adult to desired object
			Regression of language and social skills between 12–18 months in some (~25%)
				Decreased visual pursuit of objects or people
				Poor shifting of attention between:
				  Novel and familiar stimuli
				  Human and object stimuli
				Delayed object permanence—early sign of possible comorbid cognitive deficits
				Delayed ability to solve glass frustration test—early sign of possible comorbid cognitive deficits
				Decreased facial expression—masked faces
				Persistent sensory motor play
				Delayed functional play

Toe-walking
Rocking
Head banging
Whirling without dizziness
Finger-flicking
Sensory stereotypies— sniffing and licking
Proto-SIB with true SIB >5 yr of age
Hypo- or hyperactivity
Perseverative movements
Apraxia/dyspraxia
Clumsiness

Withdraws from environmental stimulation
Engages in self-stimulation
Preoccupied with spinning objects
May suddenly cease activity and stare into space, often with neck hyper-extended
May crave deep pressure or stroking

Uses adult's hand like a tool
Lack of or delayed joint attention
Insists on sameness and ritualized routines
Unable to identify with another's feelings or point of view
Failure to make friends
Lack of proto-declarative pointing (to direct another's attention to interesting object/event)

Regression may also occur after 18 months
Immediate echolalia
Delayed echolalia unrelated to social context
Pronoun reversal
Voice atonal, hollow, rhythmic
Lack of pointing for naming
Neologisms
Idiosyncratic language
Precocious counting, ABCs
Fails to use previously learned words
Oral motor dyspraxia
Poor pragmatics
Dissociation between form and function of language

Primitive (re-enactment) pretend/representational play; good constructional play
Little appropriate play of typical popular toys
Hard comfort items
Delayed matching novel items on demand, but advanced rote matching of shapes, colors, letters and/or numbers
Inability to solve "false belief" problems (Sally and Anne test at 4 yr of age)
Absent or weak ToM skills
Poor executive functioning
Poor central coherence
Inability to understand idioms, metaphors, and humor
Hyperlexia

ToM, theory-of-mind.

proportionate to language skills including the correct use of I and you pronouns (18,19). In one longitudinal study, its emergence was shown to be a significant predictor of functional language development approximately 1 year later (9,20). In this regard, many researchers consider joint attention a "pivotal skill"; that is, its mastery leads to collateral changes in a broader range of deficits within the autism phenotype. This recognition has led to important advances in early intervention strategies. Several groups are developing intervention strategies that target the development of joint attention and prelinguistic communication skills (21). In one study (22), interventionists presented children with unpredictable or predictable social stimulation. In the unpredictable condition, the teacher played with toys that did not match the toy play activities of the child. In the predictable condition, the teacher imitated the toy play of the child. Children with ASD displayed more joint attention in the predictable (imitated) condition than in the unpredictable condition. Another study (23) revealed that children with ASD are more likely to learn new words when the parent "tunes in" to (or joins attention with) what the child is looking at than when parents attempt to direct the child's gaze to an object that the parent is focusing on and labels. Said differently, language comprehension seemed to be proportional to the frequency of maternal follow-in and not to maternal-directed language (24). Once language is established, the older child is able to maintain joint attention with pure conversation regardless of visual or gestural cues (e.g., telling a parent about what happened in school) (25). The importance of joint attention as a core deficit in ASD was further substantiated in a larger study that demonstrated limitations in joint attention as linked to not only communication but also to deficits in play, emotional responsiveness, and peer interactions (26). Other studies have shown that joint attention is a necessary precursor for the development of theory of mind (see below) (27). Joint-attention deficits also appear to be specific to ASD. In one study, joint-attention skills were evaluated in children with Down syndrome and autism (matched for nonverbal cognitive ages of 18 months). Children with Down syndrome performed normally (as predicted by their mental age); those with autism did not. Joint-attention deficits reliably differentiate children with ASD from children with other neurodevelopmental disorders (28) and is a core DSM-IV criteria for autism. Currently deficits in joint attention is believed to be associated with abnormalities in the amygdala.

B. Social Orienting

Social orienting is the ability to orient to social stimuli, in particular, turning to respond to one's own name (29,30). Although it was recognized as a core deficit in ASD somewhat later than joint attention, social orienting emerges earlier in typical development and may actually influence the emergence of gestural joint attention (31). Most children will turn preferentially when their name is called at about 8–10 months of age. Although some children with ASD might sporadically respond, most do not do so consistently. In fact, one of the early concerns of parents of children with ASD is a potential hearing impairment. They are puzzled because their child seems to hear quite well in some situations but not in others. This dichotomy occurs because children with ASD often attend to environmental sounds extremely well but tend to ignore sounds generated by humans such as calling the child's name and other speech utterances (32). Again, using children with Down syndrome as a control group, it was found that children with ASD more often failed to orient to both social (name being called) and nonsocial stimuli (a musical jack-in-the-box being played or rattle being shaken); however, the difference was significantly more extreme for social stimuli. Furthermore, it was found that social orienting, but not object orienting, was significantly related to joint attention among the children with autism (33).

Several studies have evaluated infant behavior, especially in regard to responding to name. These have involved the retrospective evaluation of 1-year-old birthday videos in children later diagnosed as having ASD.

The original study demonstrated that blinded viewers could retrospectively diagnosis ASD with 91% accuracy (34). The symptoms identified by professionals had not caused parental concerns at the time of filming. Normally developing children without ASD comprised the control group. The distinguishing characteristics were decreased: (1) orienting to name, (2) looking at the faces of others, (3) showing objects, and (4) pointing. The single best distinguishing factor at 8–10 months of age was failure to orient to name since showing and pointing skills may not yet be universally present in typically developing children at 1 year. A later study (35) added a second control group consisting of children with mental retardation. Although less dramatic, responding to name still differentiated the two groups. The two groups were similar in that they both used gestures less and repetitive motor actions more than the normal group.

However, another study that also used blinded observers and home videos filmed at 9–12 months of age (36) failed to demonstrate that children with ASD could be reliably distinguished from children with other types of developmental delays based on such characteristic behaviors. This study did, however, document that parents of autistic children called their child's name more frequently, which is actually an indirect measure of orienting to name.

Finally, Maestro et al. (37) used blinded professionals to view home videos from the first 6 months of life of children later diagnosed with ASD and normal controls. They identified several behaviors that were discriminating. These included all items regarding social attention (looking, smiling, and vocalizing to people), especially orienting to human voices. The common thread that weaves these behaviors together was the seeking of or response to "attention." All nonsocial attention measures were equal in both groups.

Although these studies demonstrated that trained professionals recognized deficits in "responding to name" in videos, asking parents whether or not their child consistently responds to his name has not been found to be as reliable. Instead, a more distinguishing question for parents is asking them whether their child responds to neutral statements, such as, "Oh no, it's raining again!" without specific prompting or calling the child's name first (38).

C. Pretend (Symbolic) Play

Although pretend play is significantly correlated to receptive and expressive language (39), facilitates and requires communication, and is listed as one of the communication criteria in the DSM-IV, it is also a social skill. Lack of or very delayed pretend play (using pretend actions with objects) appears to discriminate children with autism from other children matched for mental age. In a typically developing child, play evolves in a predictable manner. Once the child can grasp objects (about 4 months), his play (exploration) is sensorimotor in nature. He mouths and manipulates objects. The 8–10-month-old will throw them, bang them on the table, or, with one in each hand, bang them together. This evolves into a more functional type of play as he becomes aware, usually through observation, of the actual intended use of the object. At about 12–14 months, using this new understanding plus his imitation skills, he attempts to build a tower with them.

Pretend play begins with simple and, later, more complex play scenarios. "Simple pretend play" usually begins at approximately 16–18 months, when children begin to use miniature representative items, for example, a plastic bottle or brush, to feed the doll or brush her hair, or a toy telephone to talk into. Very soon after this skill is mastered, the child begins to engage in "complex pretend play." There are two types of complex pretend play: (a) the use of a generic item to represent another or (b) two-step pretend play that is spontaneous. In the first situation, the child might be given a miniature plastic telephone and encouraged to "talk to grandma" (simple pretend play). Once this is accomplished, one might then take the plastic phone away and give the child a wooden dowel. Again the child is encouraged to "talk to grandma." Most typically developing children will use a generic object to pretend at approximately 18–20 months of age. Two-step play may be implemented with either miniatures or generic items or a combination of items. Use of generic items, however, represents a more mature form of play. In this situation, the child might feed the doll with a miniature plastic bottle and then, spontaneously, lie the doll down and cover her with a cloth. Depending on the child's language level, she might even say, "all done," "night night" (examples of giant words), or "baby tired" (true two-word phrase). Both types of complex pretend play represent a higher order of play that is consistently absent in 18-month-old children with ASD. When one evaluates a child's ability to engage in pretend play, using tiny pieces of real food or a play bottle containing an outer layer of milky liquid that appears to pour is discouraged since this might not represent true symbolic play. Additionally, some children already in intervention might have been "taught" to engage in certain pretend play "routines." These activities might be done repetitiously during daily therapy sessions. However, until a "pretend play routine" can be generalized to other situations, it should not be scored as "mastered." Although, children with ASD can be taught to imitate pretend play, no 20-month-old with ASD in at least one study produced spontaneous pretend play (40). Novelty is important when assessing a child's skills, especially when he or she is already receiving formal intervention services.

Imaginative play is the next level of play and is more sophisticated. True imaginative play is not usually evident until well after the second birthday. Emergence of this stage of play is more variable. When evaluating a child's ability to engage in imaginative play, no concrete representative or generic object is used to engage the child. For example, as described in one evaluation tool (ADOS), the child is asked to pretend to brush his teeth (41). The examiner draws an imaginary circle with her finger on the tabletop to represent a sink. She then points to an imaginary toothbrush and tube of toothpaste and says to the child, "Show me how you would brush your teeth." The typically developing child would then "pretend" to pick up the imaginary brush and the tube of toothpaste, open the lid, squeeze the paste out onto the brush, turn the water on, and brush his teeth. Although some children with high-functioning ASD eventually master this skill, albeit at a later age, many children with ASD never do.

Many children with severe autism never progress past the sensorimotor play stage. They mouth and manipulate objects in stereotypic ways. They may also twirl, bang, and throw objects. Often their favorite play toys are not typical popular toys, but are instead string, sticks, rocks, ballpoint pens, books (for carrying around, not reading), etc. Perhaps the only popular real toy is the puzzle, especially shape-matching puzzles. Some children with ASD are quite proficient in constructive play (e.g., using objects in combination to create a product, such as stacking blocks, nesting cups, putting puzzles together, or solving computer "puzzle" games) (42). Constructive play mastery depends on trial-and-error problem solving and not imitation or observation of others. Children with ASD excel at behaviors that do not depend on social interaction but can be instead learned through trial and error. It is not uncommon for parents to state that the child is an unusually "good" child, content to play by himself for hours, requiring little or no attention from the parent. Often this "play" is either constructive (puzzles, computer games, blocks), ritualistic (lining objects up or sorting/ matching shapes or colors), or sensorimotor in nature.

In addition to classifying play according to its developmental level, play can be described in several other ways that are helpful in differentiating children with ASD:

> Play logistics: Is the child's play ritualistic, functional, or creative?
> Communicative aspects of play: Through play, is the child attempting to communicate in some way?
> Social characteristics of play: Is the play done in isolation, parallel to other children, or is it interactive?

Children with autism often engage in ritualistic play with little or no communicative or social intent. It is carried out in isolation of other children or in parallel (side-by-side another child) with little interaction. However, these children often do like (and may appear to even be interactive during) chase games and roughhousing. It is the sensorimotor aspects of these active games that are appealing to the child and not the interactive or social aspects.

D. Additional Social Deficits

Although there are some additional deficits, the following are not as discriminating as the deficits in joint attention, social orienting, and pretend play. No single theory explains all types of dysfunction; they are often interrelated and there is much overlap. Some seem to be cognitive-dependent and involve the frontal cortex. Others seem to be functions of the limbic system, specifically the amygdala, the cerebellum, and/or the brainstem. Although cognitive development may somewhat influence emergence of skills, there is often a discrepancy between social (and usually language) development and development of skills in other domains. Of the following deficits described below, the first five appear to be more specific to persons with ASD. Some of the following deficits, particularly theory of mind, may not be recognizable or measurable until later childhood and are, therefore, not helpful in the early recognition of ASD.

1. Poor Social Referencing

Social referencing (17) is the ability to recognize the emotional significance of stimuli and includes the earlier-appearing ability to orient toward social stimuli (see above). Persons with ASD have a poor understanding of and a decreased responsiveness to the feeling of others. They rarely use an adult's facial expressions to influence their own behavior with novel objects or events (43). When faced with a novel situation, a normal infant might look to his mother for an indication of fear in her facial expression. His facial expression will usually mimic hers although he may not understand the full implication of the situation. A child with ASD often fails to look at his mother's facial expression and even so, if he does, he engages in less imitation. Children with ASD are less likely to imitate social behaviors of others overall. Such deficits in social referencing and orienting have been found to correlate with measured deficits in joint attention. Children who display a greater capacity to coordinate and imitate affect (social referencing) are more likely to communicate for social reasons (44).

2. Poor Shifting of Attention

The ability to shift one's focus of attention from one stimulus to a competing one is a very basic skill that can be measured in normally developing 4-month-olds. In the late 1980s Courchesne and his colleagues (45–48) developed a model that views attention as a critical and basic deficit in autism. Attention deficits are hypothesized to be present from early development and to contribute to the atypical development of social skills, particularly deficits in joint attention. Joint social attention relies on the ability to shift attention from the object to the partner and back again. As noted above, significant deficits exist and are thought to be responsible, in turn, for perseverative symptoms and later-developing language and social abnormalities. Functional MRI and PET studies have demonstrated that the cerebellum, particularly the vermis, is activated during attention-shifting tasks (49). Additionally, hypoplasia of these same areas has been correlated with functional deficits. Individuals with acquired cerebellar damage demonstrate similar abnormalities. These studies, along with others using normal subjects, have uncovered the relatively new role of the cerebellum in behavior, sensory processing, and cognition (50).

In one form or another, shifting of attention has been used as the basis for tests of visual acuity and nonverbal intelligence for many years. When presented with two stimuli of differing resolution (thickness of alternating black and white lines), the infant will shift his attention to the stimulus that is within the range of his visual capability. It is well known that infants prefer novel stimuli and will predictably shift their attention from a familiar image to a novel one. This assumption has been used in numerous study paradigms to measure infant intelligence and predict mental deficiency at very early ages. Such testing paradigms were used in the mid-1980s in the development of the revised Bayley Scales of Infant Development II.

Studies involving children with ASD examined two related behaviors: spontaneous shifting of attention and structured, investigator-provoked attention shifting. Children with ASD demonstrated distinct patterns in both conditions:

Spontaneous shifting of attention (51): In this study, observations were made regarding the quantity and quality of spontaneous shifts in attention in 20-month-old children who were autistic, developmentally delayed, or developmentally normal. Three types of shifting were studied: between two objects, between an object and a person, and between two persons. Whereas the two control groups shifted attention between an object and a person most often, the autistic group more often shifted attention between two objects. The autistic group spent less overall time looking at people and when they did look, they did so only briefly. They looked at objects longer than did controls.

   Structured investigator stimulated shifting of attention (52): In a novel stimulus paradigm, children matched for mental age faced screens where one, two, or three stimuli could be projected simultaneously. When presented with stimulus (A), children with autism, Down syndrome, and controls attended to it equally well. In the next situation stimulus (A) is turned off at the same time a new stimulus (B) is projected onto a screen adjacent to where (A) had been. All three groups shifted their attention to (B) equally well. Finally, in the third situation, (A) is shown for a period of time before stimulus (C) is shown. This time (A) remains on the screen and (C) is projected side by side simultaneously. Normal controls and children with Down syndrome both shifted their attention to the novel (C) stimulus; children with ASD did not. The authors state that adults with ASD also demonstrated difficulty with this task.

Since shifting of attention to a novel stimulus can be observed in very young infants (4–7 months of age), it has been postulated that this test paradigm might be used to detect early signs of ASD. As was discovered in the pilot testing of the revised Bayley, measuring eye movement is fraught with logistical challenges. Additionally, infants with severe cognitive delays who are not autistic may have difficulty in detecting novel stimuli. Nevertheless, it seems promising.

3. Decreased Facial Recognition

Even at a very young age, normal infants appear to recognize familiar faces. This has been confirmed with PET studies. However, both younger and older individuals with ASD have difficulty recognizing faces. Dawson (53) studied this phenomenon with event-related brain potentials (ERP) in 3-year-old children with and without ASD. Four stimuli were used in the testing paradigm: photo of mom's face, photo of a stranger, photo of the child's favorite toy, and photo of an unfamiliar toy. Control children showed differential ERPs to both photos of mom and his/her favorite toy. Autistic children showed differential ERPs *only* to his/her favorite toy. Furthermore, the degree of abnormality in ERPs during face-looking was correlated with the degree of deficit in joint-attention skills. Thus ability to recognize faces might yet be another skill that is contingent on joint-attention skills. It is not presently known whether the deficit is congenital or acquired. Children with ASD might primarily lack the neural components necessary to recognize faces or, on the other hand, these synapses and circuitry may not develop as a secondary consequence of their failure to attend to such stimuli. If secondary, then it is hypothesized that early stimulation might promote growth of neural pathways and result in some improvement. Curricula have been developed using a tangible reward system that may be effective in motivating children to look at and attend to faces.

4. Weak Central Coherence

Although not a true social skill, impairment in central coherence can lead to atypical social interactions. Central coherence is the ability to interpret stimuli in a relatively global way, taking context into account (54–56). Persons with ASD tend to make less use of context and to focus on parts rather than wholes; processing is piecemeal. These persons have difficulty integrating component features into a cohesive unit and seeing the "big picture." Consider this analogy. One enters a dark room, turns on the light switch, and scans the room taking in its contents. Within seconds, one is able to form a mental image of the entire room. On the other hand, one might enter a dark room, shine a flashlight on the different areas of the room, and store these images separately. When trying to form a composite image of the entire room, difficulty is encountered if a deficit in central coherence exists. In computer lingo, it is as if the child with ASD has multiple files on a topic but is unable to merge them. Their exceptional ability to attend to the details rather than the gestalt results in exceptional abilities in finding hidden figures embedded in a larger, more naturalistic picture (57). Their focus on detail also makes them less susceptible to visual illusions and may account for inflated block design scores on the WISC. It is felt by some that this splinter skill might reflect a deficit in corpus callosum functioning. PET studies have demonstrated reduction in coordinated brain activity that may require an intact corpus callosum. However, this skill in not specific to ASD and some studies have actually failed to demonstrate problems in central coherence (58).

5. Theory-of-Mind (ToM) Deficits

The theory-of-mind (ToM) skill (59,60) enables one to take the perspective of another and is based on the realization that others have thoughts and emotions that are independent from one's own. Because ToM ability is basic to perspective taking, children with ASD have difficulties with social emotional behaviors such as empathy, sharing, and comforting. ToM is important in achieving acceptable social functioning to maintain social relationships. Prior to the 1990s, it was felt that children were largely unaware of the existence of states of mind until they achieved a mental age of approximately 7 years; however, now it is generally accepted that children have some beginning awareness of the mental states of others around 3–4 years of age (61). Although some feel it is one of the core deficits defining ASD, its late appearance cannot explain the earlier deficits in joint attention, social orienting, social referencing, etc. Instead these deficits seem to be primary and likely contribute to subsequent impairments in ToM (62). Its late appearance also prevents it from being helpful in the diagnosis of ASD in the very young child, but may indeed be helpful, even critical, in the diagnosis of the later-appearing Asperger's syndrome. Besides being dependent on the development of cognitive skills at approximately a 4-year-old level, demonstration of intact ToM skills requires some language.

Hypothetically, ToM skills are dependent on a special type of cognition called metarepresentation. Metarepresentational ability allows one to mentally depict the psychosocial status of others: it involves the capacity of one individual to mentally represent the mental representations of another individual. According to the ToM theory, a disturbance in this metarepresentational thought process gives rise to pragmatic language deficits seen in persons with ASD. This is also linked to difficulties with understanding figures of speech (idioms like "two heads are better than one") and/or the communicative intent of an author who might write headlines stating, "Iraqi Head Seeks Arms." Without mastery of ToM, one would also have difficulty gauging the constraints of discourse and perceiving the informational needs of others. The fact that ToM skills are closely linked to pragmatic functioning is also evident in very early prelinguistic gestural language development. Whereas normal children develop requesting and commenting skills concurrently, children with ASD develop the more social commenting pointing skills significantly later than requesting ones (63). Commenting skills are dependent on the ability to attribute attention to others.

ToM deficits are not specific to children with ASD. They have also been found to be delayed in children with severe hearing impairment and in some children with Down syndrome (64). However, it is important to note that neither group demonstrated deficits in joint attention or social referencing. Unlike persons with hearing impairment or Down syndrome, who eventually develop some degree of ToM as their social experiences and mental age increase, adults with autism and intelligence in the average range retain their inability to decouple or segregate their own thoughts from others. Because ToM is the ability to infer states of mind based on external behavior, Baron-Cohen (65) coined the term "mindblindedness" to represent the most severe level of ToM deficit as seen in persons with ASD.

Numerous experimental studies support the hypothesis that children with autism have difficulty on ToM measures. Several mental-age-specific test paradigms have been used to measure stages of ToM development:

False belief paradigms: One of the most popular test paradigms for 4–5-year-olds is the Sally-Anne Disbelief Test (Fig. 1). In this test situation, a child is asked to watch "Sally" hide a toy in a box. Sally then leaves the room, and Anne enters. She then moves the toy from the box and puts it in a different covered container. Sally is then asked to return and the child

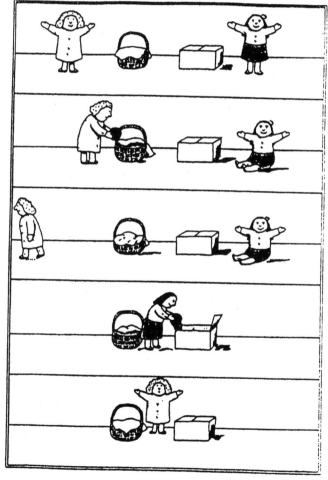

Figure 1   Sally-Anne Disbelief Test.

is asked, "Where will Sally look for the object?" To answer this question correctly, the child must be able to disregard or set aside his own knowledge about where the toy really is and think about where Sally thinks the toy is. People with ASD manifest robust difficulty with false belief and related ToM tasks as compared to language- and IQ-matched controls (65). An alternative false belief task simply requires a Band-Aid box, Band-Aids, and wrapped strips of chewing gum. It is logistically less complex and does not require a "Sally" or "Anne," which makes it easier to implement in clinical practice. The clinician asks the parents to leave the room momentarily. He/she then shows the box containing Band-Aids to the child. He removes the Band-Aids, substitutes them with strips of gum, and closes the lid. He gives the box to the child and says, "Let's bring the box to your parents and ask them what's inside the box! What do you think they will say?" Whereas most typically developing 4-year-old children will realize that their parents would expect to find Band-Aids, the child with ASD is more likely to say "gum."

Strange stories: Individuals are read short stories depicting each of the following: pretend, joke, lie, white lie, double bluff, figure of speech, irony persuasion, and a control (physical story). Afterward one is asked if the story is true and why the person said what he/she did (66). Persons with ASD often give quite different answers than other populations owing to their inability to understand humor or idioms. A mental age of at least 6 years is required.

Faux pas vignettes: A series of stories have been developed for children with mental ages of 9 years and above. For example, one story describes a mother and her daughter making an apple pie as a gift to welcome a new neighbor. When it is baked, they box it and visit the neighbor. The neighbor very graciously accepts the gift, saying, "A pie, how very thoughtful of you. I just love pies, all except apple pies that is." A set of questions follows each vignette to determine whether or not the listener understood the faux pas (67).

Judging mental states: One is asked to interpret the mental or emotional state of others by observing their facial expression in photos of pairs of eyes. He/she must choose the word from a list of four that most accurately describes the person's emotional state (i.e., angry, serious, happy, afraid) (68).

Using single-photon-emission computerized tomography data, it has been demonstrated that solving ToM vignettes involves cortical activity in the left medial frontal gyrus (Brodmann area 8) (69). Although these testing paradigms may be helpful in differentiating children with ASD, adequate performance on them does not necessarily mean that persons with high-functioning autism are able to always use this skill functionally in real-life situations (70).

6. Decreased Facial Expression and/or Animation

Often children with ASD are described as having a "flat affect" or "masked facies." Their facial expression is rather bland and monotonous and lacks the animation commonly seen in typically developing children during joint-attention activities when the child presents something that is interesting or that he is proud of to his parent in the act of "showing." Such functional deficits are similar to the neurological abnormalities seen in Möbius syndrome. Although an autopsy study revealed a hypoplastic cranial nerve VII nucleus in the brain of one adult with autism (52), this deficit seems to be more often psychophysiological and possibly associated with abnormal functioning of the amygdala.

7. Attachment

Attachment does not seem to be primarily impaired in children with ASD, though at one time it was thought to be a core feature. Occasionally children with primary attachment disorders are confused with those having ASD. In a study of a Romanian orphanage where children received less than optional attention from multiple-shiftwork caregivers, several children demonstrated quasi-autistic features and actually met full criteria based on the ADOS (71). However, symptoms improved once the child was adopted into a nurturing family environment. In an Ainsworth Strange Situations paradigm, it was demonstrated that children with ASD seek proximity and contact with their mothers as often as normal children matched by mental age (72).

8. Summary

The above discussion provides a broad overview of the social deficits in ASD. Some of these deficits are consistently seen in young children with ASD; others are not. The goal of this chapter is to help raise the clinician's awareness of these characteristics since they are more subtle and/or more difficult to evaluate than failure to attain language milestones. Hopefully, a better understanding will allow the clinician to recognize ASD at a younger age and to refer the child to an appropriate intervention program earlier. It is thought that earlier intervention utilizing strategies that address these social deficits as well as the more obvious language deficits and behavior problems will result in better functional outcomes. Recent outcome studies support this approach (7–9).

III. DEFICITS IN LANGUAGE DEVELOPMENT

Traditionally, delays and deviancies in language development have been the presenting sign in children heretofore diagnosed with ASD. Although studies during the past two decades revealed that approximately 50% of children with autism are nonverbal, the remainder have some degree of speech, and in a few, speech may "appear" to be advanced due to echolalia. Children with Asperger's syndrome may not demonstrate obvious speech delays but instead have more subtle abnormalities in language pragmatics. As more and more children are being diagnosed with milder conditions on the spectrum, those with speech represent a growing proportion of children with ASD. For a much more in-depth discussion of language development in children with ASD, the reader is referred to Chapter 6 in *Autism Spectrum Disorders*, edited by Amy Wetherby and Barry Prizant (73).

A. Absent or Delayed Speech

Delayed or absent speech is the most common presenting concern of parents. Although most parents will admit that they sensed something was wrong by 18 months of age, they often do not share these concerns with the clinician until after the child turns 2 years old (73,74). They may delay raising a concern about absent or delayed speech because they rationalize that the delays are due to the child's temperament (shy, slow to warm up), or that the child may be spoiled because either they themselves or older siblings have overanticipated the child's needs thereby eliminating any reason to speak. When the child is an "only child," parents may rationalize that the delays are due to the absence of peers to stimulate speech. The gravity of the problem is often not realized until a younger sibling "passes the child up" or a Sunday school or preschool teacher raises a concern.

However, delay in recognition and diagnosis of ASD may also be due to the lack of realization on the physician's part that the parental concerns are significant and merit further evaluation and/or intervention. Parents commonly complain that in response to verbalizing their concerns about speech delays, their physician gave false reassurance and took a "wait and see" approach. This is often followed by resentment when the parents learn about the availability of early intervention and its possible impact on prognosis. Indeed, several national parent-directed organizations have embraced the challenge to educate physicians in an effort to prevent ongoing delays in diagnosis and referral. Their fervent and intense advocacy activity has also been directed at various state and federal governing bodies and, if successful, may eventually effect changes in physician practices and increase funding for infant and school-age educational programs.

B. Loss of or Inconsistent Use of Previously Acquired Words

Approximately 25–30% of children with ASD lose previously mastered words between the ages of 18 and 24 months. However, the loss of language skills is not pathognomonic of ASD; it occurs in Rett's syndrome and other neurodegenerative disorders as well. Loss of speech associated with seizures is characteristic of Landau-Kleffner syndrome; however, onset is later, and the language regression is typically not associated with parallel regression in social skills. In other children with ASD, previously learned words seem to lose their communicative function and appear to "pop up" for no apparent reason. The words are said inconsistently and out of context. These "pop-up words" should be distinguished from meaningful words that are consistently said with intention (not merely parroted), are functional, and are used in appropriate contexts for at least a month (73,75). Sometimes a particular "pop-up word" is said frequently for a short period of time before it disappears. Occasionally the utterances may be phrases or entire sentences, also said out of context. Parents might report these words and sentences as mastered skills when, in fact, they have little or no communicative intent. On the other hand, the words and phrases might indeed be prompted by some yet unrecognizable motive. Although generally more obvious than speech delays, loss of skills may also be rationalized. Such regression is sometimes attributed to a family event such as the birth of a new sibling or a move to a new house.

C. Echolalia

The vast majority of children with ASD who eventually demonstrate functional symbolic language go through a period of using echolalia. Echolalia is classified as immediate (child's parroting occurs immediately after the partner's vocalization) or delayed (child's parroting occurs at a time remote from the original vocalization). Although a child with ASD may demonstrate both kinds of echolalia, the delayed form is more distinguishing. Most typically developing children go through a stage where they imitate other's speech, particularly the last one or two words of a sentence. It is usually immediate and occurs when children are rapidly gaining new words during the "vocabulary burst stage" (73). Autistic echolalia should be differentiated from normal imitation that occurs during this period of rapid language acquisition. The echolalia is more exact, has a monotone quality, and includes larger "chunks" of verbal utterances. It is also associated with reversal of I and you pronouns since the child repeats the phrase or sentence exactly as he himself hears it. For example, he may say, "Do you want a drink?" when he actually is requesting a drink for himself. Additionally delayed echolalia in children with ASD may include recitation of songs, advertisement jingles, ABCs, etc. to a degree that far exceeds the child's functional language ability. These abilities are sometimes viewed as an indication of genius on the part of parents and observers.

Echolalia may serve as a verbal type of reenactment (see discussion above in the section on joint attention) whereby the child repeats a phrase or sentence to make the event happen again. For example (73): "A 4-year old boy with ASD repeatedly approached his teacher and stated, 'Do ahhh' while opening his mouth. It was clear by his nonverbal behavior that he was trying to communicate something, but his teacher was at a loss to understand his meaning. After school, the teacher called the boy's mother and explained the dilemma. Without hesitation, his mother explained that when her son is not feeling well, she tells him to open his mouth and 'Do ahhh' so that she can observe whether his throat is inflamed. Recently, he had begun to initiate interactions with her using this same phrase to 'tell' her that he was not feeling well. Thus, he used this rather unconventional gestalt language form that he had come to associate with feeling ill." Often these and other reenactments might not be understood if the listener does not know the history of how the behavior evolved. Reenactments are performed with some sense of anticipation and may serve as building blocks to symbolic communication.

In the past, echolalia was considered deviant and not to play a role in the development of functional language. It is now recognized that most verbal children with ASD go through a stage of using both immediate and delayed echolalia. It may be a necessary first step for children with ASD in their unique journey to meaningful language; they use echolalia to communicate rather than just parrot. Parents are now encouraged to acknowledge it and help functional language development by providing context and meaning to echolalic phrases and sentences. Transforming seemingly meaningless echolalia into functional language appears to take place in five stages (76):

First the child simply repeats the phrase spontaneously without understanding its meaning or use.

Then, the child gradually learns the meaning of the phrases by using them repeatedly and finding out how they "work." In the example above, once the parent deduces that "Do you want a drink?" might actually mean that the child wants a drink, he/she may stop answering "no" and, instead offers the child a drink while saying, Oh, so [name], you want a drink. Here is a drink for you, [name], and here is a drink for me, too.

This, in turn, reinforces the utterance and the child begins to use the sentence/phrase purposefully, yet the pronoun reversal persists since he can only repeat it as he has heard it.

Next the child starts to break the sentence down into chunks... smaller meaningful units that he might mix and match in various contexts.

Finally he transforms it into a rule-governed language system and he is able to substitute I for you and make it a personal request: "Can I have a drink?"

Children with ASD who eventually develop functional language tend to develop grammatical skills in the same general progression as normal children. However, they lag far behind and, in fact, may never develop an understanding of the social rules, how to take turns in conversation or how to "read" the listener's interest or response to what is being said. These are all aspects of pragmatic language (see below).

D. Preoccupation with Labeling

Some children are quite obsessed with labeling colors, shapes, numbers, and letters of the alphabet, yet they are unable to use these in functional language or point to them upon request. Unlike typically developing children, they demonstrate less interest in common everyday objects or pictures in books and rarely point to them to request new words from the listener. In recognizing their child's advanced interest in letters and numbers, parents will sometimes purchase flashcards and other educational materials to promote spelling and written word recognition. This may lead to hyperlexia or advanced oral reading without accompanying comprehension skills. Such skills are out of sync with the child's functional use of symbolic language. However, since written words are coded and processed in a different manner than verbal words, these splinter skills are sometimes used in an effort to bridge the gap in oral-verbal abilities (73).

E. Idiosyncratic Use of Language

Children with ASD may utter unique words that have meaning only to them (neologisms). They may use these words in a series of utterances that represents a unique form of jargoning. Unlike typically developing children this jargoning does not eventually evolve into a more mature jargoning style whereby recognizable words are sporadically inserted and provide some meaning to the listener. Additionally the intonation, inflection, rate, and rhythm may be idiosyncratic and unlike more typical jargoning. It appears that the child has developed a unique language schema that is uttered without any attempt to make the listener understand. Finally, it may be associated with laughing out loud for no apparent reason, at least to the observer. In the higher-functioning child with some degree of fluent, symbolic language, recognizable words may be used in very unique ways. For example, one high-functioning 6-year-old (nonverbal IQ of 143, verbal IQ of 86, and a seventh-grade reading level) in a conversation with his 12-year-old sister who was complaining about how hard her homework was, said in reply, "That isn't so hard, it's just medium."

F. Advanced Expressive Language Relative to Receptive Language

It has been said, "Comprehension is the power that fuels expression" (77). Comprehension is basic to and a building block for expressive communication. In a child learning his first language or in an older individual learning an additional language, expressive language development usually trails behind receptive. Some children with ASD and exceptionally good memory and articulation skills may demonstrate advanced speech relative to comprehension. This results in an apparent disconnect from the typical receptive-expressive relationship just described. However, their word combinations (giant words or multiword echolalic utterances) really function as single words and thoughts rather than as a true phrase or sentence. Comprehension at the one-word stage on testing should confirm this observation. The rather sophisticated long utterances actually function as single words and thoughts and should be scored as such. In so doing the more typical receptive-expressive relationship is preserved (73).

G. Preverbal Language Abnormalities

The language deficits described above are those that are more typical of older children with ASD. To facilitate *earlier* diagnosis of children with ASD, the clinician must also be familiar with the earlier-appearing prelinguistic language deficits that characterize the disorder. These are often more subtle receptive milestones, include gestural deficits, and go unnoticed by parents. Some are communicative manifestations of joint attention or other social deficits described above. It takes an astute clinician to probe with pointed questions to determine if these earlier signs are present. Some of these include:

  Lack of the usual alternating to-and-fro pattern of vocalizations between baby and parent that usually occurs at approximately 5 months (i.e., vocalizations continue to overlap without regard for the partner's vocalization)

  Lack of recognition of mother's (or father's or consistent caregiver's) voice

  Disregard for vocalizations, yet keen awareness for nonlanguage or environmental sounds

  Lack of interest in babbling to and/or patting one's own reflection in a mirror

  Delayed onset of babbling past 9 months of age

  Decreased or absent use of prelinguistic gestures (pointing, showing, waving, nodding head)

  Lack of expressions such as "oh oh," "huh," etc.

  Lack of interest or response to neutral statements (e.g., "Oh no, it's raining again!")

  Lack of any attempt to compensate for lack of language

Often the parent is unaware of these deficits, and may not be able to answer the clinician's questions decisively. However, once brought to their attention, parents often become very vigilant and later notice them.

H. Pragmatic Deficits

Some high-functioning children with ASD may have mild or very limited speech delays and actually demonstrate rather fluent symbolic speech patterns. The only defining abnormality may be in speech delivery and/or in the social use of language (pragmatics). Their language may seem odd and not listener-responsive. Early diagnosis of (later-appearing) Asperger's syndrome might be missed unless the clinician and parents have a good understanding of language pragmatics. The description of the pragmatic components of language came relatively late to the accumulated fund of knowledge on language development (78). First described by Bates in 1976, the study of pragmatics revolutionized language-learning literature (79). (For a comprehensive discussion of pragmatics, the reader is referred to Chapter 10, in *Autism Spectrum Disorders*, edited by Amy Wetherby and Barry Prizant (78). Pragmatics rest on three premises:

1. Speech acts have function; they express intentionality to accomplish a given purpose. Simple functions might include making requests or protests; more complex functions include negotiating and expressing opinions. Although verbal children with ASD may learn to use language for simple functions, they have much more difficulty with more complex ones, especially those that require abstract reasoning and discussion of thoughts and opinions of others.

2. Competent communication requires the speaker to make judgments about what the listeners already know and what new facts they need to be given in order to comprehend the intentions of the speaker. For most people this is automatic and effortless. For those with ASD it is not. For example, one teen with ASD simply exclaimed, "Florida!" Not knowing what he meant, his teacher approached him and discovered he was concerned about a lesion on his leg. It looked like a map of Florida. Persons without pragmatic deficits would intuitively know that they needed to provide more information to the listener than simply "Florida" (80).

3. To engage in cooperative conversational exchanges, one must speak according to the "rules of discourse." This may include such things as: how to choose a topic of conversation, understanding and producing appropriate facial expression and body language during conversation, politeness, recognizing when the partner has lost interest in a topic, knowing when to start, sustain, and end a conversation based on listener cues, knowing when and how to repair a communication breakdown, and appropriate tempo and turn taking (78). For example, a teen with Asperger's syndrome suffered a minor injury at a fund-raising event. The physician on duty approached him to inquire of his status. Instead of answering the inquiries regarding the injury, the teen

delivered a monotone oration comparing and contrasting different makes of automobile motors (his particular obsession at the time). The doctor attempted repeatedly to redirect his interest to the presumed injury. After each attempt, the boy stopped briefly, momentarily looked bewildered, and then resumed his oration. Finally, he said, "That will be all. You are dismissed."

In these children there appears to be dissociation between the *form* and the *function* of language. Whereas the *form* (syntax, tense, grammar, articulation, and vocabulary) is intact, *function* (pragmatics and semantics or word meaning) is significantly impaired. This disconnect may not be helpful in the early diagnosis of classic autism but it can be very helpful in the early recognition of Asperger's syndrome.

Mastery of pragmatic skills depends on competence in ToM and executive function. ToM ability allows one to mentalize or understand the intent of the speaker so that one, in turn, can understand metaphors, irony, lies, jokes, faux pas, and deception (59,65). Individuals with ASD and deficient ToM abilities will have difficulty with statements like "Put your money where your mouth is," "Eyes on the board," "Two heads are better than one," or a news caption such as "Iraqi Head Seeks Arms" (78). Finally, fluent children with ASD may demonstrate unique delivery of speech in regard to intonation, volume, rhythm, and pitch that also tend to disregard listener needs.

IV. STEREOTYPIES AND REPETITIVE, RESTRICTIVE PLAYS

Children with ASD often demonstrate little interest in the usual popular childhood toys, often preferring everyday items such as string, rocks, dirt, feathers, and chains. They may play with them in a stereotypic, sensorimotor manner for hours at a time without seeking attention. Sometimes parents will state that the child is exceptionally "good" and can entertain himself indefinitely, requiring little or no supervision. Depending on the child's developmental stage, he may line objects up, put objects in and out of containers, complete board puzzles, turn pages of books, or play for hours with constructive toys or computer games. Sometimes children with ASD are, indeed, interested in typical toys but in unusual ways or in only their parts. For example, rather than playing with a miniature truck in the typical way, they instead turn it upside down and spin the wheels repeatedly. Still others are intensely interested, even obsessed, with certain unusual items such as fans, light switches, electric cords, etc. Although most children, at some time during their early development, form attachments with a stuffed animal, a special pillow, or a "blankee," children with ASD often prefer hard items (ballpoint pens, chains, fast-food giveaway toys, etc.). Moreover, the attachment is much more robust; they may even insist on holding the object most of the day, even during meals, and protest violently when the object is removed. Children may violently protest other types of transitions as well, insisting on "sameness" in regard to events and routines. When forced to change to a different activity or toy, they may become extremely angry and quickly escalate to a prolonged temper tantrum characterized by aggression or self-injurious behaviors.

Many children with ASD develop stereotypies (e.g., hand flapping, twirling, finger movements, rocking, head nodding etc.). Although stereotypies are often very distinctive and obvious, they are not specific to children with ASD. They often do not occur until after 3 years of age and thus they are not helpful in the early diagnosis of ASD. Normal toddlers, especially prior to the onset of fluent language, sometimes flap briefly when they are excited or frustrated and children with profound mental retardation and/or severe visual deficits also demonstrate stereotypies. Somewhat unique to children with ASD, however, is the demonstration of habitual toe walking and/or sensory stereotypies such as persistent sniffing and licking of nonfood items.

V. SELF-INJURIOUS BEHAVIOR

It is estimated that 5–17% of persons with ASD, especially those with comorbid mental retardation, demonstrate some form of self-injurious behavior (SIB). SIB is a symptom expressed in many different syndromes and in various forms. It is also thought to have several etiologies: operant, metabolic, neurochemical (dopa, serotonin, opioid, and GABA neural transmitter systems have all been implicated), or anatomical. True SIB usually does not appear until after 5 years of age. A proto-SIB (head banging that is not injurious and, occasionally, self-biting without breaking skin) occurs prior to 5 years. Reasons for SIB include (81):

Frustration with skill deficits, primarily in language, whereby the SIB serves a social-communication function.

Reaction to a stimulus where SIB is used to obtain a tangible, to cope with an under- or overstimulating environment, to escape from an anxiety-provoking situation (encroachment on one's personal space or a requirement to transition from one activity/toy to another); an endogenous neurochemical abnormality in dopa, serotonin, opioid, or GABA neural transmitter systems.

A trait that makes up the behavioral phenotype in specific genetically determined syndromes (self-picking in Prader-Willi and self-hugging in Smith-Magenis syndromes).

A chronic health problem: pain, illness, pruritus, sleep deprivation, etc.

SIB is often the most challenging behavior that caregivers encounter. Management is best accomplished with a functional analysis of behavior to determine the stimulus for the SIB. The stimulus may be obvious when it immediately precedes the behavior and is consistent (e.g., hand biting each time a transition is attempted). However, it is more elusive when the stimulus does not consistently produce the SIB, when it is rarely considered noxious by nonautistic persons, or when it occurs well in advance of the SIB (e.g., a delayed response to running water in a distant bathroom). Additionally, the antecedent may not be readily evident when it is associated with an ongoing condition (sleep deprivation, illness, pain).

VI. COGNITIVE AND EXECUTIVE FUNCTION DEFICITS

In the past, cognitive deficits were thought to be extremely common in children with ASD. Most studies published prior to 1990 report a prevalence of mental retardation in 90% or more of individuals. More recently, the prevalence has been commonly reported as 75%. This figure continues to drop and, in one study, was as low as 26% (82). Better ascertainment of children with milder disorders, more effective strategies for evaluating cognitive abilities in children with ASD, and early intense intervention in integrated settings have all been cited as possible reasons for the decreasing prevalence of comorbid mental retardation. The presence or absence of mental retardation in a child with ASD may be the most important factor in determining long-term functional prognosis (83).

EF abilities have been traditionally "housed" in the frontal lobe and enable one: to process information, plan, organize, and regulate one's behavior; to monitor one's own performance and make use of feedback; and to think about and organize one's own thoughts. It was not until the mid-1980s that empirical work directly assessing executive function (EF) in persons with high-functioning autism were conducted, some with conflicting results. Until that time the main cognitive deficits known to be associated with persons with ASD included difficulties with abstract thinking, tendencies toward preservative response patterns, and stimulus overselectivity. EF skills also include the ability to disengage from external context to inhibit an inappropriate response and to disregard a false literal meaning in favor of a correct nonliteral inference. Although many children with ASD are unable to understand humor, jokes, sarcasm, and figurative speech (e.g., "Two heads are better than one"), these are not specific to ASD. One longitudinal study of high-functioning children with autism demonstrated consistent deficits in EF performance with little improvement over time, thus indicating a possible developmental ceiling on this type of ability (84).

VII. ABNORMAL SENSORY PROCESSING

Although not at all specific for ASD, "sensory integration" problems have received much attention in the recent years. [For a comprehensive review of sensory and motor processing in ASD, the reader is referred to Chapter 6 in this book and/or Chapter 7 (Understanding the Nature of Communication and Language Impairments) in *Autism Spectrum Disorders*, edited by Amy Wetherby and Barry Prizant (85).] Children with ASD tend to demonstrate simultaneous hyposensitivities and hypersensitivities for different stimuli even within the same sensory modality. For example, the slightest sound of water dripping may provoke a negative response, yet the child seems oblivious to his mother calling his name loudly. Although part of the explanation may be rooted to the tendency of children with ASD to selectively tune out social (human) sounds (see above discussion of social orienting), some degree of physiological deficit might also be responsible. As noted earlier in this chapter, often one of the first concerns the parents have is the possibility of deafness. Yet they eventually deny that the child has a hearing problem since he seems to hear environmental sounds exceptionally well. Vision does not seem to be as problematic, but parents will often report that their child explores toys visually in unusual ways. He may hold the object very close to his eyes, look at the object out of the corners of his eye, or demonstrate an unusual head tilt (which would typically raise concerns about visual impairment and/or strabismus). Additionally, some children seem annoyed with fluorescent lights and if verbal, they might complain that the light makes things "jump around." Although motor stereotypies are seen in other disabilities, particularly severe mental retardation and blindness, children with ASD demonstrate somewhat unique sniffing and licking stereotypies. On the other hand, children with ASD may have oral aversions and intolerance to certain textures that contribute to self-imposed restricted diets. In addition to oral aversions, many children demonstrate "tactile defensiveness" and are intolerant of soft touch and various clothing textures. Conversely, they may be indifferent to significant injuries and other noxious stimuli that would typically be quite painful to children without ASD. The dichotomy is puzzling, but most experts feel that it is due to an abnormal arousal level or sensory gating system in the cerebellum and/or brainstem. Recently, the frontal cortex has been the focus of attention for its abnormal minicolumns possibly resulting in less "insulation" of neural transmissions thus causing overstimulation (86). Abnormalities in the gating of stimuli are thought to account for two patterns of children with autism: (a) the hyporeactive child with a high sensory threshold requiring excessive sensory input to achieve activation of the system and (b) the hyperreactive child with a low sensory threshold who is often overly focused on detail. Understanding these patterns has implications for medical intervention, with SSRIs possibly being more helpful in the former and stimulants in the latter (87).

VIII. MOTOR ABNORMALITIES

One isolated video study of very young infants who were later diagnosed with ASD (88) demonstrated unusual movement abnormalities of the mouth, trunk, and extremities. Some investigators feel that these abnormalities may herald the praxic deficits noted to be present in many older children with ASD. Praxis refers to the planning, execution, and sequencing of movements (89). Apraxia (severe deficits) and dyspraxia (milder deficits) are linked to deficits in imitation and cannot be linked to neuromotor pathology. Praxic deficits affect the imitation of speech, facial expressions, play, and/or motor patterns of the extremities. Most children with ASD exhibit less imitation. In those children with comorbid praxic deficits, imitation quality as well as quantity is impaired; the movements appear awkward and inaccurate. The children are often labeled as clumsy and uncoordinated, which seems to contradict earlier reports that children with ASD usually had advanced gross motor skills. Dyspraxia is not unique to ASD; oral-motor dyspraxia has long been known to be a contributing factor to speech delay in children without ASD. Both groups have difficulties imitating sequenced oral-motor movements (e.g., imitating "da-pa-ka" rapidly) necessary for fluent speech in spite of intact neurological and oral cavity exams. Praxis problems also prevent automatic, smooth synchronous, continuous motor matching of a partner and result in problems in timing, speed, and grading of movements (90). Praxia has been conceptualized as encompassing three steps: (1) ideation (formulating the goal), (2) motor planning (figuring out how to accomplish the goal), and (3) execution (the actual carrying out of the planned action) (85). Deficits can occur at any step and result in failure. For example, when faced with the task of playing in a carpeted play tunnel, a child must first develop some concept that it is possible to crawl through a tunnel. Children with ASD often had difficulty with this first step, ideation. They have little idea of the goal for play in a tunnel. Others may have a deficit in the next step, motor planning; although they desire to go through the tunnel, they cannot figure out how to accomplish the task owing to a poor sensorimotor awareness. Still others will be unable to execute the activity owing to poor motor control and coordination. These children may also demonstrate gross and fine motor delays.

In addition to abnormal quality of motor actions, children with ASD may demonstrate abnormal amounts of activity. Some may appear to be "hyperactive" and motor-driven with an exterior focus of attention. Others may be hypoactive, move little, seem to have an interior focus of attention, and are withdrawn. This may impact decisions regarding medication management at a later time. Whereas the former may respond to stimulants, the latter may more likely respond to a selective serotonin reuptake inhibitor.

IX. PHYSICAL CHARACTERISTICS

As noted in the introduction to this chapter, ASD is not associated with a classic physical phenotype. Fewer than 25% of children will have a comorbid genetic syndrome and thus will manifest the physical signs that are characteristic for that syndrome (91) (see Chapter 6). Most children have idiopathic autism and are not dysmorphic. Approximately 25–30% of children develop postnatal-onset macrocephaly that is not associated with ventricular pathology (92). A few studies have reported children with slightly posterior rotated ears.

X. AUTISM REGRESSION SYNDROME

Although the majority of children with ASD present with abnormalities as described above, 25–35% will appear to develop normally until 12–24 months at which point they regress in both language and social skills (93). Parents report that the children were smiling, waving "bye-bye," and saying a few words, when they either suddenly or gradually stopped speaking and "withdrew into a shell." Although the underlying mechanism is unknown, several hypotheses, such as immune dysfunction and stress, have been proposed (94,95). A detailed discussion of these hypotheses is beyond the scope of this chapter. Home videos recorded prior to the onset of regression have revealed that, in at least some children, subtle early signs were present before the apparent regression (35–38). Some investigators have reported an increased incidence of seizures and/or abnormal EEG in regressive form; otherwise, physical, medical, or neurological characteristics appear to be very similar (93).

XI. CONCLUSION

If the pediatrician is to be successful in detecting the early signs of ASD, he/she must be knowledgeable and extremely vigilant. Owing to the increased prevalence of ASD and its broader phenotype, an even higher degree of vigilance is warranted in the younger siblings of children already diagnosed with ASD. Ascertainment of deficits in very early social skills and in preverbal language skills is critical. Although a variety of screening tools target these skills, no current one can be singled out as superior (see Chapter 6). Newer tools, as well as modifications of the current, are being studied to improve sensitivity and specificity. Hopefully, the ideal tool will emerge soon. In the meantime, pediatricians are encouraged to have a high index of suspicion, use one of the tools (realizing its limitations), and, most important, *listen to the parents*. Again most parents become concerned by 18 months. At that point, if the clinician does not feel qualified to conduct a comprehensive evaluation, he/she should *immediately refer* to a specialist or, ideally, to an autism team. Additionally, the pediatrician should refer the child to the local early-intervention program. It is not necessary to have a definitive diagnosis, or an etiological one, for the child to qualify for early-intervention services. Most programs have multidisciplinary teams that can conduct a developmental evaluation and provide a profile of the child's strengths and weaknesses. This developmental profile can then assist the physician in making a diagnosis especially if it demonstrates language and social skills that are significantly below the child's overall level of functioning.

REFERENCES

1. Rogers SJ, Pennington BF. A theoretical approach to the deficits in infantile autism. Dev Psychopathol 1991; 3:137–162.
2. Rogers SJ, Benneto L. Intersubjectivity in Autism. In: Wetherby AM, Prizant BM, eds. Autism Spectrum Disorders. Baltimore: Paul H. Brookes Publishing Co., 2000:79–107.
3. Mundy P, Sheinkope S. Social behavior and the neurology of autism. Int Pediatr 1993; 8:205–210.
4. Travis L, Sigman M. Social deficits and interpersonal relationships in autism. Ment Retard Dev Disabil Res Rev 1998; 4:65–72.
5. Minshew N, Goldstein G. Autism as a disorder of complex information processing. Ment Retard Dev Disabil Res Rev 1998; 4:129–136.
6. Stone WL. Can autism be diagnosed accurately in children under 3 years? J Child Psychol Psychiatry 1999; 40:219–226.
7. Dawson G, Osterling J. Early intervention in autism. In: Guralnick JM, ed. The Effectiveness of Early Intervention. Baltimore, MD: Paul H Brookes Publishing Co., 1997:307–326.
8. Hurth J, Sahw E, Izeman SG, Shaley K, Rogers SJ. Areas of agreement about effective practices among programs serving young children with autism spectrum disorders. Infants Young Child 1999; 12:17–26.
9. Committee on Education Interventions for Children with Autism (Chair: Catherine Lord). Educating Children with Autism. Washington, DC: National Academy of Science, 2001.
10. Howlin P, Moore A. Diagnosis of autism: a survey of over 1200 patients in the UK. Autism 1997; 1:135–162.
11. Howlin P, Asgharian A. The diagnosis of autism and Asperger syndrome: findings from a survey of 770 families. Dev Med Child Neurol 1999; 41:834–839.
12. Fombonne E. The epidemiology of autism: a review. Psychol Med 1999; 29:769–786.
13. Zwaigenbaum L. Baby sibs studies expanded. Narrative 2002; Fall:7.
14. Bailey A, Le Courteur A, Gottesman I. Autism as a strongly genetic disorder: evidence form a British twin study. Psychol Med 1995; 25:63–77.

15. Folstein S, Tagge-Flusber H, Jseph R. Current directions in research on autism. Ment Retard Dev Disabil Res Rev 2001; 7:21–29.
16. Rogers SJ, Benneto L. Intersubjectivity in autism. In: Wetherby AM, Prizant BM, eds. Autism Spectrum Disorders. Baltimore: Paul H. Brookes Publishing Co., 2000:97.
17. Wetherby AM, Prizant BM, Hutchinson TA. Communicative, social/affective and symbolic profiles of young children with autism and pervasive developmental disorders. Am J Speech Lang Pathol 1998; 7:79–91.
18. Mundy P, Markus J. On the nature of communication and language impairment in autism. Ment Retard Dev Disabil Res Rev 1997; 3:343–349.
19. Wetherby A, Prizant B, Hutchinson T. Communicative, social-affective and symbolic profiles of young children with autism and pervasive developmental disorders. Am J Speech Lang Pathol 1998; 7:79–91.
20. Mundy P, Sigman M, Kasari C. A longtime study of joint attention and language development in autistic children. J Autism Dev Disord 1990; 20:115–120.
21. Bondy A, Frost L. Education approaches in preschool: behavior techniques in a public school setting. In: Schopler E, Mesibov G, eds. Learning and Cognition in Autism. New York: Plenum Press, 1995:311–334.
22. Lewy A, Dawson G. Social stimulation and joint attention in young autistic children. J Abnorm Child Psychol 1992; 20:555–566.
23. Baron-Cohen S, Baldwin D, Crowson M. Do children with autism use the speaker's direction of gaze strategy to crack the code of language? Child Dev 1997; 68:48–57.
24. Wetherby AM, Prizant B, Schuler AL. Understanding the nature of communication and language impairments. In: Wetherby AM, Prizant BM, eds. Autism Spectrum Disorders. Baltimore: Paul H. Brookes Publishing Co., 2000:25.
25. Tomasello M. The role of joint attentional processes in early language development. Lang Sci 1988; 10:69–88.
26. Wetherby AM, Prizant B, Schuler AL. Understanding the nature of communication and language impairments. In: Wetherby AM, Prizant BM, eds. Autism Spectrum Disorders. Baltimore: Paul H. Brookes Publishing Co., 2000:111.
27. Rogers SJ, Benneto L. Intersubjectivity in autism. In: Wetherby AM, Prizant BM, eds. Autism Spectrum Disorders. Chapter 5. Baltimore: Paul H. Brookes Publishing Co., 2000:93.
28. Wetherby A, Prizant BM, Guthinson TA. Communicative, social/affective, and symbolic profiles of young children with autism and pervasive developmental disorders. Am J Speech Lang Pathol 1998; 7:79–91.
29. Dawson G, Meltzoff A, Osterling J. Children with autism fail to orient to naturally occurring social stimuli. Paper presented at the meeting of the Society for Research in Child Development, Indianapolis, IN, March 1995.
30. Mundy P. Joint attention, social-emotional approach in children with autism. Dev Psychopathol 1995; 7:63–82.
31. Carpenter M, Tomasello M. Joint attention, cultural learning, and language acquisition. In: Wetherby AM, Prizant BM, eds. Autism Spectrum Disorders. Baltimore: Paul H. Brookes Publishing Co., 2000:31–54.

32. Leekam S, Lopez B. Attention and joint attention in preschool children with autism. Dev Psychol 2000; 36:261–273.

33. Dawson G, Meltzoff A, Osterling J. Children with autism fail to orient to naturally occurring social stimuli. Paper presented at the meeting of the Society for Research in Child Development, Indianapolis, IN, March 1995.

34. Osterling J, Dawson G. Early recognition of children with autism: a study of first birthday home videotapes. J Autism Dev Disord 1994; 24:247–257.

35. Osterling J, Dawson G. Early recognition of infants with autism versus mental retardation. Poster presented at the meeting of the society for research in child development. Albuquerque, NM, 1999.

36. Baranek GT. Autism during infancy: a retrospective video analysis of sensory-motor and social behaviors at 9–12 months of age. J Autism Dev Disord 1999; 29:213–224.

37. Maestro S, Muratori F, Cristina M, Pei F, Stern D, Golse B, Palacia-Espasa F. Attentional skills during the first 6 months of age in autism spectrum disorder. J Am Acad Child Adolesc Psychiatry 2002; 41:1239–1245.

38. Lord C. Follow-up of two year-olds referred for possible autism. J Child Psychol Psychiat Allied Discipl 1995; 36:1365–1382.

39. Mundy P, Sigman M, Ungere J, Sherman T. Nonverbal communication and play correlates of language development in autistic children. J Autism Dev Disord 1987; 17:349–364.

40. Charman T, Wettenham J, Baron-Cohen S. An experimental investigation of cognitive abilities in infants with autism: clinical implications. Infant Mental Health J 1998; 19:260–275.

41. Lord C, Risi S, Lambert L, et al. The Autism Diagnostic Observation Schedule–Generic: a standard measure of social and communication deficits associated with the spectrum of autism. J Autism Dev Disord 2000; 30:205–223.

42. Wetherby AM, Prizant BM, Hutchinson T. Communicative, social-affective, and symbolic profiles of young children with autism and pervasive developmental disorder. Am J Speech Lang Pathol 1998; 7:79–91.

43. Dawson G, Hill D, Spencer A, Galpert L, Watson L. Affective exchanges between young autistic children and their mothers. J Abnorm Child Psychol 1990; 18:335–345.

44. Greenspan SI, Wieder S. Developmental patterns and outcomes in infants and children with disorders in relating and communicating: a chart review of 200 cases of children with autistic spectrum diagnoses. J Dev Learning Disord 1997; 1:87–114.

45. Courchesne E, Yeung-Courchesne R, Press G, Hesselink JR, Jernigan TL. Hypoplasia of cerebellar vermal lobules VI and VII in infantile autism. N Engl J Med 1988; 318:1349–1354.

46. Courchesne E. Infantile autism. Part 2. A new neurodevelopmental model. Int Pediatr 1995; 10:155.

47. Courchesne E, Hesselink JR, Jernigan TL, Yeung-Courchesne R. Abnormal neuroanatomy in a non-retarded person with autism: unusual findings with magnetic resonance imaging. Arch Neurol 1987; 44:335–341.

48. Courchesne E, et al. Impairment in shifting attention in autistic and cerebellar patients. Behav Neurosci 1994; 108:848–865.

49. Townsend J, Singer-Harris NS, Courchesne E. Visual attention abnormalities in autism: Delayed orienting to location. J Int Neuropsychol Soc 1996; 2:541–550.

50. Akshoomoff NA, Courchesne E. A new role for the cerebellum in cognitive operations. Behav Neurosci 1992; 106:731–738.

51. Swettenham J, Baron-Cohen S, Charman T, Cos A, Baird G, Drew A, Rees L. The frequency and distribution of spontaneous attention shifts between social and nonsocial stimuli in autistic, typically developing, and nonautistic developmentally delayed infants. J Child Psychol Psychiatry 1998; 39:747–753.

52. Rodier PM. The early origins of autism. Sci Am 2000; February:56–63.

53. Dawson G. Facial recognition in children with autism. Mol Psychiatry 2002; 7(suppl 18):36–39.

54. Frith U, Happé F. Autism: beyond the "theory of mind." Cognition 1994; 50:115–132.

55. Happé F. Studying weak central coherence at log levels: children with autism do not succumb to visual illusions. A research note. J Child Psychol Psychiatry 1996; 37:873–877.

56. Briskman J, Happé F. Exploring the cognitive phenotype of autism: weak "central coherence" in parents and siblings of children with autism. II. Real life skills and preferences. J Child Psychol Psychiatry 2001; 42:309–316.

57. Rinehart N, Bradshaw JL, Moss SA, Breeton AV, Tonge BT. Atypical interference of local detail on global processing in high functioning autism and Asperger's disorder. J Child Psychol Psychiatry 2000; 41:769–778.

58. Rumsey J, Ernst M. Functional neuroimaging of autistic disorders. Ment Retard Dev Disabil Res Rev 2000; 6:171–179.

59. Baron-Cohen S, Leslie AM, Frith U. Does the autistic child have a "theory of mind"? Cognition 1985; 21:37–46.

60. Twachtman-Cullen D. More able children with autism spectrum disorders. In: Wetherby AM, Prizant, BM, eds. Autism Spectrum Disorders. Baltimore: Paul H. Brookes Publishing Co., 2000:225–246.

61. Astington JW, Barriault T. Children's theory of mind: how young children come to understand that people have thoughts and feelings. Infants Young Child 2001; 13:1–12.

62. Wetherby AM, Prizant BM. Understanding the nature of communication and language impairments. In: Wetherby AM, Prizant BM, eds. Autism Spectrum Disorders. Baltimore: Paul H. Brookes Publishing Co., 2000:123.

63. Wetherby AM. Ontogeny of communicative functions in autism. J Autism Dev Disord 1986; 16:295–316.

64. Yirmiya N, Erel O, Shaked M, Solonimca-Levi D. Meta-analysis comparing theory of mind abilities of individual with autism, individuals with mental retardation, and normally developing individuals. Psychol Bull 1998; 124:283–307.

65. Baron-Cohen S. Mindblindness. Cambridge, MA: MIT Press, 1995.

66. Happé F. An advanced test of theory of mind: understanding of story characters' thoughts and feelings by able autistic, mentally handicapped, and normal children and adults. J Autism Dev Disord 1994; 24:129.

67. Baron-Cohen S, O'Tiordan M, Stone V, Jones R, Plaisted K. Recognition of faux pas by normally developing children and children with Asperger syndrome or high-functioning autism. J Autism Dev Disord 1999; 29(5):407–418.

68. Baron-Cohen S, Wheelwright S, Hill J, Raste Y, Plumb I. The "Reading the Mind in the Eyes" test revised version: a study with normal adults, and adults with Asperger syndrome or high-functioning autism. Presented at the Association for Child Psychology and Psychiatry, 2000.

69. Fletcher P, Happé F, Frith U, Baker S, Sloan R, Frackowiak P, Frith C. Other minds in the brain: a functional imaging study of ToM in story comprehension. Cognition 1995; 57:109–128.

70. Gillberg C, Ehlers S. High-functioning people with autism and Asperger syndrome: a literarture review. In: Scholpler E, Mesiboc GG, Kunce LJ, eds. Asperger Syndrome or High-Functioning Autism? New York: Plenum, 1998:79–106.

71. Rutter M, Andersen-Wood L, Bekett C, Bredenkamp D, Castle J, Groothues C, Kreppner J, Keaveney L, Lord C, Oconner TG, English and Romanian Adoptees Study Team. Quasi-autistic patterns following severe early global privation. J Child Psychol Psychiatry 1999; 40:537–549.

72. Rogers SJ, Ozonoff S, Maslin-Cole C. A comparative study of attachment behavior in young children with autism or other psychiatric disorders. J Am Acad Child Adolesc Psychiatry 1991; 30:483–488.

73. Wetherby AM, Prizant BM. Understanding the nature of communication and language impairments. In: Wetherby AM, Prizant BM, eds. Autism Spectrum Disorders. Baltimore: Paul H. Brookes Publishing Co., 2000:109–141.

74. Mundy P, Markus J. On the nature of communication and language impairment in autism. Ment Retard Dev Disabil Res Rev 1997; 3:343–349.

75. Lord C. Follow-up of two year-olds referred for possible autism. J Child Psychol Psychiatry Allied Discipl 1995; 36:1365–1382.

76. Wetherby AM, Prizant BM, Schuler AL. Understanding the nature of communication and language impairments. In: Wetherby AM, Prizant BM, eds. Autism Spectrum Disorders. Baltimore: Paul H. Brookes Publishing Co., 2000:113–114.

77. Twachtman-Cullen D. Comprehension: the power that fuels expression. Morning News, 1997; 9–11.

78. Twachtman-Cullen D. More able children with autism spectrum disorders. In: Wetherby AM, Prizant BM, eds. Autism Spectrum Disorders. Baltimore: Paul H. Brookes Publishing Co., 2000:225–249.

79. Bates E. Language and Context: The Acquisition of Pragmatics. San Diego: Academic Press, 1976.

80. Twachtman-Cullen D. Methods to enhance communication in verbal children. In: Quill KA, ed. Teaching Children with Autism: Strategies to Enhance Communication and Socialization. New York: Delmar Publishers Inc., 1995:133–162.

81. Schroeder SR. Self-injurious behavior. Ment Retard Dev Disabil Res Rev 2001; 7:3–11.

82. Chakrabarti S, Fombone E. Pervasive developmental disorders in preschool children. JAMA 2001; 285:3093–3099.

83. Szatmari P, Mérette C, Bryson SE, Thivierge J, Roy MA, Cayer M, Maziade M. Quantifying dimensions in autism: a factor-analytic study. J Am Acad Child Adolesc Psychiatry 2002; 41:467–474.

84. Ozonoff S, McEvoy RE. A longitudinal study of executive function and theory of mind development in autism. Dev Psychopathol 1994; 6:415–431.

85. Anzalone ME, Williamson G. Sensory processing and motor performance in autism spectrum disorders. In: Wetherby AM, Prizant BM, eds. Autism Spectrum Disorders. Baltimore: Paul H. Brookes Publishing Co., 2000:143–166.

86. Casonova P. Abnormal mini-columns in individuals with autism spectrum disorder. Neurology 2002; 58:438–444.

87. Anzalone ME, Williamson G. Sensory processing and motor performance in autism spectrum disorders. In: Wetherby AM, Prizant BM, eds. Autism Spectrum Disorders. Baltimore: Paul H. Brookes Publishing Co., 2000:148–149.

88. Teitelbaum P. Movement analysis in infancy may be useful for early diagnosis of autism. Proc Natl Acad Sci 1998; 95:1–6.

89. Rogers SJ, Benneto L. Intersubjectivity in autism. In: Wetherby AM, Prizant BM, eds. Autism Spectrum Disorders. Baltimore: Paul H. Brookes Publishing Co., 2000:84.

90. Rogers SJ, Benneto L. Intersubjectivity in autism. In: Wetherby AM, Prizant BM, eds. Autism Spectrum Disorders. Baltimore: Paul H. Brookes Publishing Co., 2000:101.

91. Gilberg C, Coleman M. Autism and medical disorders: a review of the literature. Dev Med Child Neurol 1996; 38:191–202.

92. Bailey A. Luthert P, Bolton P, Le Courteur A, Rutter M, Harding B. Autism and megalencephaly. Lancet 1993; 341:1225–1226.

93. Tuchman RF, Rapin I. Regression in pervasive developmental disorders: seizures and epileptiform electroencephalogram correlates. Pediatrics 1997; 99:560–566.

94. van Gent T, Heijnen CJ, Treffers PD. Autism and the immune system. J Child Psychol Psychiatry Allied Discipl 1997; 38:337–349.

95. Cook EH Jr, Perry BD, Dawson G, Wainwright MS, Leventhal BL. Receptor inhibition by immunoglobulins: specific inhibition by autistic children, their relatives, and control subjects. J Autism Dev Disord 1993; 23:67–77.

6

Screening and Diagnosis for Autistic Spectrum Disorders

Pasquale J. Accardo
Virginia Commonwealth University, Richmond, Virginia, U.S.A.

I. INTRODUCTION

Several clinical practice guidelines for the screening and diagnosis of autism and autistic spectrum disorders are fairly similar in their components, and any variations in the process reflect their target audience. Guidelines drafted by the American Academy of Pediatrics (1) are intended for pediatricians; those by the American Academy of Neurology (2,3), for child neurologists; those by the American Academy of Child and Adolescent Psychiatry (4), for child psychiatrists; and those by the New York State Department of Health (5), for professionals from diverse disciplines as well as for parents. The present chapter will assume some familiarity with such protocols and attempt to provide a rationale for the major steps in this clinical process. Familiarity with the more traditional components of routine pediatric health care provision as well as with child developmental surveillance will also be assumed. The emphasis will be on how the medical practitioner can most effectively contribute.

The American Psychiatric Association's DSM-IVTR (6) and the American Academy of Pediatrics DSM-PC (7) place autism within the category of pervasive developmental disorders (PDD). This category includes five separate conditions:

Autism occurs when the child displays significant impairment in all of three separate areas of functioning: communication, socialization, and repetitive, self-stimulatory, and restrictive behaviors, and these impairments have their onset before the age of 3 years (Table 1).

Table 1 DSM-IVTR/DSM-PC Criteria for Autism

Six of the following 12 items with onset prior to 3 years:

Socialization—at least two of the following four behaviors:
1. Impaired nonverbal interactive behaviors (e.g., eye contact, facial expression)
2. Poor peer relationships
3. No spontaneous sharing (e.g., joint attention)
4. No social reciprocity

Communication—at least one of the following four behaviors:
5. Delayed language (including nonverbal communication): the communication delay may be part of a more generalized delay in developmental competency; since children with autism may have mental retardation, children who present with global cognitive delay should be assessed for the presence of autism.
6. Conversational (pragmatic) difficulties
7. Stereotyped (echolalia) or idiosyncratic use of language
8. Lack of symbolic or social imitative play

Repetitive, stereotypic, restrictive behaviors—at least one of the following four behaviors:
9. Intense or narrowed focus of interest
10. Rigidity with regard to routines or schedules
11. Stereotypic and repetitive mannerisms (e.g., hand flapping or hand regarding)
12. Preoccupation with parts of objects

Children with autism may present with signs and symptoms of developmental delay, developmental coordination disorder, expressive and receptive language delay (5), impulsive/hyperactive or inattentive behaviors, obsessive, compulsive behaviors (9,11,12), sleep disorders, constipation, restrictive diets or extreme sensitivity to food texture/odors (10), self-stimulatory behaviors (11), and social interaction behavior problems (1–4,6,8). Difficulties with social interaction can present as variations (overly sensitive to social interaction such as the slow-to-warm-up child), problems (shy and solitary), and autistic disorders (absence of most basic interactional behaviors such as eye contact).

The numbers in the last paragraph do not refer to footnotes but to the table.
Source: Refs. 6, 7.

Pervasive developmental disorder–not otherwise specified (PDD-NOS) occurs when the child exhibits many of the features of autism but is not severely impaired in all three areas of functioning. Age of onset may be later than 3 years of age. PDD-NOS is sometimes referred to as atypical autism. It is not necessarily accurate to describe it as a milder form of autism since associated developmental problems (such as intellectual deficiency) may render a child with PDD-NOS and severe global cognitive impairment more severely involved than a child with autism but without any intellectual disability. The lower boundary for PDD-NOS remains unclear: how few autistic-like symptoms will qualify for a diagnosis of PDD-NOS?

Asperger's syndrome occurs when the child exhibits typical communication skills development up to 3 years of age but later in life is found to have autistic-like behaviors in addition to significant problems with pragmatic language. (This behavioral pattern can be mimicked by right-brain-deficit learning disabilities.) Outcome research is finding it increasingly difficult to distinguish between Asperger's syndrome and high-functioning autism. The presence/absence of language difficulties prior to age 3 years seems to have little impact on prognosis in high-functioning autism.

Rett's syndrome occurs only in girls who exhibit a dramatic regression in language, motor, and social skills before the age of 2 years. This regression is fairly permanent and accompanied by an acquired microcephaly and two strikingly autistic-like behaviors: hand wringing and severe gaze aversion. Since Rett's syndrome has now been identified as a specific genetic defect (an MECP2 mutation), it will probably be removed from the PDD category in the next DSM revision.

Childhood disintegrative disorder (Heller's syndrome) has its typical onset in children between 5 and 10 years of age when they undergo a severe generalized deterioration in cognitive functioning so that they go from normal intellectual functioning to moderate mental retardation. The presence of several autistic-like features does not strongly support the placement of disintegrative disorder within the PDD classification; it is more properly conceptualized as a neurodegenerative disorder that needs a comprehensive neurological assessment rather than educational and behavioral services appropriate to children with autism.

To streamline an approach to this family of neurodevelopmental disorders, (1) the last two conditions (Rett's syndrome and disintegrative disorder) will be removed from the PDD category, (2) Asperger's syndrome will be considered to be the equivalent of high-functioning autism (the person with autism with normal to superior intellectual capabilities and relatively intact language skills), and (3) the distinction between autism and PDD-NOS will be considered essentially irrelevant for the purposes both of diagnostic-biomedical assessment and of educational-behavioral intervention in infants and young children (5). PDD can then be condensed to autism—PDD-NOS—high-functioning autism with this new triad being referred to as autistic spectrum disorders (ASD).

Since early identification is imperative, any discussion of the diagnostic process must focus on 18–36 months of age, or younger. There can be no acceptable approach to late diagnosis. When some variant of ASD presents outside this age window, it should not be difficult for the clinician to extend the following rationale to older age groups and analogous presentations.

II. SCREENING IN THE PRIMARY CARE SETTING

All children who are receiving well-child health care have their developmental progress routinely evaluated at each visit. The physician is less concerned to be intimately familiar with all aspects of a given child's developmental progress than to identify significant developmental delays and neurological diagnoses that warrant biomedical assessment and both general and specific intervention strategies. From this perspective, screening procedures can be situated within a larger framework that rationally delineates their use.

Focusing on which conditions can be diagnosed at specific ages can help further to limit the investment of time needed to screen for different conditions. With the partial effectiveness of early (prior to age 60 months) intensive behavioral intervention strategies in the treatment of ASD (8), the importance of early identification is increasingly recognized. Nevertheless, it is not unusual still to encounter a child with developmental problems in whom the diagnosis of ASD was not considered or confirmed until after the age of 60 months (9). Parents usually become concerned by 18 months of age, but do not present to the primary care provider with these concerns until 6 months later and considerable time lapses between first parental concern and the final definitive diagnosis (10). In the current state of knowledge, failure to diagnose ASD earlier is unacceptable. While researchers pursue the diagnosis of ASD into the age group prior to 18 months (see Chapter 5), the clinician needs to be comfortably familiar with the presentation of ASD between the ages of 18 and 36 months. Most children who will qualify for a diagnosis of ASD will actually develop sufficient signs and symptoms between 18 and 24 months, and the remainder will do so between 24 and 36 months of age. Eager to initiate therapy by 24 months of age, there is concern that the age for diagnosis be lowered to 24 months. The average age of diagnosis in Europe has, indeed, decreased to 30 months from 4 years (11). It has been suggested that DSM criteria be modified for younger children to include social skills deficits, such as decreased use of nonverbal behaviors, lack of social and emotional reciprocity, and lack of seeking to share enjoyment, to account for unreliability of some DSM criteria in children less than 3 years of age (12). However, some children with ASD will simply not be diagnosable until closer to age 36 months, the upper age limit as defined by DSM-IVTR.

Until the development of a screening tool based on the early social signs of autism (see Chapter 5), it is acceptable for a working approach to screening for this group of conditions to rely on the DSM system's characterization of ASD as disorders with significant impairments in communication, socialization, and repetitive, stereotypic behaviors. Since the specific and often striking stereotypies are not pathognomonic, and social interaction is difficult to assess in the pediatric office setting, the screening process can best start with universal prospective surveillance of communication skills in children.

III. SCREENING COMMUNICATION IN INFANTS AND YOUNG CHILDREN

Some degree or type of communication disorder occurs in 20–25% of all children (13). With such a high incidence of problems in communication, routine detailed surveillance of language development in infants and young children can and should be universal. There are many different tools for screening language in children. It is less important which instrument is used than that an instrument be used, be used routinely, and be interpreted consistently in accordance with the specific developmental diagnoses under consideration. Thus although the physician may routinely ask about the child's acquisition of language milestones, if any reported delays are then attributed to willfulness, personality (shy, quiet child), older siblings talking for the child, grandparental spoiling, or even genius ("Einstein didn't talk until he was 5 years old"), then the whole purpose of the screening process will be vitiated. Significant delays need to be taken seriously and considered as markers for potentially treatable developmental problems.

Three early language instruments are appropriate for the pediatric office setting: the MacArthur Communicative Developmental Inventories (CDI, with Infant and Toddler versions), Early Language Milestone Scale—Second Edition (ELMS-2), and the Clinical and Linguistic Milestone Scale (CLAMS). The CLAMS, the language component of the Capute Scales, is an assessment instrument specifically devised for use by the physician in the medical office setting (Table 2). Using such instruments, children with ASD will be found to present around age 24 months with impaired communication according to one of three patterns:

1. *Mute:* The child has no expressive spoken language—no words. Technically, any child at 18 months who has no words should be evaluated further or immediately referred for in-depth assessment of a developmental problem. Some children with ASD will have had several (or more) words at 18 months but will then have regressed and lost them by 24 months of age or later (one component of "autistic regression"). While not diagnostic, such loss of previously acquired expressive language skills is highly suggestive of ASD.

2. *Delayed expressive language milestones:* The child has a less-than-50-word vocabulary and no two-word combinations at 2 years of age. These two milestones are associated or linked; they occur or fail to occur together. If a child has more than 50 words, he will almost certainly be putting two words together; if a child is putting two words together, his vocabulary is almost certainly greater than 50 words. If a parent reports the presence of one of these milestones without the other, there is usually an error in the reporting. Thus the child with a 10-word vocabulary and several two-word phrases will often have

Table 2 Selected CLAMS Milestones

Expressive		Receptive
12 mo	1 word	One-step command with gesture
14 mo	3 words	
	Immature jargoning	
16 mo	4 words	One-step command without gesture
18 mo	6 words	Points to one picture
		Points to one body part
	Vocabulary explosion	
22 mo	2 word phrases	
24 mo	50 words	Points to a half-dozen body parts
	2–3-word sentences	Two-step command
30 mo	Pronouns	Points to a half-dozen pictures

"bye-bye" and "ice cream" as examples of the "two-word phrases." The child with valid two-word phrases and a vocabulary of only 30 or so words will be found actually to have a larger vocabulary when the parent is asked to record all the child's different words as used over a 2-week period.

3. *Typical expressive language milestones:* Occasionally children who might qualify for a diagnosis of ASD will present at around 24 months of age with a greater-than-50-word vocabulary and several two-word phrases. If, however, an additional question is used to supplement the CLAMS language milestones, the artificiality of this attainment can be discovered: "Is any..., how much of your child's spoken language is merely being repeated (echoed, parroted, either immediately or delayed) rather than being spontaneous to the situation and with relatively novel combinations?" If a significant percentage (>20%) of the child's spoken utterances are echolalic, then the child's language achievement needs to be adjusted to whatever part is not just repeated. Expressive language delay will then often be recognized. Although echolalia is often both prominent and prolonged in children with ASD, it is neither diagnostic nor pathognomonic. Many children with other (and much more common) communication disorders along with some children with mental retardation will also exhibit significant echolalia. Along with the expressive language delay, this specific finding merely invites further investigation.

With the identification of expressive language delay, the primary care physician can either refer the child on for more detailed developmental assessment or utilize further screening steps to narrow the range of diagnostic possibilities. Caution should be observed if the child is to be referred to a state early-intervention program. In some state programs there is a reluctance to diagnose ASD, so that children who when assessed are found to exhibit significant delays in communication and socialization as well as stereotypic and repetitive behaviors will have designed for them an intervention program that addresses each and every area of delay and problematic behavior without ever grouping the findings into a specific "diagnosis" of an ASD. The recommended treatment for the specific ASD diagnosis is often much more intense than the proposed intervention strategies for the separate parts that comprise the syndrome.

Even if the child is being referred for more in-depth assessment elsewhere, it is often helpful and productive for the primary care physician to take steps to remain an integral component of the diagnostic and evaluation process that follows. Any differential diagnosis achieved at this stage will be subject to clarification and refinement (but not contradiction) according to more detailed discipline assessments. Further developmental assessment gives the primary care physician "hands on" experience with the strengths and weaknesses of the child that will be the subject of future assessment and intervention, and a baseline from which to measure later progress in response to various interventions.

IV. DIFFERENTIAL DIAGNOSIS OF EXPRESSIVE LANGUAGE DELAY

Children who present with delayed expressive language delay will typically fall into one of the following broad diagnostic categories:

1. Isolated expressive language delay, slow talkers
2. Communication disorder with delays in both expressive and receptive language
3. Global cognitive impairment (intellectual deficiency, mental retardation)
4. Hearing impairment
5. ASD

There are a number of clinical observations by which these conditions might be distinguished in the primary care setting (14). Although such clinical clues might seem to adequately differentiate one condition from another, it is generally accepted that any child who presents with some variant of expressive language delay needs to have a formal audiological assessment and never just a hearing screening.

Isolated expressive language delay is the single most common developmental problem in children. It can be distinguished from all the other items in the above differential diagnosis list by the presence of intact receptive language abilities. The child who is not talking at an age-appropriate level but who understands what is said to him at an age-appropriate level cannot have global communicative or cognitive impairment and is unlikely to have a significant hearing problem. The child who demonstrates age-appropriate receptive language abilities is also very unlikely to have ASD.

The problem in the primary care setting is to effectively assess receptive language skills. Even in a formal speech/language evaluation, receptive language is considered rather difficult to assess adequately in the second year of life. Typically one expects 12-month-old children to begin to follow single-step commands (with accompanying gesture by 12 months and without an accompanying gesture by 16 months of age), and 24-month-old children to respond to two-step commands. Obtaining such cooperation in the pediatric office setting is, however, quite difficult, and even parent history for the child's ability to follow two-step instructions at home is fraught with difficulties. Typically developing 2-year-old children are frequently very much into a negativistic or "no" phase (15) and are rarely very cooperative in routinely doing what they otherwise might be able to do.

Table 2, however, presents several alternative receptive milestones that are more easily elicited either in the office setting or by parental history. Between 12 and 18 months of age, children begin to point to what they want; between 18 and 24 months of age they begin to point in order to identify things. Protodeclarative pointing (pointing to elicit shared interest) also comes in between 18 and 24 months of age. Starting at around 18 months of age most children can point to one or more body parts as well as one or more pictures in a book. By 24 months of age a number of pictures and body parts should be in the child's receptive (with pointing responses) repertoire. These pointing milestones provide a very useful probe for tapping receptive language.

When the child has both expressive and receptive language delays, then global developmental delay (cognitive impairment, intellectual deficiency, mental retardation) and ASD must be specifically ruled in or out.

V. SCREENING FOR AUTISM VERSUS GLOBAL COGNITIVE IMPAIRMENT

The child with delayed expressive but intact receptive language milestones has some version of isolated expressive language disorder. The child with expressive and receptive language delays may have a more severe combined communication disorder, global cognitive impairment such as mental retardation, or ASD.

To differentiate communication disorder from cognitive impairment requires some measure of nonverbal intelligence. The Clinical Adaptive Test (CAT) component of the Capute Scales or formal psychometric testing by a child psychologist [using the Bayley Scales of Infant Development, Second Edition (BSID-II) or the Stanford-Binet Intelligence Scale, Fourth Edition (SB-FE)] might be used for this purpose (16).

Alternatively, clinical observation and history can be used to ascertain the child's major or preferred ways of interacting with toys and other objects in the environment. This preference can be converted to an approximate mental age level (Table 3). The child who is significantly delayed in expressive language, receptive language, and problem-solving abilities probably has global cognitive delay rather than just a communication disorder. However, whether or not the child appears to have global cognitive impairment does not appreciably help to decide the presence or absence of ASD since the latter may occur along with global cognitive delay. In other words, nonverbal-problem-solving abilities will be in the normal range in a significant percentage of children with ASD while a significant percentage of children with ASD will exhibit delayed nonverbal-problem-solving abilities and will also be mentally retarded. (The issue of exactly what these percentages might be is under active discussion.) If global cognitive limitation is present (with or without ASD), then the appropriate biomedical assessment will focus on that neurodevelopmental disorder (17).

Suspected because of the presence of language delay, the diagnosis of ASD will now depend on the additional presence of atypical features of the language delay (such as echolalia and pronominal ["I/me"—"you"] reversal), impairment in socialization (out of proportion to the language or other developmental delays), and stereotypical or repetitive behaviors. Whenever a child is shown to have a severe communication disorder, behavioral screening for ASD should follow. The DSM-IVTR criteria can be used. Various listings of specific behaviors associated with each of the deficit areas can be helpful (Table 4). One of the problems in listing autistic-like behaviors is deciding exactly how to classify a

Table 3 Patterns of Object Interaction

Visual tracking	0–3 months
Reaching/grasping	3–6 months
Mouthing	6–9 months
Banging/noisemaking	9–12 months
Throwing/receptacle play	12–15 months
Stacking blocks	15–18 months
Puzzle/shape fitting	18–21 months
Scribbling with pencil	21–24 months

Table 4 Autism Features

Qualitative impairment in social interaction	Qualitative impairment in communication	Deviant (restrictive, repetitive) behaviors
No/poor eye contact	Language delay	Water play
In own little world	Echolalia, immediate and	Lines up/groups toys
No peer interaction	delayed	Perseverative
No reciprocity or sharing	Equinus gait (toe walking)	Preservation of sameness
Doesn't read faces	Acts as if deaf	Stereotypies
Treats people like	No protodeclarative	Rocking
furniture	pointing ("joint	Spinning/twirling
Laughs for no reason	attention")	Likes fans
	Language regression	Stiff/noncuddly baby
	(18–24 months)	Splinter skills
	Refers to self in third	Inflexible routines/rituals
	person	Tone abnormalities
	Pronominal reversal	Arching
	Good rote memory	Flapping
	Poor pragmatic language	Absence of pretend play
	No communicative intent/	Preoccupation with parts
	lack of frustration over	of objects
	failure to communicate	Insensitivity to pain
		Olfactory
		Hyperactivity (ADHD)

specific behavior. Thus, is poor eye contact a communicative or socialization item? Is toe-walking a communicative or stereotypical behavior?

It is interesting to note that children with ASD exhibit several communicative behaviors that are not typically found in other children with severe communication disorders. These more specific behaviors all seem to relate to a failure in the development of the desire to communicate (communicative intent). Although children with ASD will tantrum when their wants are not met, they rarely get upset when other communicative efforts fail—usually because there are no other communicative efforts. Children with other types of communication disorder and those with hearing impairments frequently grow increasingly frustrated as they approach the age of 24 months because they recognize that others are trying to verbally interact with them and they want to respond—but cannot. This failure of communicative intent characterizes children with ASD and some with severe to profound mental retardation.

There are no physical findings specific to ASD (18). If an equine gait (persistent toe walking) is present, the child should be checked for heel-cord tightness (shortened tendo Achillis). Even with a persistent equinus gait, the heel cords usually reduce past neutral (19). While global cognitive limitation and most other neurodevelopmental disabilities are frequently associated with some degree of microcephaly, ASD is more often found with macrocephaly (20,21).

One screening test for ASD that has been proposed is the CHAT (22). While statistics do not support its general usage, it does highlight several key behaviors that can be used to help diagnose ASD (Table 5). An obvious weakness in the construction of the CHAT is simply that many of the items are not specific to ASD but rather are common to global cognitive impairment or mental retardation. As the percentage of ASD children with mental retardation decreases, so does the utility of the test. The CHAT behaviors more specific to ASD are those that involve pretend play and joint attention (protodeclarative pointing). (For a more detailed discussion of these behaviors see Chapter 5.) The use of these markers can help discriminate ASD from other types of communication disorders. Apart from issues with sensitivity and specificity, the CHAT may be too long for routine use in the primary-care office setting, particularly in the American managed-care setting.

Table 5 Checklist for Autism in Toddlers (CHAT)

Parent questions
  1. Does your child enjoy being swung, bounced on your knee, etc.?
  2. Does your child take an interest in other children?
  3. Does your child like climbing on things such as up stairs?
  4. Does your child enjoy playing peek-a-boo/hide-and-seek?
  5. Does your child ever pretend, e.g., to make a cup of tea using a toy cup and teapot, or pretend other things?
  6. Does your child ever use his/her index finger to point, to ask for something?
  7. Does your child ever use his/her index finger to point, to indicate interest in something?
  8. Can your child play properly with small toys without just mouthing, fiddling, or dropping them?
  9. Does your child ever bring objects over to you to show you something?

Professional observations
  1. Has the child made eye contact with you?
  2. Get the child's attention, then point across the room at an interesting object and say, "Oh look! There's a...!" Watch the child's face. Does the child look across to see what you are pointing at? [and not just at your finger]
  3. Get the child's attention, then give a miniature toy cup/teapot, and say, "Can you make a cup of tea?" Does the child pretend to pour out tea, drink it, etc.?
  4. Say to child, "Where's the light?" or "Show me the light." Does the child point [with his/her index finger] to the light?
  5. Can the child build a tower of bricks? (If yes, of how many bricks?)

VI. FORMAL DIAGNOSTIC EVALUATION

There is no single accepted diagnostic evaluation process for ASD. To answer the question as to what such a battery should contain, the specific goal of the diagnostic evaluation must be clarified. Specialists are often looking to answer questions of little concern to the parents, while parents are often asking questions that the most extensive test batteries do not address. There are four separate questions that a diagnostic assessment might attempt to address:

1. Does this child have ASD or not?
2. If the child has ASD, how severe is the condition?
3. What tests are appropriate to investigate possible etiologies for the ASD?
4. What are the interventions appropriate to this specific child?

1. The response to the first question is a straightforward clinical one. The clinician familiar with the diagnostic criteria for ASD can usually answer it with reasonable certainty after a developmental history and a period of observation and interaction taking something on the order of 1–2 hr. Not infrequently in more classic cases the diagnosis can be strongly entertained after only several minutes of observation. Needless to say, the diagnosis should never be based on such a quick glance but rather such an initial impression needs to be supported by a developmental history that confirms such behaviors to be pervasive across settings and chronic in duration—in other words, that this atypical behavior is actually typical for this child.

A number of formal ASD screening tools exist: Autism Behavior Checklist (ABC), Autism Screening Questionnaire (ASQ), Checklist for Autism in Toddlers (CHAT), Pervasive Developmental Disorder Screening Test (PDDST) Stage 1, Social Communication Questionnaire (SCQ), and Screening Tool for Autism in Two-year-olds (STAT) (Table 6). Since it is usually not practical to screen the general population of young children for autism using a specific autism screening test, it is recommended instead to look for clinical clues (5). The clinical decision tree outlined here does not allow a major role to the routine employment of screening instruments.

Formal diagnostic instruments include: Autism Diagnostic Interview–Revised (ADI-R), Autism Diagnostic Observation Schedule–Generic (ADOS-G), Behavioral Summarized Evaluation (BSE), Childhood Autism Rating Scale (CARS), Diagnostic Instrument for Social and Communicative Disorders (DISCO), Gilliam Autism Rating Scale (GARS), Parent Interview for Autism (PIA), Pervasive Developmental Disorder Screening Test (PDDST) Stages 2 and 3, Pre-Linguistic Autism Diagnostic Observation Schedule (PL-ADOS) (Table 7). The ADI-R and ADOS-G are considered the "gold standard" for such diagnostic instruments and the CARS has the longest history and the widest use. No single

Table 6 Autism Screening Instruments

Autism Behavior Checklist (ABC): Originally intended more for designing educational placement and monitoring progress as part of a broader tool, the Autism Screening Instrument for Educational Planning (ASIEP), rather than for diagnosis, the ABC is sometimes used for screening. 57 dichotomous items are scored across five domains (sensory, relating, body and object use, language, social and self-help). Total scores >67 indicate a high probability of autism, between 53 and 67 are questionable for autism, and <53 make autism unlikely.

Autism Screening Questionnaire (ASQ, formerly Social Communication Questionnaire, SCQ): A brief 40-item dichotomous behavioral questionnaire that addresses reciprocal social interaction, language and communication, and repetitive, stereotypical behaviors. One version is for children under age 6, and another version is for children 6 and older.

Checklist for Autism in Toddlers (CHAT): A screening test for autism in children from 18 to 36 months of age; it contains 9 parent questions and 5 behavioral observation items. Absence of three items is considered critical: protodeclarative pointing, gaze monitoring, and pretend play (administration time: 15 min). MCHAT: A revision of the CHAT with 23 parent questions and no behavioral observation items.

Pervasive Developmental Disorder Screening Test (PDDST) Stage 1: A parent questionnaire for use in the primary care setting; 3 affirmative answers support further diagnostic consideration for autism.

Screening Tool for Autism in Two-Year-Olds (STAT): An interactive play instrument designed for children 24–25 months old. Failure in 2 of 3 areas (play, motor imitation, and nonverbal communication) differentiates autism from other developmental problems (administration time: 20 min).

---

instrument should be used as the sole basis for diagnosing ASD (5). On the one hand, the better formal instruments require extensive training and experience; on the other hand, the instruments are intended for use by practitioners not clinically experienced in the diagnosis of ASD (3).

The confirmation of the clinical diagnosis of ASD by a formal instrument is strongly recommended but will be subject to the reasonable availability of professionals with the requisite training in the administration of such scales. Reasonable availability can also refer to the fact that a diagnostic medical evaluation by a child neurologist, child psychiatrist, or developmental pediatrician may be covered by the family's health insurance, but the performance of an ASD rating scale by a child psychologist or other certified professional is rarely covered. Neither is the requisite training expertise universally available through either early-intervention programs or the public school system.

Table 7 Autism Diagnostic Instruments

Autism Diagnostic Interview–Revised (ADI-R): A comprehensive semistructured parent interview with behavioral items scored on a 0 (none) to 4 (extreme) point Likert scale. Three domains (communication and language, reciprocal social interaction, and restrictive, perseverative, and stereotypical behaviors) have different cutoffs (administration time: 60 min).

Autism Diagnostic Observation Schedule–Generic (ADOS-G): Four modules (for use in persons with different developmental levels: preverbal/single words, phrased speech, fluent speech child-adolescent, fluent speech adolescent-adult) administer structured standardized situations to assess communication, social interaction, and play/imaginative use of objects (30–45 min). The Pre-Linguistic Autism Diagnostic Observation Schedule (PL-ADOS) is derived from the ADOS to be used with nonverbal children under the age of 6 years (administration time: 30–45 min).

Behavioral Summarized Evaluation (BSE): A set of French instruments that includes the 20-item BSE Likert scale, the 29-item BSE-R scale, and the 23-item IBSE (Infant Behavioral Summarized Scale).

Childhood Autism Rating Scale (CARS): In the most widely used autism diagnostic instrument, 15 items are scored on a 7-point Likert scale. It combines parent report with direct observation. Scores <30 make autism unlikely; scores between 30 and 36 suggest mild to moderate autism, and scores >36 suggest moderate to severe autism (administration time: 30 min).

Gilliam Autism Rating Scale (GARS): A behavioral checklist to estimate the severity of autistic symptoms in persons aged 3 years to adult.

Parent Interview for Autism (PIA): A semistructured parent interview with 118 items grouped into 11 domains and scored on a Likert scale from 1 (almost never) to 5 (almost always) to assess autism in preschool children (administration time: 45 min).

Pervasive Developmental Disorder Screening Test (PDDST) Stage 2 and 3: A parent questionnaire in which 4 or more affirmative answers on Stage 2 (Developmental Disorders Clinics version) or 6 or more affirmative answers on Stage 3 (Autism/PDD Clinic version) indicate further diagnostic consideration for autism.

Pre-Linguistic Autism Diagnostic Observation Schedule (PL-ADOS): A version of the Autism Diagnostic Schedule (ADOS) that uses a semistructured assessment of play, interaction, and social communication to diagnose autism in children under 6 years of age. 12 brief play activities are scored on a Likert scale from 0 (no abnormality consistent with autism) to 2 (response consistent with autism) and generate 17 individual and 31 overall ratings (administration time: 30 min).

While the usefulness of formal scales to help confirm a diagnosis of ASD is readily conceded, the ability of such instruments to discriminate ASD from whatever borders on the milder end of the autistic spectrum remains controversial. Such difficulty resembles the quite similar problem that occurs when attempting to discriminate a slow learner from a person with mild mental retardation by the use of an intelligence test score alone. The psychometric properties of the test can be excellent, but is the instrument being used to discover or to create a cutoff? Psychometric instruments are similar to blood tests in that quantitative results are always subject to clinical interpretation. There is no perfect test that will obviate the need for clinical judgment.

2.   The severity of the ASD does not necessarily relate to the incidence or frequency of various autistic-like behaviors but rather to the degree to which these behaviors interfere with more typical functioning. Thus children with many striking autistic behaviors may sometimes be able to be easily drawn out to interact with others. The presence of associated dysfunctions such as cognitive limitation may render a child with milder autistic-like features much more impaired. Scores on formal autism rating scales may be used to quantitate the degree of severity and to provide a baseline for treatment efficacy. Nevertheless, with the exception of the degree of associated mental retardation, degrees of severity of autistic-like symptoms have not been shown to correlate with the long-term responsiveness to intervention. Measuring global cognitive impairment in ASD, however, presents its own set of assessment problems.

A measure of general intellectual level should always be attempted in the assessment of children with ASD. Since it is not unusual to find such children very difficult to engage in the testing situation, the evaluation should be performed by a professional skilled in working with children with ASD. Although many children with ASD will test out in the intellectually deficient range, significant dissociation is often observed. Thus, while the overall IQ may be in the retarded range, there is often a verbal-performance discrepancy such that verbal skills are much more delayed than nonverbal skills. ASD performance on the verbal or communication sections of various intelligence tests is often impaired by limitations in language usage or by deviance in communicative and social interaction. On the other hand, selected verbal items or subtests may be inflated by their rote language or sometimes excellent memory skills.

Most children with ASD will perform much better on the nonverbal sections of intelligence tests or on those items that are defined as more classically right brain (nonlanguage or nondominant hemisphere) dependent. It is therefore not surprising to find that whenever these children exhibit savant skills (isolated isles of superior ability), these are almost always derived from right-brain skill areas such as mathematics, numerical calculation, music, memory, and graphic art. Similarly, when one groups genetic syndromes associated with different learning disability patterns, those syndromes with the strongest association with

ASD are all found within the syndrome group with verbal skills more impaired than nonverbal skills. Therefore, any attempt to measure general intellectual ability in ASD children should always use instruments with a strong nonverbal component such as the Leiter International Performance Scale–Revised (Leiter-R), the Griffiths Mental Development Scale, the Raven's Progressive Coloured Matrices, the Seguin Formboard, and the Clinical Adaptive Test (CAT) of the Capute Scales. The finding of nonverbal-problem-solving superior to verbal abilities (e.g., a CAT score above the CLAMS score) should be considered typical for ASD.

When a child with ASD tests out globally delayed with low scores in both the verbal and nonverbal areas, the problem will be to differentiate an associated mental retardation from difficulties in obtaining the cooperation of a child who is not socially reciprocating. How can one differentiate superior nonverbal skills that equate with overall better nonverbal intelligence from an isolated "splinter skill" or two? Sometimes the examiner can note test behaviors that make one of these two interpretations more probable, but it will often take time for the picture to sort itself out. The difficulties in interpreting such data should not dissuade one from obtaining such baseline information. Sometimes the use of the Vineland Adaptive Behavior Scales can help in this differential diagnosis by providing developmental age levels for several other functional areas. Modifications in the use of the Vineland with ASD persons have been published, and this population will be specifically addressed in the next revision of the instrument. Rating scales for repetitive, obsessive compulsive, stereotypic, and tic behaviors (23) are less diagnostic than treatment oriented by providing baseline measures for targeted behaviors.

3.   The pediatric medical evaluation for ASD should review and explore all those prenatal, perinatal, and postnatal factors associated with the entire spectrum of neurodevelopmental disabilities.

Since the incidence of seizures is increased in children with ASD (and tends to increase further with age), *electroencephalography* needs to be considered in the diagnostic medical assessment. Children with obvious or suspicious seizure episodes should receive an electroencephalogram (EEG). This recommendation does not support the routine use of the EEG.

Concern remains that even in the absence of overt seizure activity, epileptiform discharges might represent a deleterious influence on certain brain areas. The classic example of such an association is the *Landau-Kleffner syndrome* (or acquired epileptic aphasia) (24). In this syndrome, children develop a seizure focus directly over the language areas of the brain and lose previously acquired speech (they develop aphasia). Most cases of Landau-Kleffner syndrome occur later than the upper age limit for the onset of ASD (3 years), and most have obvious clinical seizures. There are, however, some cases of Landau-Kleffner syndrome with only electric discharges and no clinical seizure activity. A key distinction between the regression that typically occurs in ASD and the regression that occurs in acquired epileptic aphasia relates to the accompanying impairment of social interaction and relatedness. In children who are developing some form of ASD, the language loss is contemporaneous with the onset of social withdrawal. In children with an acquired epileptic aphasia, the emotional withdrawal will occur only after the language impairment has had time to exert a secondary impact on socialization. In this latter case, the effect and its time course are similar to the socialization difficulties that occur with significant hearing impairment.

No consistent *neuroimaging* findings are associated with ASD. The criteria for obtaining an MRI or CT scan should be the same as with children without ASD: abnormalities of the head (other than mild macrocephaly), facial dysmorphology (e.g., midface hypoplasia), positive or localizing findings on neurological examination, or significant global developmental delay (mental retardation) (17,25). The last reflects the importance of attempting an assessment of general intelligence in ASD. Otherwise neuroimaging cannot be considered routine in ASD.

ASD has been associated with a number of genetic syndromes (Table 8). Often such syndromes will have been identified prior to the development and diagnosis of the ASD. For a long time ASD was thought to be relatively uncommon in children with Down syndrome (trisomy 21). Recent research supports an incidence of ASD in Down syndrome on the order of magnitude of 10% (26,27).

Sometimes the diagnosis of ASD will lead the clinician to search more closely for a genetic etiology (Table 9). The most common genetic disorder associated with autism is *fragile X syndrome*. In fact it would be more correct to say that fragile X syndrome is strongly associated with the presence of autistic-like features and less so with ASD. And more importantly, the primary developmental association of fragile X syndrome is with mental retardation and not with ASD. A child who qualifies for a diagnosis of ASD but who is not mentally retarded rarely needs to be screened for fragile X syndrome. Using a checklist in which each of six items (mental retardation, family history of mental retardation, ADHD, large ears, elongated face, autistic-like behaviors) is scored 0 (absent), 1 (borderline), or 2 (present), scores of 5 or more will identify all cases of fragile X syndrome (28,29).

The accumulation of various trace elements and *heavy metals* in the body has been claimed to be associated with ASD, and attempts have been made sometimes to measure their levels in hair, blood, and urine for the purpose of recommending chelation therapy. With the exception of lead, there is no scientific support for either the validity of these measures, their association with ASD, or any responsiveness to the proposed therapy.

Lead poisoning (plumbism) is a disorder most commonly found in children who engage in pica in settings where interior lead-based paint is flaking from the walls or ceiling. Children with ASD often engage in pica and are therefore at

Table 8   Genetic Syndromes Associated with Autism

Angelman
Bardet-Biedl
Coffin-Siris
Cornelia de Lange*
Down*
Duchenne muscular dystrophy*
Fragile X*
Gilles de la Tourette
Goldenhar
Hurler
Hypomelanosis of Ito
Joubert
Laurence-Moon-Biedl
Lugan-Fryns (X-linked mental
    retardation with marfinoid habitus)
Möbius
Myotonic dystrophy
Neurofibromatosis I*
Noonan
Oculocutaneous albinism
Phenylketonuria*
Prader-Willi
Rett*
Rubella, congenital
Sanfillippo
Smith-Magenis
Tuberous sclerosis*
Velocardiofacial syndrome*
Williams
XYY

These syndromes have all had several case reports of their occurrence with autism; those with an asterisk (*) have had data to support more than an incidental association with autism. Syndromes with a strong association with ASD are detailed in Table 9. Sites on more than half a dozen genes have been reported to have some association with autism.

greater risk of developing lead poisoning. Generally the relationship with lead is considered to be secondary rather than causative, but the possibility remains that some cases of ASD might be caused or (more likely) exacerbated by toxic levels of lead (30). Lead screening should be entertained in any medical assessment for ASD in children with pica and possible exposure to lead-based paint. In addition, such lead screening may need to be periodically repeated in ASD children with persistent pica.

Table 9 Genetic Syndromes Strongly Associated with Autism

Cornelia de Lange syndrome: A syndrome of severe mental retardation, hirsutism, microcephaly, prenatal-onset short stature, micromelia, thin downturning upper lip, small nose with anteverted nostrils. The hirsutism is especially prominent in the synophrys (bushy eyebrows that tend to meet in the middle).

Down syndrome (trisomy 21): A chromosomal disorder with mental retardation, hypotonia, short stature, flat facial profile, microcephaly, epicanthal folds, upslanting palpebral fissures, small ears, simian creases, and cardiac and duodenal defects.

Duchenne muscular dystrophy: An X-linked muscular disorder that typically presents with motor loss progressing from around 4 years of age until death by respiratory compromise.

Fragile X syndrome: A form of X-linked mental retardation caused by an increased number of trinucleotide repeats at the fragile site on the X chromosome. It includes mild to profound mental retardation, macrocephaly, large, prominent ears, prognathism, and (postpubertal) large testes. The typical behavioral pattern comprises hyperactivity, poor eye contact, and autistic-like features.

Neurofibromatosis I: An autosomal dominant (chromosome 17) neurocutaneous syndrome with café au lait spots, axillary freckling, neurofibromata (tumors of the skin, brain, optic and auditory nerves), with mental retardation in only 10% of cases.

Phenylketonuria (PKU): An autosomal recessive inborn error of metabolism resulting in elevated blood phenylalanine levels. Untreated PKU causes microcephaly, mental retardation, seizures, and atypical behaviors.

Tuberous sclerosis: A hereditary neurocutaneous syndrome with mental retardation, a facial rash, and seizures.

Velocardiofacial syndrome: Shprintzen syndrome, or 22q deletion syndrome, is comprised of cleft palate and structural heart defects, and associated with learning disabilities, psychiatric disturbances, and mild mental retardation.

A wide variety of *immunoglobulin* abnormalities have been reported in ASD. The patterns have been inconsistent and unrelated to any clinical symptoms of either the ASD or any diagnosable immunological disorder.

There have been inconsistent reports of an increased rate of *gastroenterological symptoms* in children with ASD. These symptoms include diarrhea, constipation, and stomach cramps. While such symptoms should be inquired after, no routine gastroenterological work-up is indicated. Many children with ASD are placed on dairy-free or gluten-free diets on the basis of a supposed association between ASD and some variant of a gastroenterological disorder such as celiac disease. Recent reports of an association between various neurological and neurodevelopmental disorders in children with celiac disease (31,32) have supported the possibility of an atypical central nervous system response to gluten. The presence of diarrhea or constipation in a child with ASD who also has growth parameters (height and weight) below the tenth percentile for age would represent a reasonable indication to test for celiac disease. Serological screening should include total IgA, antigliadin IgA, tissue transglutaminase, and antiendomyseal IgA. In the presence of ASD one's index of suspicion for celiac disease should be heightened, and the criteria for further investigation loosened. A diagnosis of celiac disease and the prolonged commitment to the use of a gluten-free diet should not, however, be undertaken without confirmation of the diagnosis by an intestinal biopsy.

Biochemical studies of serum and urine amino acids and organic acids as well as other *metabolic* and *endocrine tests* should be considered in the presence of relevant family history, atypical growth pattern, specific physical findings, fluctuating symptoms of lethargy, episodic vomiting, or severe global cognitive delay. In other words, the indication for such studies is similar to their indication in the medical assessment of mental retardation (17).

4. There is no definite listing of disciplines that need to be involved in the diagnostic and evaluation process for a child with suspected autism. A number of different professionals from a variety of disciplines may be appropriate to help in assessing the strengths and weaknesses of any given child. Which would be appropriate for this child may depend on the specific behavioral pattern and problems presented by the child as well as the expertise and experience of the various professionals with children with ASD. There should be no routine assessment process but rather the process should be tailored to the needs of each individual child and family. Assessments and tests should be performed to answer specific questions of diagnosis, differential diagnosis, and treatment planning, and to obtain baselines for follow-up measures used to monitor progress. Parents should be informed whenever more extended testing is being administered predominantly to complete research databases.

A medical assessment by a specialist (child neurologist, child psychiatrist, developmental or behavioral pediatrician) should be performed and can help decide whether any further medical assessments (such as genetics) are warranted. A child psychologist with experience with ASD should confirm the diagnosis with a formal autism rating scale, attempt a measure of general intelligence, and perhaps review problem behaviors and possible interventions.

Speech language assessments can provide detailed levels for communicative abilities, verbal, nonverbal, and pragmatic language. These levels of functioning can be used to plan intervention strategies and to serve as baselines for measuring treatment progress.

In those children with ASD who also exhibit problems with sensory processing, an assessment of sensory-integration dysfunction may be indicated.

Feeding selectivity and tactile aversion are specific behaviors for which desensitization procedures may be helpful.

VII. CASE EXAMPLE

At his 18-month well-child checkup a boy has a vocabulary of six words, is following one-step commands, and is beginning to point to body parts; additionally mother has no concerns about the child's social relatedness. At his 2-year visit mother reports that in the interval he has lost all his vocabulary and has withdrawn socially so that he is no longer making eye contact or even seeming to want to communicate. He no longer responds to his name or to commands and often appears deaf. She also notes, however, that his interest and skill in solving puzzles have increased significantly. The pediatrician asks about several other autistic behaviors (including perseverative and reciprocal social interaction items), strongly suspects autism, and refers the child to a local child psychiatrist with expertise in ASD and to the state's early-intervention (EI) program. Using DSM-IVTR criteria, the child psychiatrist clinically confirms a diagnosis of autism and refers the child to a geneticist for a medical investigation. The EI program team assessment includes formal audiological testing (hearing intact), a speech language assessment (expressive and receptive language delays and communicative deviance), and psychological testing (Bayley Scales of Infant Development–II, Childhood Autism Rating Scale, and Vineland Adaptive Behavior Scales). A diagnosis of mild developmental delay with moderate autism is confirmed, and the child is placed in an ABA program with the intensity scheduled to increase over the next year. The geneticist screens the child for fragile X (negative) but does not consider further biomedical tests warranted. The EI case manager links the family to a parent support group and maintains close contact with them through the initial stages of adjustment to the diagnosis and treatment.

VIII. CONCLUSION

Because of the many uncertainties that cloud the field of autism, there is a tendency to rush to conclude that the latest research finding, instrument, test, suspected cause, or even risk factor is the final key to having it all make sense. The vast amount of clinical data that needs to be restructured by new interpretations cannot yet be jettisoned by an oversimplification of the complex phenomena that can present as ASD.

Despite the wide prevalence of out-of-home caregiving settings for infants and young children (e.g., nursery, day care, preschool), the primary-health-care provider remains the mainstay for early diagnosis of ASD. Given the importance of early diagnosis for early intervention, the primary-care physician should specifically rule out ASD at the 18–36-month checkups. Expressive language screening accompanied by several probes into social reciprocity can effectively rule out most cases of ASD and alternately identify those children who need to be referred for more in-depth assessment. It would also be appropriate for the primary care physician to raise the possibility of autism with those patients otherwise identified with various communication disorders or other patterns of nonspecific developmental delay since it is not unusual for children with ASD to be identified with neurodevelopmental problems but incorrectly categorized.

Although ASD is a serious neurodevelopmental disorder, the only formal assessment that is routinely indicated in every case is a careful and comprehensive audiological assessment. Every other possible medical test and procedure needs some other specific indication. ASD by itself is not sufficient to justify an expensive battery of biomedical and behavioral tests. When accompanied by significant global developmental delay (mental retardation), ASD becomes open to a much larger range of biomedical considerations. Measured clinical judgment needs to collaborate with informed parents to select the best approach to a comprehensive diagnosis.

REFERENCES

1. American Academy of Pediatrics, Committee on Children with Disabilities. The pediatrician's role in the diagnosis and management of autistic spectrum disorder in children (RE060018). Pediatrics 2001; 107:1221–1226.
2. Filipek PA, Accardo PJ, Baranek GT, Cook EH Jr, Dawson G, Gordon B, Gravel JS, Johnson CP, Kallen RJ, Levy SE, Minshew NJ, Prizant BM, Rapin I, Rogers SJ, Stone WL, Teplin S, Tuchman RF, Volkmar FR. The screening and diagnosis of autistic spectrum disorders. J Autism Dev Disord 1999; 29:437–482.
3. Filipek PA, Accardo PJ, Ashwal S, Baranek GT, Cook EH Jr, Dawson G, Gordon B, Gravel JS, Johnson CP, Kallen RJ, Levy SE, Minshew NJ, Ozonoff S, Prizant BM, Rapin I, Rogers SJ, Stone WL, Teplin S, Tuchman RF, Volkmar FR. Practice parameter: screening and diagnosis of autism: report of the Quality Standards Subcommittee of the American Academy of Neurology and the Child Neurology Society. Neurology 2000; 55:468–479.
4. Volkmar F, Cook EH Jr, Pomeroy J, Realmunto G, Tanguay P. Practice parameters for the assessment and treatment of children, adolescents, and adults with autism and other pervasive developmental disorders. J Am Acad Child Adolesc Psychiatry 1999; 38:32S–54S.
5. Clinical Practice Guideline: Autism/Pervasive Developmental Disorders: Assessment and Intervention for Young Children (Age 0–3 Years): The Guideline Technical Report. Albany: New York State Department of Health Early Intervention Program, 1999.

6. American Psychiatric Association. Diagnostic and Statistical Manual of Mental Disorders. 4th edition, text revision; DSM-IVTR. Washington, DC: American Psychiatric Association, 2000.
7. American Academy of Pediatrics. The Classification of Child and Adolescent Mental Diagnoses in Primary Care: Diagnostic and Statistical Manual for Primary Care (DSM-PC), Child and Adolescent Version. Elk Grove, IL: American Academy of Pediatrics, 1996.
8. Lovaas OI. Experimental design and cumulative research in early behavioral intervention. In: Accardo PJ, Magnusen C, Capute AJ, eds. Autism: Clinical and Research Issues. Timonium, MD: York Press, 2000:133–161.
9. Stone WL, Hoffman EL, Lewis SE, Ousley OY. Early recognition of autism: parental reports vs clinical observation. Arch Pediatr Adolesc Med 1994; 148:174–179.
10. Howlin P, Asgharian A. The diagnosis of autism and Asperger syndrome: findings from a survey of 770 families. Dev Med Child Neurol 1999; 41:834–839.
11. Fombonne E. The epidemiology of autism: a review. Psychol Med 1999; 29:769–786.
12. Stone WL, Lee EB, Ashford L, Brissie J, Hepburn SL, Coonrod EE, Weiss BH. Can autism be diagnosed accurately in children under 3 years? J Child Psychol Psychiatry 1999; 40:219–226.
13. Clinical Practice Guideline: Communication Disorders: Assessment and Intervention for Young Children (Age 0–3 Years): The Guideline Technical Report. Albany: New York State Department of Health Early Intervention Program, 1999.
14. Accardo PJ. The child who does not talk: a pediatric overview. In: Accardo PJ, Rogers BT, Capute AJ, eds. Disorders of Language Development. Baltimore: York Press, 2002:113–124.
15. Spitz RA. No and Yes: On the Genesis of Human Communication. New York: International Universities Press, 1957.
16. Accardo PJ. Diagnostic issues in autism. In: Accardo PJ, Magnusen C, Capute AJ, eds. Autism: Clinical and Research Issues. Timonium, MD: York Press, 2000:103–131.
17. Battaglia A, Carey JC. Diagnostic evaluation of developmental delay/mental retardation: an overview. Am J Med Genet 2003; 117C:3–14.
18. Gilberg C, Coleman M. The Biology of the Autistic Syndromes. Clinics in Developmental Medicine Number 126. London: MacKeith Press, 1992.
19. Accardo PJ, Whitman BY. Toe walking: a marker for language disorders in the developmentally disabled. Clin Pediatr 1989; 28:347–350.
20. Fidler DJ, Bailey JN, Smalley SL. Macrocephaly in autism and other pervasive developmental disorders. Dev Med Child Neurol 2000; 42:737–740.
21. Gilberg C, deSouza L. Head circumference in autism, Asperger syndrome, and ADHD: a comparative study. Dev Med Child Neurol 2002; 44:296–300.
22. Baron-Cohen S, Allen J, Gillberg J. Can autism be detected at 18 months? The needle, the haystack, and the CHAT. Br J Psychiatry 1992; 161:839–843.
23. Lewis MH, Bodfish JW. Repetitive behavior disorders in autism. Ment Retard Dev Disabil Res Rev 1998; 4:80–89.
24. Mantovani J. Autistic regression and Landau-Kleffner syndrome: progress or confusion? Dev Med Child Neurol 2000; 42:349–353.

25. Filipek PA. Neuroimaging in the developmental disorders: the state of the art. J Child Psychol Psychiatry 1999; 40:113–128.

26. Kent L, Evans J, Paul M, Sharp M. Comorbidity of autistic spectrum disorders in children with Down syndrome. Dev Med Child Neurol 1999; 41:153–158.

27. Rasmussen P, Borjesson O, Wentz E, Gillberg C. Autistic disorders in down syndrome: background factors and clinical correlates. Dev Med Child Neurol 2001: 43:750–754.

28. Giangreco CA, Steele MW, Aston CE, Cummings JH, Wenger SL. A simplified six-item checklist for screening for fragile X syndrome in the pediatric population. J Pediatr 1966; 129:611–614.

29. Accardo PJ, Shapiro LR. FRAXA and FRAXE: when to test or not to test. J Pediatr 1998; 132:762–764.

30. Accardo PJ, Whitman BY, Caul J, Rolfe U. Autism and plumbism: a possible etiological contribution. Clin Pediatr 1988; 27:41–44.

31. Bostwick HE, Berezin SH, Halata MS, Jacobson R. Celiac disease presenting with microcephaly. J Pediatr 2001; 138:589–592.

32. Gordon N. Cerebellar ataxia and gluten sensitivity: a rare but possible cause of ataxia, even in childhood. Dev Med Child Neurol 2000; 42:283–286.

7

Informing, Educating, and Supporting the Family

Alfred L. Scherzer
Joan and Sanford I. Weill Medical College, Cornell University, New York, New York, U.S.A.

I. THE FAMILY AS THE FOCUS OF TREATMENT

While the family plays an important role in the subsequent development of all children with developmental disabilities, it has a unique and multifaceted position when the child has autism. The interactive relationship involving communication and behavior between the family and child is fundamental and unique in the autistic spectrum disorders (ASD). It serves both as a basis for alerting the family that something is awry, and an opportunity for involvement in treatment and management. That a special kind of relationship exists between the family and the child with ASD is apparent in the literature. Comparison with family references to other major developmental disabilities from the National Library of Medicine (PubMed) indicates that only mental retardation approaches the frequency of ASD entries (Table 1).

The special relationship between a child with ASD and his or her family has led to the widespread practice of direct parental involvement in the treatment and management of ASD. The family is specifically an integral part of all the currently described model treatment programs for children with autistic spectrum disorder (1,2).

The unique interactive parent involvement in the subsequent development of the child with ASD can greatly influence outcome. For example, there is a relation between the development of communication skills of the child and parents' ability to synchronize interaction with the child's attention and activity (3). At the same time, the greater severity of the child with autism may have considerable impact on

149

Table 1 References to Family and Disability in PubMed

Developmental disability	Frequency of citations
Autism	6928
Mental retardation	5270
Learning disabilities	1186
Down syndrome	1185
ADHD	1174
Cerebral palsy	515
Spina bifida	443

parental stress (4). In turn, this can be related to less social responsiveness as the child develops. On the other hand, more mutual play and positive feedback by the parent is seen with more highly communicative children who have ASD (5).

The parents, therefore, are in a pivotal position with respect to the child with autism. They are involved early because of the fundamental deviations in behavior and communication, and have a role in identification by bringing their concerns to the primary care provider. They have a major team role in the very nature of the therapy and treatment processes that have evolved. At the same time, it is clear that their interaction with the child in itself may significantly influence the treatment process and ultimate development. Finally, parental coping ability, stress, and mental health are all intimately intertwined in the process.

II. COMMUNICATING THE DIAGNOSIS

Regardless of whether a family has preexisting concerns about their child's development, how they are told about the diagnosis will have profound effects on their emotional adjustment, interaction with the child, and subsequent relationships with professionals (6). Estimates of satisfaction with the informing process by parents of children with developmental disabilities vary greatly (7–10). Many factors have been identified that influence its effectiveness, including: medical versus educational setting (11); availability of both parents or caregivers (12); giving appropriate attention to cultural considerations (13); language and technical terms used and amount of information given (9); provision of a written report for later reference (14,15); as well as the tone and empathy of the physician (16,17).

Communicating the diagnosis is an active, highly charged process (18). Either through direct discussion or more subtle body language, there is often a seesaw effect in discussions. Professionals generally use labels rather than emphasizing function, whereas the parent wants to know how the child will be able to perform now and in the future. The process can be a kind of unstated active negotiation about pessimism versus optimism, on either side, out of which evolves a jointly constructed diagnosis. Though the physician or other professional controls the interaction, there is great need to allow parents to freely express feelings, doubts, and concerns during this informing process and at any subsequent meetings (16). Parental dissatisfaction with how the diagnosis is disclosed is not inevitable (19–21). Success requires appropriate understanding, sensitivity, and technical skill on the part of the physician (9).

Training in "breaking the news" needs to be given much more emphasis in the medical curriculum, and is increasingly essential in continuing medical education programs (CME) (7,8). Targeted communication training programs can be effective in changing physician attitudes (22,23).

In general, the broad steps to guide planning for a successful informing experience include the following:

1. Planning the setting
2. Assessing the family's background knowledge and experience
3. Individualizing the strategy of informing
4. Evaluating the family's understanding

From a consensus of several studies, Table 2 summarizes specific guidelines to follow in developing optimum conditions to achieve an effective parent/professional communication process for discussing the child's diagnosis.

Table 2 Guidelines for Communicating the Diagnosis

1. Arrange for a *private setting* to ensure confidentiality and reduce distraction;
2. Include *both parents* or caregivers together;
3. Have a *colleague* present if possible;
4. *Individualize* the information given, specifically related to the particular child;
5. Use simple, *direct language*;
6. Be open and *sympathetic*;
7. *Avoid* medical jargon;
8. *Be sensitive* to cross-cultural, and language considerations;
9. Discuss both *strengths and weaknesses* of the child;
10. Provide *professional empathy* and support;
11. *Share* one's own anxiety in the situation;
12. *Allow time* for questions;
13. Provide a *written report* for later parental reference;
14. Arrange for *follow-up* sessions for ongoing parental questions or concerns.

Of course, these guidelines should also provide the basis for all subsequent communication with parents, and can help to develop the kind of rapport necessary for long-term care. Remember that initial disclosure represents but the first of many opportunities for communicating with parents. Subsequent contacts will need to keep in mind the strategies outlined above, particularly when further clinical contacts with the child may result in revisions in prognosis concerning degree of involvement, functional capability, the presence of comorbidity, or even the diagnosis itself.

III. FAMILY STRESS AND COPING

Once the diagnosis of autism is confirmed, irrespective of the effectiveness of initial communication, there is bound to be initial stress in the family, and some degree of mourning for the loss of a normal child that was anticipated (24). Guilt and blame are common feelings, especially in the mother (25), and often a source of later poor adaptation (26). Other factors that may affect initial stress include race and ethnicity, as well as lower socio-economic status (27).

Family stress can be expected to continue in every subsequent stage of the child's development. Data suggest that stress is significantly greater in families of children with any type of developmental disability compared to normal (26,28), but is more frequent in autism than in mental retardation (29), Down syndrome (30,31), or cystic fibrosis (32).

Factors influencing ongoing family stress include severity, especially of communication problems, and changes or limitations that become apparent as the child ages (33). However, the availability of resources and support in managing the child, and positive personality beliefs of the parent, seem to be more predictive of positive adaptation than severity alone (34,35).

Greater stress is found in mothers than fathers (36), and is related to more responsibilities in management, and perceived position of dependency (37). Moreover, preexisting psychopathology is seen more frequently in the mother and may be an important factor in adjustment (38).

Siblings may be equally affected. More stress is suggested in the ASD group compared to children with mental retardation or the nondisabled. Siblings with autism were seen as a burden; there were more peer problems, concerns about the future, and feelings of loneliness (39). However, sibling adjustment appears to be strongly influenced by degree of understanding of the disorder (40).

It should also be noted that *preexisting* stress and psychopathology might be seen in some parents of children with ASD. However, it is essential to emphasize that there is no evidence to indicate that parental mental health is causally related to autism, or that the parent is responsible for the autistic condition of the child. (For discussion see Section IV, "Mental Health Issues.")

The wide range of strategies used by parents for coping with the child and dealing with stress includes: authoritarian versus permissive discipline (31), variable sharing of responsibility with spouse and siblings (41), partnering with the professional team (42), and even becoming a community advocate (43).

Heightened anxiety relating to unanticipated or delayed changes as the child develops can also greatly affect both parents and professionals as the child develops (6). Open exchange on each side is needed when this occurs. The clinician must be sensitive to the tensions that appear and encourage expression of concerns by the parent, yet be able to share his own feelings of uncertainty and anxiety. Where there is need for emotional assistance or treatment of existing psychopathology, counseling or psychiatric intervention should be strongly recommended.

Periodic respite care also provides an important alternative to ease the constant demands of daily management, and can greatly relieve the stress to which many families are often subjected (44).

IV. MENTAL HEALTH ISSUES

To begin with, the stress of adjusting to life with a child who has autism, and coping with long-term care and management, may be associated with significant psychopathology in some families (38). Compared to normal populations and those with Down syndrome, mothers of children with autism show depression (36%), anxiety (46%), or both (9%) (25). Established maternal coping styles, attitudes, and philosophy are found to be important determinants in later adjustment (26).

On the other hand, fathers are said to show relatively good adaptation, comparable to those raising children with Down syndrome, but are frequently under significant stress as well (45). Both parents of children with autism are reported to experience significantly lower marital intimacy, associated with greater stress and depression, than those with Down syndrome, or normal children (46).

Siblings, likewise, are at greater risk for emotional and behavioral problems (47). In addition, *preexisting* personality abnormality and even psychopathology is reported in some parents and families of children with autism (48–50). Parents have been noted to be more aloof, untactful, and less responsive than those with children who have Down syndrome (51). Fathers are considered to have more schizoid and intellectual traits (52,53). Compared to a normal population, mothers of children with autism showed a greater degree of family problems during the pregnancy (54). Lifetime prevalence rates for anxiety disorder and major depressive disorder were likewise found to be greater in the group whose children have autism (55).

These findings are reported in an effort to alert and sensitize professionals to potential family mental health issues, rather than in any way to suggest an etiological relation to autism. In fact, it is concluded in studies reported that there is no evidence of an association between preexisting family mental health and autism (49). Indeed, parents must be constantly reassured that neither their own prior or current mental health is *the cause* for the condition of their child. This must be emphasized wherever professionals come into contact with the family.

With these mental health concerns in mind, it is essential that the professional be sensitive to and identify early any emotional problems and psychiatric disorders in parents and siblings of children with autism, and help provide the necessary timely intervention. Management of the child with autism requires addressing the needs of the family as a whole, and not simply targeting the affected child.

Emotional needs should be brought to the attention of the family at any point in the course of professional contact. In early-intervention programs for children up to age 3, for example, the staff can help the family build an awareness of the need for emotional support in the course of developing the individual family service plan (IFSP). At whatever point providers identify emotional issues, the family should be informed tactfully so that parents do not feel responsible for the condition of their child, and are enabled to recognize the need for assistance. All professionals who deal with children who have autism should be involved with *the entire family*. If they suspect significant stress, adjustment and coping problems, or overt psychopathology, they must take the responsibility for timely referral of the family for counseling, networking, support groups, or direct psychiatric care. Follow-up is equally essential to determine ongoing needs and assure adequate provision of appropriate services.

V. PARENTAL EDUCATION AND TRAINING

Children with ASD have fundamental needs in the areas of communication, socialization, and behavior that set them apart from those with other developmental disabilities. The home is obviously the primary setting in which development and change in these areas is routinely influenced on a daily basis by parents, siblings, and other caregivers. In addition, the home environment is essential for follow-through and transfer of the communication skills training, social maturation activities, and behavior change treatment programs in which the child is participating. Recognition of the important place of the home and the parental role led to a strong partnering relationship with professionals in the early design of treatment programs (56). Today, all of the existing and most frequently used educational and behavioral treatment programs offer training to parents either in direct involvement or in follow-up at home, including a major role in management (57). Available information concerning training methods of parents showed that skills were obtained equally through the use of professionals or peers (58). Studies involving training of parents to participate in treatment programs for their children indicate a favorable attitude to involvement, but many expressed difficulty with the responsibilities required (59).

Data have generally confirmed positive effects of parent involvement in school/education programs conducted outside the home (60–64). Participation of parents in the treatment process itself has also shown reduction in stress (63), and more positive parent-child interaction (65).

Specific benefits from a totally home-based program provided by parents with outside professional assistance appear to be mixed. On the one hand, higher posttreatment IQ scores are reported using ABA methodology at home compared to those receiving conventional school-based interventions (66). In contrast, the results obtained when families used methods from various consultants were not comparable to professionally directed programs (67). Significant gaps exist in the available data, with the need for better documentation of family interaction, use of training materials, change in attitudes and practice, and research design using control groups (68). Effectiveness of primary parent leadership in a home-based program clearly needs further and more uniform evaluation (69).

VI. INFLUENCE OF THE MEDIA

The universal availability of information (and misinformation) has powerful effects on conceptualization of the entire field of autism, its etiology, pathogenesis, management, and treatment (70). Much of the information can be completely accurate and helpful. However, a barrage of stories and theories often surround both the lay public and professionals with quasi-scientific breakthroughs that may confuse, misinform, and misdirect. The print media frequently give daily access to sensationalist articles and case histories without objective review. The Internet places at the fingertips a vast amount of information that is but a click away (71). This swirling amount of data and ideas has a profound effect on how families deal with professionals, and with interrelationships among professionals themselves. Add to this the impact of "secondhand" information, advice, and recommendations gleaned from the media by relatives and friends, which is imparted to families with the best of intentions.

The public information that is constantly being accessed may have an adverse effect on families that can influence acceptance of the diagnosis, increase stress, reduce coping ability, and possibly heighten the presence of anxiety and depression. Witness the media flurry concerning secretin as a treatment alternative (72), or the continuing controversy about immunizations (73–75).

Conflicting views expressed with scientific certainty and conveyed by articles in the press on these topics, for example, present continuous challenges to the clinician both to keep up with relevant scientific data and to maintain sensitivity to the background of information to which parents are exposed. At every level of professional contact, it is essential to enquire directly about parental information and attitudes in an open and candid manner. This approach can set the stage for a mutual interchange of ideas and help separate out the factual from the hearsay. It is this kind of interaction that is especially relevant in the field of autism, where etiology, pathogenesis, and treatment are in an active evolving stage, and where there is no cure for this lifelong chronic condition. Without such an approach, the rapidly increasing flight to poorly established, or even harmful, alternative medical protocols will continue (76).

A special case exists with the media influence on coprofessionals. There is a wide and varying range of understanding and acceptance among physicians, educators, and therapists concerning the field of developmental disabilities in general, and autism in particular. Many pediatricians, for example, have limited interest or background and may respond subjectively to media prejudice or misinformation. How they deal with parents who turn to them for guidance about what they have been told by specialists in the field may greatly affect all of the issues of accepting the diagnosis, family stress, coping ability, and mental health. The clinician in this field needs to reach out to coprofessionals at all levels of contact to engage in dialogue about information in the media, to answer concerns on the basis of current knowledge, and to allay prejudicial ideas that may not have a basis in established fact. It is an important educational task that falls to those of us dealing with this condition in its present state of rapid change.

VII. THE ATTRACTION OF ALTERNATIVE TREATMENTS

Discussion elsewhere (see Chapter 12) reviews the major issue of complementary/alternative medicine (CAM). The use of CAM has been increasing in the United States over the past 50 years, and today is said to involve more than one-third of the population (77). A burgeoning number of websites now provide extensive information on CAM, and are easily accessible (78). The use of CAM is common and significant among pediatric patients with acute illness seen in primary care practices, and includes herbs/homeopathic medicines, prayer healing, high-dose vitamin therapy, nutritional supplements, folk/home remedies, massage therapy, chiropractic care, biofeedback, self-help groups, relaxation, hypnosis, and acupuncture or acupressure (79–81). It is estimated that up to 50% of families of children with autism are using CAM (82). Among the family factors identified in this practice is maternal age over 31, foreign-born caretakers, religious affiliation, and the use of CAM by parents (79). And more than 50% of pediatricians in practice also reported using CAM (83). The extent to which caretakers inform physicians about their use of CAM is estimated variously (80,84).

While there are many theories concerning the widespread use of CAM in autism, the clinical basis of the (sometimes changing) diagnosis, massive amounts and diverse quality of available information, and influence of well-meaning person-to-person and family contacts are all factors in play. Perhaps most important is inadequate or failed communication between physician and family. In one respect it goes back to the initial diagnostic interview when trust, sharing, and mutual acceptance form the basis for an ongoing relationship. If successful it will help to shield the family effectively from turning to alternatives that either may be of little value or are possibly expensive and even harmful.

Particularly with the child who has autism, there needs to be a medical home setting that provides compassionate, family-centered care. An atmosphere of mutual participation is essential between clinician and family, in which the range of options for care is mutually explored, and a collaborative decision about management is based on informed consent (84). This has been termed "shared decision making and relationship-centered care" (85).

One principle to keep in mind is that the family has the *right* to choose CAM, yet it is the *physician's obligation* to be aware of any untoward effects and to communicate them effectively (86). There may not be complete agreement, but such discussions and how they are handled provide opportunities for developing positive relationships (87).

Another principle is that coincidental use of both traditional medicine and CAM may be acceptable provided the risks and benefits are well understood. The bottom line is not whether one or the other is used exclusively, but rather finding a solution acceptable to the family that is best for the child. The process of arriving at such a plan is the essence of truly good medicine (85).

VIII. THE PARENT AS ADVOCATE

Assuming a major parental role as advocate at many levels flows naturally from the unique involvement and relationship of the family with a child who has autism. This often initially begins with the discussions and negotiations concerning services for the infant under age 2, when the IFSP is formulated (88,89). At that point the parent has the opportunity to express concerns regarding available treatment and support services, and to press for additional or more targeted programs. The process continues into the preschool level with the parent-professional team preparation of the individual education plan (IEP). Opportunities for parental involvement in influencing awareness of the unique needs of their child, and the provision of relevant services, continues throughout the entire subsequent school experience during periodic updating of the IEP. In the course of participating in the school setting, many parents become knowledgeable about their legal rights and are better able to initiate requests for special services or a Section 504 Plan that will better meet their child's needs.

Parents may also become involved when there are concerns about availability and adequacy of medical, social, and mental health services. Either individually or through the efforts of support groups, parents may bring their concerns to government at various levels, help in fund raising, and work toward changing or adopting needed legislation. This can result in stimulating the community to influence legislation, organizing advocacy groups to educate the public, and heighten awareness of the medical profession to the needs of children with autism (90,91).

One area of special concern is the transition from school to employment, and eventual integration into the adult world. For those children who will remain totally dependent, parents will be stimulated to work for residential and day-care services in a group setting where dignified and compassionate management is available at a community level. The more challenging advocacy issue relates to integration into the workplace, changing attitudes of employers, and ensuring fair and equitable employment practices. Mobilization of parents to achieve these goals will take on more immediacy as children with autism increasingly age into the workforce.

The extent to which parents become personally involved in advocacy issues will depend on many variables: education, socioeconomic status, gender, religion, perceived local needs, and mental health status. Fostering a partnership with professionals as a team member in caring for the child with autism will greatly assist in developing a more realistic and productive advocacy role. Much-needed research is essential to better understand parental involvement in advocacy, and

Table 3   Potential Opportunities for Parental Advocacy

1.	During the initial disclosure diagnostic interview;
2.	At subsequent contacts with clinicians and other professionals;
3.	At early-intervention individual family service plan (IFSP) conferences;
4.	As a team member at the annual (or more frequent) school individual education plan (IEP) review;
5.	Organizing and participating in parent support groups, local, state, and national voluntary organizations;
6.	Developing and participating in speakers' bureaus for education of the lay public and as a means of informing professionals;
7.	Partnering with local business groups, industry, chambers of commerce for employment opportunities for adults with autism;
8.	Helping raise funds for services and research;
9.	Campaigning for legislation to improve services and facilities;
10.	Working in the political process on behalf of candidates for elective office.

how best to channel and educate to achieve maximum effectiveness. Table 3 summarizes some potential opportunities for parental involvement in advocacy.

IX. SUMMARY

Children with autism differ from those with other developmental disabilities in that they have aberrations in the basic, fundamental areas of communication, behavior, and social interaction that affect their function. These are the areas normally nurtured within the family context from the earliest age, and when they have gone awry place both burdens and opportunities on the family for resolution. For this reason it was early recognized that the family should have a pivotal place in treatment programs and strategies as they evolved. No wonder, then, that the family of the child with autism is perhaps more at the center of early diagnosis and management than all the other major childhood disabilities.

At the same time, there is likely to be a unique sensibility of the family when their child is diagnosed with autism. Disclosure can greatly influence their subsequent relationship with the child, other family members, and siblings, as well as caregivers. The procedure for communicating the diagnosis, therefore, requires careful planning and a sensitive, caring process.

Since the disabilities in autism are so basic to development, it is not surprising that the family is likely to experience significant stress when the diagnosis is confirmed, and subsequently as daily care and treatment progress. In addition, data currently available indicate that in some cases parents of children with autism have preexisting personality abnormalities and emotional disorders. Sensitive professional caregivers must assure families that their emotional or psychiatric status is *not a cause* of the child's condition, and help to provide necessary mental health services where indicated. Management of the child with autism must focus on family needs as a whole, and not simply target the affected child.

The vast amount of information on autism through news media and the Internet to which families are exposed can greatly affect their involvement with the child, participation in treatment programs, as well as their use of complementary/alternative therapies. This places great responsibility on professionals to maintain close communication with families to help interpret information and develop a partnership relationship in which there is shared decision making in care of the child.

Finally, families that initially work to improve facilities and services for their own affected child may go on to assist other parents through discussion groups, attempt to educate professionals, work toward improving employment opportunities for adults with autism, campaign for needed funds and legislation, or even become involved in the political process itself. The opportunities are extensive; the challenges are great, for there is much more yet to be learned about this family-centered condition.

REFERENCES

1. Lord C, McGee JP, eds. National Research Council: Educating Children with Autism. Washington, DC: National Academy Press, 2001:140–172.
2. Rogers SJ. Empirically supported comprehensive treatments for young children with autism. J Clin Child Psychol 1998; 27:168–179.
3. Siller M, Sigman M. The behaviors of parents of children with autism predict the subsequent development of their children's communication. J Autism Dev Disord 2002; 32:77–89.
4. Kasari C, Sigman M. Linking parental perceptions to interactions in young children with autism. J Autism Dev Disord 1997; 27:39–57.
5. Kasari C, Sigman M, Mundy P, Yirmiya N. Caregiver interactions with autistic children. J Abnorm Child Psychol 1988; 16:45–56.
6. Bax MCO. Disclosure. Dev Med Child Neurol 2002; 44:579.
7. Sloper P. Determinants of parental satisfaction with disclosure of disability. Dev Med Child Neurol 1993; 35:816–882.
8. Garwick AW, Patterson J, Bennett FC, Blum RW. Breaking the news: how families first learn about their child's chronic condition. Arch Pediatr Adolesc Med 1995; 149:991–997.
9. Hasnat MJ, Graves P. Disclosure of developmental disability—a study of parent satisfaction and determinants of satisfaction. J Paediatr Child Health 2000; 36:32–35.
10. Baird G, McConachie H, Scrutton D. Parents' perceptions of disclosure of the diagnosis of cerebral palsy. Arch Dis Child 2000; 83:475–480.
11. Bartolo PA. Communicating a diagnosis of developmental disability to parents—multiprofessional negotiation frameworks. Child Care Health Dev 2002; 28:65–71.
12. Ahmann E. Review and commentary: two studies regarding giving "bad news." Pediatr Nurs 1998; 24:554–556.
13. Krauss-Mars AH, Lachman P. Breaking bad news to parents with disabled children—a cross-cultural study. Child Care Health Dev 1994; 20:101–113.
14. Partridge JW. Putting it in writing: written assessment reports for parents. Arch Dis Child 1984; 59:678–681.
15. McConachie H, Lingam S, Stiff B, Holt KS. Giving assessment reports to parents. Arch Dis Child 1988; 63:209–210.
16. Sharp MC, Strauss RP, Lorch SC. Communicating medical bad news: parents' experiences and preferences. J Pediatr 1992; 121:539–546.
17. Jan M, Girvin JP. The communication of medical bad news to parents. Can J Neurol Sci 2002; 29:78–82.
18. Abrams EZ. Diagnosing developmental problems in children: parents and professionals negotiate bad news. J Pediatr Psychol 1998; 23:87–88.

19. Krahn GL, Hallum A, Kime C. Are there good ways to give "bad news"? Pediatrics 1993; 91:578–582.

20. Cottrell DJ, Summers K. Communicating an evolutionary diagnosis of disability to parents. Child Care Health Dev 1990; 16:211–218.

21. Cunningham CC, Morgan PA, McGucken RB. Down's syndrome: is dissatisfaction with disclosure of diagnosis inevitable? Dev Med Child Neurol 1984; 26:33–39.

22. Vaidya VU, Greenberg LW, Patel KM, Strauss LH. Teaching physicians how to break bad news: a 1-day workshop using standardized parents. Arch Pediatr Adolesc Med 1999; 153:419–422.

23. Greenberg LW, Ochsenschlager D, O'Donnell R, Mastruserio J, Cohen GJ. Communicating bad news: a pediatric department's evaluation of a simulated intervention. Pediatrics 1999; 103:1210–1217.

24. Fajardo B. Parenting a damaged child: mourning, regression, and disappointment. Psychoanal Rev 1987; 74:19–43.

25. Shu BC, Lung FW, Chang YY. Mental health of mothers with autistic children in Taiwan. Kaosiung J Med Sci 2000; 16:308–314.

26. Dunn ME, Burbine T, Bowers CA, Tantliff-Dunn S. Moderators of stress in parents of children with autism. Community Ment Health J 2001; 37:39–52.

27. Kalyampur M, Rao SS. Empowering low-income black families of handicapped children. Am J Orthopsychiatry 1991; 61:523–532.

28. Dyson LL. Fathers and mothers of children with developmental disabilities—stress. Am J Ment Retard 1997; 102:267–279.

29. Donavan AM. Family stress and ways of coping—maternal perceptions. Am J Ment Retard 1988; 92:502–509.

30. Holroyd J, McArthur D. Mental retardation and stress on the parents—a contrast between Down's syndrome and childhood autism. Am J Ment Defic 1976; 80:431–436.

31. Holmes H, Carr J. The pattern of care in families of adults with a mental handicap: a comparison between families of autistic adults and Down syndrome adults. J Autism Dev Disord 1991; 21:159–176.

32. Bouma R. Impact of chronic childhood illness on family stress: autism vs cystic fibrosis. J Clin Psychol 1990; 46:722–730.

33. Henderson D, Vandenberg B. Factors influencing adjustment in families with autism. Psychol Rep 1992; 71:167–171.

34. Bristol MM. Mothers of children with autism or communication disorders: successful adaptation and the double ABC X model. J Autism Dev Disord 1987; 17:469–486.

35. Hastings RP, Johnson E. Stress in UK families conducting intensive home based behavioral intervention for their young child with autism. J Autism Dev Disord 2001; 31:327–336.

36. Moes D, Koegel RL, Schreibman L, Loos LM. Stress profiles of mothers and fathers of children with autism. Psychol Rep 1992; 71:1272–1274.

37. Koegel RL, Schreibman L, Loos LM, Dirlich-Wilhelm H, Dunlap G, Robbins PR, Plienis AJ. Consistent stress profiles in mothers of children with autism. J Autism Dev Disord 1992; 22:205–216.

38. Firat S, Diler RS. Comparison of psychopathology in the mothers of autistic and mentally retarded children. J Korean Med Sci 2002; 17:679–685.
39. Bogenholm A, Gilberg C. Psychological effects on siblings of children with autism. J Ment Def Res 1991; 35:291–307.
40. Roegers H, Myoke K. Siblings of children with autism. Child Care Health Dev 1995; 21:305–319.
41. Frey KS, Greenberg MT, Fewell RR. Stress and coping among parents of handicapped children: a multidimensional approach. Am J Ment Retard 1989; 94:240–249.
42. Kolko DJ. Parents as behavior therapists for their autistic child. In: Schopler E, Mesibov GB, eds. The Effects of Autism on the Family. New York: Plenum Press, 1984.
43. Tissot C. Parental advocacy. J Autism Dev Disord 1999; 29:345–346.
44. Factor DC, Perry A, Freeman N. Stress, social support, and respite care use in families with autistic children. J Autism Dev Disord 1990; 20:139–146.
45. Rodrigue JR, Morgan SB, Geffken GR. Psychosocial adaptation of fathers of children with autism, Down syndrome, and normal development. J Autism Dev Disord 1992; 22:249–263.
46. Fisman SN, Wolf LC, Noh S. Marital intimacy in parents of exceptional children. Can J Psychiatry 1989; 34:519–525.
47. Kaminisky L, Dewey D. Siblings relationships of children with autism. J Autism Dev Disord 2001; 31:399–410.
48. DeLong R, Nohria C. Psychiatric family history and neurological disease in autistic spectrum disorders. Dev Med Child Neurol 1994; 36:441–448.
49. Piven J, Palmer P. Psychiatric disorder and the broad autism phenotype: evidence from a family study of multiple-incidence autism families. Am J Psychiatry 1999; 156:557–563.
50. Murphy M, Bolton PF, Pickles A, Fombonne E, Piven J, Rutter M. Personality traits of the relatives of autistic probands. Psychol Med 2000; 30:1411–1424.
51. Piven J, Wzorek M, Landa R, Lainhart J, Bolton P, Chase GA, Folstein S. Personality characteristics of the parents of autistic individuals. Psychol Med 1994; 24:783–795.
52. Wolff S, Narayan S, Moyes B. Personality characteristics of parents of autistic children: a controlled study. J Child Psychol Psychiatry 1988; 29:143–153.
53. Narayan S, Moyes B, Wolff S. Family characteristics of autistic children: a further report. J Autism Dev Disord 1990; 20:523–535.
54. Ward AJ. Comparison of analysis of the presence of family problems during pregnancy of mothers with autistic vs. mothers of normal children. Child Psychiatry Hum Dev 1990; 20:279–288.
55. Piven J, Chase GA, Landa R, Wzorek M, Gayle J, Cloud D, Folstein S. Psychiatric disorders in the parents of autistic individuals. J Am Acad Child Adolesc Psychiatry 1991; 30:471–478.
56. Lovaas OI, Koegel R, Simmons JQ, Long JS. Some generalization and follow-up measures on autistic children in behavior therapy. J Appl Behav Anal 1973; 6:131–166.
57. Lovaas OI. Behavioral treatment and normal educational and intellectual functioning in young autistic children. J Consult Clin Psychol 1987; 55:3–9.

58. Neef NA. Pyramidal parent training by peers. J Appl Behav Anal 1995; 28:333–337.

59. Holmes N, Hemsley R, Rickett J, Likierman H. Parents as cotherapists: their perceptions of a home-based behavioral treatment for autistic children. J Autism Dev Disord 1982; 12:331–342.

60. Jocelyn LJ, Casiro OG, Beattie D, Boe J, Kniesz J. Treatment of children with autism: a randomized control trial to evaluate a caregiver-based intervention program in community day-care centers. J Dev Behav Pediatr 1998; 19:326–334.

61. Ozonoff S, Cathcart K. Effectiveness of a home program intervention for young children with autism. J Autism Dev Disord 1998; 28:25–32.

62. Shields J. The NAS Early Bird Programme: partnership with parents in early intervention. The National Autistic Society. Autism 2001; 5:49–56.

63. Salt J, Shemilt J, Sellars V, Boyd S, Coulson T, McCool S. The Scottish Centre for autism preschool treatment programme. II. The results of a controlled treatment outcome study. Autism 2002; 6:33–46.

64. Panerai S, Ferrante L, Zingale M. Benefits of the Treatment and Education of Autistic and Communication Handicapped Children (TEACCH) programme as compared with a non-specific approach. J Intellect Disabil Res 2002; 46:318–327.

65. Koegel RL, Bimbela A, Schreibman L. Collateral effects of parent training on family interactions. J Autism Dev Disord 1996; 26:347–359.

66. Sheinkopf SJ, Siegel B. Home-based behavioral treatment of young children with autism. J Autism Dev Disord 1998; 28:15–23.

67. Bibby P, Eikeseth S, Martin NT, Mudford OC, Reeves D. Progress and outcomes for children with autism receiving parent-managed intensive interventions. Res Dev Disabil 2001; 22:425–447.

68. Helm DT, Kozloff MA. Research on parent training: shortcomings and remedies. J Autism Dev Disord 1986; 16:1–22.

69. Boyd RD, Corley MJ. Outcome survey of early intensive behavioral intervention for young children with autism in a community setting. Autism 2001; 5:430–431.

70. Berney TP. Autism—an evolving concept. Br J Psychiatry 2000; 176:20–25.

71. Risdon C. Cybersearch. Quick clicks to answer clinical questions. Can Fam Physician 2001; 47:1183.

72. Patel NC, Yeh JY, Shepherd MD, Crismon ML. Secretin treatment for autistic disorder: a critical analysis. Pharmacotherapy 2002; 22:905–914.

73. Ramsay S. UK starts campaign to reassure parents about MMR-vaccine safety. Lancet 2001; 357:290.

74. Fischman J. Vaccine worries get shot down but parents still fret. US News World Rep 2001; 130:61.

75. Allen A. The not-so-crackpot autism theory. NY Times Magazine. 2002; Nov 10:66.

76. American Academy of Pediatrics, Committee on Children with Disabilities. The pediatrician's role in the diagnosis and management of autistic spectrum disorder in children. Pediatrics 2001; 107:1221–1226.

77. Kessler RC, Davis RB, Foster DF, Van Rompay MI, Walters EE, Wilkey SA, Kaptchuk TJ, Eisenberg DM. Long-term trends in the use of complementary and alternative medical therapies in the United States. Ann Intern Med 2001; 135:262–268.

78. Elliott B, Elliott G. Complementary or alternative medicine and the Internet. Del Med J 1998; 70:479–484.
79. Sawni-Sikand A, Schubiner H, Thomas RL. Use of complementary/alternative therapies among children in primary care pediatrics. Ambul Pediatr 2002; 2:99–103.
80. Pitetti R, Singh S, Hornyak D, Garcia SE, Herr S. Complementary and alternative medicine use in children. Pediatr Emerg Care 2001; 17:165–169.
81. Straus SE. Herbal medicines—what's in a bottle? N Engl J Med 2002; 347:1997–1998.
82. Nickel RE. Controversial therapies for young children with developmental disabilities. Infants Young Child 1996; 8:29–40.
83. Sikand A, Laken M. Pediatricians' experience with and attitudes toward complementary/alternative medicine. Arch Pediatr Adolesc Med 1998; 152:1059–1064.
84. American Academy of Pediatrics, Committee on Children with Disabilities. Counseling families who choose complementary and alternative medicine for their child with chronic illness or disability. Pediatrics 2001; 107:598–601.
85. Perlman AI, Eisenberg DM, Panush RS. Talking with patients about alternative and complementary medicine. Rheum Dis Clin North Am 1999; 25:815–822.
86. Clark PA. The ethics of alternative medicine therapies. Public Health Policy 2000; 21:447–470.
87. Cauffield JS. The psychosocial aspects of complementary and alternative medicine. Pharmacotherapy 2000; 20:1289–1294.
88. Seligman M, Darling RB. Ordinary Families, Special Children. 2nd ed. New York: Guilford Press, 1997.
89. Schopler E. Will your journal support parents advocating for intensive behavior therapy (the Lovaas Method) as an entitlement under Part H of the IDEA? J Autism Dev Disord 1999; 29:345–346.
90. Aylott J. Understanding and listening to people with autism. Br J Nurs 2001; 10:1676–172.
91. American Academy of Pediatrics, Committee on Children with Disabilities. Pediatrician's role in the development and implementation of an individual education plan (IEP) and/or an individual family service plan (IFSP). Pediatrics 1992; 89:340–342.

8

Behavioral and Educational Interventions for Young Children with Autism

John M. Suozzi
Children's Hospital, Richmond, Virginia, U.S.A.

I. INTRODUCTION

Behavioral and educational interventions are the mainstay of management of individuals with autism (1–7). A wide array of such "treatments" is available for young children with autism. While there is empirical evidence for the efficacy and effectiveness of some of these interventions, many have gained support in the absence of empirical data to verify their effectiveness and utility. Behavioral and educational interventions, both proven and unproven, are discussed here, because the absence of a research-based demonstration of efficacy does not mean that a treatment is ineffective, only that its efficacy has not been demonstrated through objective means (8).

II. BEHAVIORAL INTERVENTIONS

A. Applied Behavior Analysis and Discrete Trial Training

Broadly defined, the body of knowledge known as applied behavior analysis (ABA) focuses on what people say and do (behavior), and utilizes experimental analyses of environmental influences on behavior to derive techniques for behavior change. The origin of the experimental analysis of behavior is credited to B.F. Skinner (9). Based on his extensive data from observation, manipulation, and analysis of animal and human behavior, Skinner hypothesized that behavior is a function of its consequences. He believed that there are rules or laws that govern all behavior, and he developed procedures from these laws that were used to produce significant changes in a number of different types of behavior. Many years of experimental research by a number of prominent psychologists of a behavioral orientation have given credence and support to Skinner's original theories.

Although skeptics feel that it is too simplistic to posit that behavior is solely a function of its consequences, and that human behavior can be controlled or changed in much the same way as animal behavior, there are enough research and clinical data to support the use of the principles and practices of applied behavior analysis in the treatment of individuals with autism. ABA techniques advise the simultaneous strengthening of adaptive behaviors and the reduction of challenging behaviors. The characteristics of individuals with autism, such as idiosyncratic behavior patterns, lack of responsiveness to social reinforcers, difficulty anticipating and/or delaying reinforcement, poor communication skills, and the presence of competing behaviors, necessitate the use of structure, repetition, and dense reinforcement schedules (all of which are advised by ABA). Moreover, ABA relies on the collection of copious data about the impact of various environmental manipulations on behavior, and provides a record of therapeutic progress to guide future treatment. Finally, ongoing inquiry and research into the factors that influence rate of behavior and the effectiveness of reinforcers (such as establishing operations, motivation, and response effort) ensure that the most effective strategies are being employed. (See Table 1.)

In ABA, the focus is on observable behavior, that is, on what the individual says and does. ABA helps us to understand how people access reinforcement for different behaviors and effectively "learn" the behaviors that provide reinforcers. Children with autism often obtain reinforcement through the display of inappropriate behavior (for a variety of reasons). To teach newer, more adaptive behaviors, reinforcement principles are utilized in a manner that increases the value of performing the newer more adaptive behaviors relative to the value of performing inappropriate behavior. To increase the value of newer, more adaptive behaviors, reinforcement must be contacted quickly, easily (i.e., with little effort), and, at first, frequently.

The first to "package" ABA principles as a treatment for individuals with autism was O. Ivar Lovaas. His "UCLA Young Autism Project" (10) is perhaps the most widely cited treatment study of individuals with autism. Lovaas reported that a percentage of his subjects achieved "normal" intellectual and educational functioning. This was popularly interpreted as a "cure" for autism. The more realistic interpretation of Lovaas' findings is that he has formulated an

Table 1 Basic Applied Behavior Principles

Reinforcement: The procedure used to increase the likelihood that a behavior will occur or to increase the rate of a behavior.

Reinforcer: The event that follows the occurrence of a behavior and increases the probability or rate of that behavior. Generally, a reinforcer is most effective if delivered immediately after the behavior occurs (immediacy) or if access to that reinforcer has been limited or denied for some time (deprivation).

Schedules of reinforcement:

Continuous reinforcement: A behavior is reinforced every time it occurs.

Ratio schedule: A behavior is reinforced after the occurrence of a number of *fixed* or *variable* responses.

Interval schedule: A reinforcer is administered after a *fixed* or *variable* period of time and after the occurrence of a response. Variable ratio schedule builds behavior most resistant to extinction.

Punishment: A procedure used to decrease the likelihood that a behavior will occur again in the future (or to decrease the rate of the behavior).

Punisher: The event that follows the occurrence of a behavior and decreases the probability or rate of that behavior. There are fixed and variable ratio and interval schedules of punishment. Forms of punishment include contingent punishment, extinction, time out, and overcorrection. Overapplication of punishments can create conditions of aversion for the learner.

Establishing operation (EO): Refers to a condition that establishes the power of a reinforcer and that evokes particular behavior(s). The effect of an EO is to change the reinforcing effectiveness of some stimulus and to change the frequency of all behavior that has been reinforced by that stimulus.

Motivation: A state of willingness to perform an action or a set of actions.

Response effort: The amount of effort that must be spent to perform a task. Familiar tasks with fewer steps require less response effort than novel tasks with several steps.

Generalization: The occurrence of a behavior in the presence of a novel stimulus. A behavior should be reinforced in different stimulus situations, such as across instructors and settings until it generalizes to other related stimuli.

Shaping: A method of teaching successive approximations of behavior by reinforcing a portion of a desired response or a behavior that approximates a desired response.

Chaining: The process of creating a sequence of two or more behaviors in which each behavior produces a result that acts as a stimulus for the next behavior to occur and in which the last behavior is reinforced.

Prompting: A process of providing an added stimulus to increase the likelihood of a correct response.

Fading: Withdrawing a prompt quickly to avoid creating a condition under which behavior occurs only when prompted. Prompts must be faded quickly from most to least restrictive in order to build behavior that occurs when environmental conditions call for its use.

Discriminative stimulus (or S^D): A stimulus associated with reinforcement of a particular behavior. Refers to the conditions under which a behavior is taught and/or is expected to occur.

---

intervention that is highly effective in some and less so in other cases of autism. Importantly, Lovaas' specific results have not been replicated universally. While the method of intensive one-to-one instruction that Lovaas described is the mainstay of several highly effective programs, some aspects of his instruction, such as the use of prompts and punishments, remain unclear. Moreover, methodological weaknesses in the design of Lovaas' study have been identified, such as nonrandom assignment of subjects to treatment groups and no indication of whether children in the treatment group received other kinds of treatment simultaneously (11).

Lovaas' method of intensive one-to-one instruction is known as discrete trial training. A discrete trial follows the basic format of presentation of an instruction or request (called a "discriminative stimulus"), an expected response from the learner, and a consequence delivered by the instructor. If required, a prompt (an additional stimulus that helps the learner to make the correct response) may be administered as well. This general format allows for several interpretations of how antecedents, learner responses, and consequents are to be rendered.

Proper training and education of individuals who provide ABA is essential because a few inappropriate and unproven applications of the format, such as the use of the "no-no" prompt, have found their way into widespread popular application. The "no-no" prompt consists of the instructor providing the verbal consequent "no" contingent on the learner giving an incorrect response, and then informing the learner that "no" reinforcement will be provided. While there are no data that support the use of the "no-no" prompt (12), research does support the use of errorless learning approaches (13) for response acquisition. In the errorless approach, the learner is prompted to make swift and correct responses that always end with delivery of a reinforcer, as opposed to the "traditional" discrete trials in which the learner obtains reinforcement only when a correct and independent response is made. A clear distinction must be made between "behavioral" and "educational" techniques that involve some element of reinforcement and those that are truly grounded in ABA. There are several effective techniques that fall under the latter category, such as discrete trial training, functional behavior assessment (FBA), functional communication training (FCT), applied verbal behavior (AVB), the picture exchange communication system (PECS), and pivotal response training (PRT). Other behavioral interventions that have shown promise include social stories and programs devoted to social skills training (including modeling strategies).

B. Applied Verbal Behavior

Skinner (14) broke down communication into seven functionally independent categories. A word and its meaning are categorized according to the conditions under which a person was taught to use them: a single word could be categorized

Table 2   Applied Verbal Behavior Communication Categories

Tact	A label, or the name of an object, an action, or an event
Mand	A request for something
Echo	Repeating what is heard
Receptive language	Following instructions
Receptive by feature, function, and class	Being able to respond to items when given some information about them
Intraverbal	Answer to "wh" question
Text	Symbolic representation of a word (e.g., written or signed)

as tact, mand, echo, receptive, intraverbal, receptive by feature, function, and class, or text. (See Table 2.)

For truly functional communication to develop, the meaning of a word needs to be taught across all categories of verbal behavior.

Verbal behavior is thus not limited to speech. It consists of vocalizations, signs, gestures, and even the use of augmentative systems for communication. Analyses of the verbal behavior of children with autism suggest that they often possess large receptive repertoires and many labels, but very few spontaneous requests and almost no conversational speech (15). Assessment of the verbal behavior of individuals with autism is typically accomplished via tools such as the Assessment of Basic Learning and Language Skills (ABLLS) (16). Although verbal behaviorists provide direct instruction to individuals with autism in accordance with the core principles of ABA—appropriate use of prompting procedures, fading, shaping, and the use of errorless learning techniques, verbal behaviorists are careful to distinguish the appearance and results of their mode of instruction from the appearance and results of "traditional discrete trial training." From the verbal behavior perspective, all of these distinctions from discrete trials are central to effective instruction of individuals with autism.

Traditional discrete trials may achieve little in the way of functional skills, because the emphasis is largely on imitation and labeling. A verbal behavior approach usually begins by pairing the instructor with reinforcement so that the child comes to see the instructor as a very powerful source of reinforcers. This is done in the absence of demands or contingencies for expected behavior. Once the child consistently approaches the instructor to obtain reinforcers, he is then taught to request reinforcing items directly. Demands for learning new tasks are increased slowly by number and by amount of effort required to complete them. Again, there is clear intent to teach across categories of verbal behavior. While instruction through traditional discrete trials appears structured because it begins by setting up response requirements to obtain reinforcement, instruction based on verbal behavior has a "natural" look to it, because careful attention is paid to build foundational skills that help the child with autism to become an effective learner. In a verbal behavior approach, the instructor is also responsible for maintaining a high rate of response from the learner, by being mindful of the rate at which the learner obtains reinforcement, the number of demands placed on the learner, and the amount of effort required of the learner to complete demands. Empirical research supports teaching verbal behavior to individuals with autism using these principles of functional and applied behavior analysis (17).

C. Functional Behavior Assessment

FBA provides a framework for investigating functional relationships between aberrant behavior and specific environmental events (18). As typically applied to developmentally disabled populations, the method promotes careful experimental manipulation of environmental events (i.e., sources of reinforcement) that apparently maintain the challenging behavior. FBA is generally directed toward determining an appropriate intervention for specific behavioral issues, rather than toward skill building. The goal is to identify antecedent conditions and the sources of reinforcement that produce and maintain behavior problems. This can be accomplished by anecdotal reports, checklists, and most effectively, analog procedure (19). In the analog procedure, first hypotheses are made about the source(s) of reinforcement that may maintain aberrant behavior (such as escape, attention, or automatic reinforcement), and real-life conditions are set up to test these hypotheses. For example, if aggressive behavior displayed by an individual is thought to be maintained by attention, then an analog condition to test that hypothesis would consist of attention being delivered after each instance of aggressive behavior. Data about the frequency of aggression would be collected during that condition. Next, data from the "attention" condition could be compared to data from a condition in which there is no consequence for aggression, and to data from a condition in which escape is permitted contingent on the display of aggression. In this way, possible conclusions can be reached about the factor that maintains aggression, and a treatment can be developed that addresses that specific factor.

D. Functional Communication Training

FCT involves teaching adaptive ("functionally equivalent") responses that serve the same purpose as the problem behavior (20). In other words, communicative responses are taught so that the individual can request and obtain the specific reinforcers that serve to maintain aberrant behavior instead of acting out. There is some evidence for the effectiveness of this technique in reducing problem behaviors such as aggression, self-injury, disruptive behavior, stereotypy, and communication problems. For example, if FBA determines that a child exhibits aggressive behavior when presented with a task because it results in the removal of demands ("escape"), an intervention advised by FCT would be to teach a communicative response that would also result in removal of demands. An FCT intervention would teach the child to request a "break," by a sign, vocalization, or other augmentative strategy that would achieve the same end as the aggressive behavior, that is, the removal of demands. The greatest advantage of FCT is that it results in a relatively rapid reduction of the problem behavior owing to the specificity of the intervention. A thorough FBA to determine the purpose of the problem behavior is a prerequisite for FCT.

A criticism of FCT is that it teaches additional behaviors that achieve the same end as the challenging behavior. To use the example above, the learner now has another behavior in his repertoire that can be used to remove demands. However, in the case of aggressive behavior (especially if the aggression is directed toward other people), it is critical to achieve a rapid reduction so that other more functional skills can be taught.

E. Picture Exchange Communication System

PECS was intended to provide nonverbal individuals with a mode of expressive communication (21). Specifically, line drawings are used to represent everyday objects, foods, and activities, and the PECS protocol begins with building simple requests. The learner delivers the picture representation of the object, food, or activity to the instructor and then receives what is represented in the picture. As the learner becomes more proficient in requesting preferred items, carrier phrases are added, such as "I want_____." Teaching the child to make a request reduces the demands associated with receptive tasks. This practice is consistent with what is observed in typical development, in which the skill of requesting is the first expressive skill to emerge. Later, more advanced skills are taught through PECS, such as calling attention to what one observes (e.g., "I see") and what one possesses (e.g., "I have"). PECS requires the child to approach a listener and initiate interaction before "communicating." The PECS system is grounded in basic behavioral principles such as shaping, differential reinforcement, and transfer of stimulus control.

Charlop-Christy et al. (22) were the first to present an empirical assessment of the efficacy of PECS in a multiple baseline design involving three children. Vocal communication and social-communicative behaviors emerged in all the three and a reduction in problem behavior was observed after they mastered the use of PECS. Some limitations of picture systems relate to problems with portability of the system, problems displaying complex words in symbol form, the lack of a natural community that uses pictures, and difficulty in emitting the appropriate communicative response exactly when it is needed (23).

F. Pivotal Response Training

PRT was developed by Robert L. Koegel and Laura Schreibman (24,25). This technique is related to incidental teaching and includes didactic instruction, modeling, role playing, and feedback. The instructor capitalizes on the learner's interests, motivation, and needs, using naturally occurring opportunities as the basis for instruction. PRT is less contrived than discrete trials, which emphasize the use of instructor-controlled reinforcers, a very highly structured environment, and repetition. It uses both naturally occurring and formally structured opportunities to teach new behaviors. The core considerations in PRT are motivation and the ability to respond to multiple cues, both of which are considered "pivotal" behaviors. Motivation is a pivotal behavior because it leads to concomitant changes in other related behaviors (24). Reinforcement is direct, and is specifically related to the behavior being taught. The behaviors most likely to change through this technique are speech and language, social behavior, and disruptive responses (25). As a more natural (or social-pragmatic) form of intervention, PRT may be more appealing to parents and educators because it does not involve the withholding of reinforcers and the structure or repetition of structured interventions that characterize discrete trials.

G. Social Stories

Social stories (26) are intended to provide individuals with autism with information about what can be expected in various social situations. Social stories can provide information about what the physical setting may look like, what other people in that setting might say and do, and offers suggestions about the behavior(s) that may be expected in that setting. Stories normally consist of words and pictures, and are rendered in a simple fashion without extraneous detail. Social stories can be written to address virtually any social situation that may arise, based on a basic "formula" that is offered. Social stories are used prophylactically or preventively; that is, they are reviewed prior to entering social situations in which the individual with autism encounters some difficulty, in an attempt to prevent the difficulty. The use of social stories is supplemented with modeling and role playing of appropriate behavior as well as corrective feedback. Through the use of social stories, individuals with autism have the opportunity to experience elements of a number of different problem settings, from a "safe" environment in which they can practice responses to social situations without negative consequences. However, social stories may not be able to capture the nuances of all social situations and environmental settings.

H. Social Skills Training

Because socialization is a core area of deficit in autism, training in social skills is of great importance in the treatment of autism. Social skills training usually entails modeling, feedback, and direct reinforcement for appropriate behavior. Very recently, a good deal of attention has been paid to the effects of video modeling on the acquisition of play and social skills. Research has revealed that children with autism are capable of acquiring complex sets of play and social skills, including verbal language, from watching videos of other individuals performing various acts (27). Video modeling has some excellent advantages, such as not requiring the learner to interact with another person during instruction, and presenting the behavior to be learned the same way each time it is viewed.

III. EDUCATIONAL INTERVENTIONS

Most educational programs for children with autism are based to varying degrees on the principles of ABA (28,29). Few educational programs have empirical support for their efficacy based on properly controlled studies. Methodological flaws in outcome studies of educational programs for children with autism often make it impossible to determine with certainty if the intervention (or some component of the intervention) truly contributed to the putative outcome. Therefore, the interventions below can strictly be considered as "unproven" (30).

A. Rutgers Autism Program

"Based upon a broad spectrum of methods derived from the principles of applied behavior analysis," the Rutgers Autism Program is geared toward helping families to develop home-based programs (31). Parents are considered an integral part of the team and have to be committed to an intensive and "pure" behavior analysis intervention. Additionally, the Rutgers Autism Program consults with schools to develop educational and behavioral programs for children with autism, and provides intensive and ongoing staff training. The primary method of instruction is through discrete trial training. Children receive 30–40 h/week of one-to-one, individualized ABA instruction.

B. UCLA Young Autism Project

This program is "based on research by Ivar Lovaas and colleagues, as well as studies from other ABA treatment programs worldwide" (32). Instruction is through discrete trials. Although Lovaas (10) claimed to normalize about 40% of his subjects, the study has been criticized for the punishment procedures. Currently more positive approaches are emphasized.

C. Children's Unit for Treatment and Evaluation (SUNY Binghamton)

This program individually selects goals for each participant, based on an individualized goal selection curriculum (IGS), and provides instruction primarily through discrete trials (33). Curriculum items are chosen from approximately 2000 individual tasks in 18 "areas" of development. The program provides a "comprehensive, integrated, and state-of-the-art behavioral model of service delivery" for children from 10 months to 11 years of age (34). Although the proponents claim that their "philosophy is derived from empirical research rather than a philosophy in search of research support," program outcomes have been reported only in non-peer-reviewed publications (35,36).

D. Denver Model

This program is based on a developmental model of autism first described by Rogers and Pennington (37). Since autism is a social disorder, building social relationships should be the core of treatment. This is done by providing opportunities for social interaction and play at home, in an integrated preschool, and during one-to-one teaching. The program is geared toward children from ages 2 to 5 years. More than 20 h/week of systematic instruction is provided with preplanned objectives and ongoing data collection. Instructional approach in this program is interdisciplinary and eclectic, including relationship-based, developmental, sensory, and discrete trials-based approaches. Curriculum emphasizes building communication, play, sensory, and motor skills, and promotes personal independence and participation in social routines. The Denver Model is a comprehensive "best practices" model without a narrow theoretical underpinning.

E. Alpine Learning Group, Paramus, NJ

This program is rooted in the teachings of ABA, and instruction is mostly given through discrete trials, although incidental teaching is also mentioned as an instructional strategy. Individualized programs are created for each student, with clearly defined and measurable objectives for learning. The initial focus of instruction is on teaching attending, imitation, receptive language, expressive language, and play skills, with additional emphasis placed on reducing challenging behavior through the use of differential reinforcement. With a very small class size (i.e., two to four children), the environment is highly structured and there is ample opportunity for individual instruction (38). Moreover, the

Alpine Learning Group utilizes visual supports in the form of daily activity schedules, a strategy made popular within Treatment and Education of Autistic and Related Communication Handicapped Children (TEACCH). Initially the program is strictly 1:1, but after mastering some prerequisite skills, the child is allowed to participate in regular education programs with typically developing peers through a supported inclusion program.

F. The Walden Early Childhood Programs

The Walden Early Childhood Programs provides "a continuum of early instruction," through a comprehensive incidental teaching approach (39). Incidental strategies derived from ABA are the only mode of instruction. Programming consists of at least 30 h/week of planned instruction to provide an inclusive experience for the young learner to develop his/her language and social skills. For the youngest learners, the initial focus is on improving social responsiveness, and overall engagement with classroom materials and activities. Development of verbal language through incidental strategies is considered a priority. The Walden Program professes that high levels of social engagement represent the surest means of avoiding challenging behaviors. Family programs and overall family involvement are considered critical to maximizing a child's potential.

G. Princeton Child Development Institute

The Princeton Child Development Institute offers a broad range of services, including early intervention for children younger than age 3, a preschool and a primary school program, family services, group homes, and career services. All services are provided through individualized programming based on applied behavior analysis (40). Teaching new learners to follow simple directions is often the starting point for instruction, because this foundational skill is a prerequisite for building other skills. Picture schedules are utilized to promote independence in navigating the events of the day, as well as to generalize skills from preschool and home to community settings. Children with autism are integrated with typically developing peers, and foundational skills that are prerequisites for integration, such as the ability to follow instructions, sustain interest and engagement with leisure materials, and generalization of skills to new settings, are developed.

H. Treatment and Education of Autistic and Related Communication Handicapped Children (TEACCH)

The basis for education at TEACCH is structured teaching, which combines cognitive and behavioral strategies to minimize problem behaviors associated with autism (41). The emphasis is on reinforcement-based procedures for behavior change, and to address skill deficits that underlie challenging behavior. Developed in the early 1970s by Eric Schopler at the University of North Carolina at Chapel Hill, TEACCH emphasizes the culture of autism, the concept that children with autism have learning and social interaction characteristics that are different from, but not necessarily inferior to, those of typically developing children. Understanding those differences allows the construction of programs and teaching tasks to optimize learning potential. Thus learning environments are structured in such a way as to capitalize on the visual-perceptual strengths of individuals with autism. The program attempts to build on the child's strengths and interests rather than drilling deficit areas. TEACCH may be categorized as an eclectic program because of its both developmental and behavioral under-pinnings (42). It is one of the most frequently replicated models for autism intervention and is especially popular among public school special education programs.

I. Douglass Developmental Disabilities Center Programs

The center-based Douglass School and outreach home-based preschool programs rely on the principles of ABA such as discrete trials, functional assessments, functional communication training, and incidental teaching strategies. The curriculum addresses domains of attention, speech and language, cognition, fine and gross motor skills, socialization, self-help, and appropriate behavior. The Douglass Center Programs believe that intensive individual work is needed before large-group integration with typically developing peers is possible. Parents are an integral part of the team and are involved in the creation of routines and strategies for use in the home setting (43).

J. Developmental, Individual Differences, Relationship (DIR) Model

This model was pioneered at the George Washington University School of Medicine. Relationship-based, the "Greenspan" approach emphasizes affect and relationships, developmental levels, and individual differences in motoric, sensory, affective, cognitive, and language functioning by targeting six developmental skills through intensive floor-time work, which is also known as "DIR" (44). These six skills include shared attention and regulation, engagement, affective reciprocity and gestural communication, social communi-cation and problem solving, symbolic use of ideas, and logical and abstract use of ideas. There is an extensive home-based component in this program in which parents are taught to follow the lead of the child in play and other interactions for

3–5 h/day. In the data supporting DIR (45), the composition of the "comparison group" raised the possibility of a significant placebo effect. The DIR approach might better be considered more a theoretical framework for intervention rather than a specific intervention: this framework incorporates a variety of approaches, each adjusted to the individual child's specific needs rather than to theoretical needs. To varying degrees the application of DIR to a specific child might therefore overlap with any number of other intervention approaches.

K. LEAP Preschool at the University of Colorado School of Education

The Learning Experiences and Alternatives for Preschoolers and Their Parents (LEAP) preschool was one of the first programs in the United States to include children with autism with typical children. It provides a preschool program for children from ages three to five, with typically developing and children with autism in a ratio of 2:1. The program also provides behavioral skill training for the parents. The curriculum at LEAP is best known for its peer-mediated social skill interventions. The individualized curriculum also targets goals in domains of social, emotional, language, adaptive behavior, cognitive, and physical skill development. LEAP blends a behavioral approach with developmentally appropriate practices (46). The model has now been replicated at several other sites but there are no efficacy studies.

L. Pivotal Response Model at the University of California at Santa Barbara

The aim of pivotal response training is to effect change in "pivotal" areas such as responsivity to multiple cues, motivation, self-management, and self-initiation. These domains are considered central or pivotal because improvements in these areas often bring about positive changes in other areas of adaptive behavior. The program provides individuals with autism with the social and educational skills necessary to participate in inclusive settings. Curriculum goals are targeted in domains of communication, self-help, academics, and social and recreational skills (47). In the beginning phase of the program, children are taught through discrete trials, and as proficiency is gained, there is a shift toward more naturalistic behavioral interventions. Also critical is a parent education component. Currently, the intervention consists of in-clinic and one-on-one home teaching. Children enrolled in the program also participate concurrently in special education services in the schools.

Table 3 Parent Questions for Treatment Programs

---

1. What kinds of services do you provide?
2. What is your philosophy or approach to working with children with autism?
3. How many hours of service per week are included in the program?
4. How many of those hours are one-on-one?
5. Can you describe a typical day?
6. What are the teachers'/therapists' qualifications/experience?
7. What is the parent role in this therapeutic program?
8. How do you manage difficult behaviors?
9. What communication system/approach do you use?
10. Is there an integration/inclusion component with typically developing children?
11. How do you measure progress?
12. Are there arrangements for transitioning to the next school/educational level?

Source: Modified from Ref. 55.

M. Higashi School (Boston, MA)

Five principles are espoused by daily life therapy at the Higashi School: group-oriented instruction, highly structured routine activities, learning through imitation, rigorous physical exercise, and a curriculum that is based on movement, music, and art (48). To date, there are no outcome studies to examine the effectiveness of this program.

IV. CONCLUSION

On the one hand, there appear to be a wide variety of intervention approaches and programs for children with autism. On the other hand, the presence of more than a few (if any) options within a given community is rare. Theoretically, many of these approaches differ significantly from one another. Practically, many programs tend to be more eclectic and diverse in content. The components common to effective programs could be derived from the above review of available approaches. Research supports the early (prior to age 5 years) application of a program with a significant component of applied behavioral analysis (49–53). A recent study found that the specific nature of the intervention is more important than merely the intensity (54). Table 3 presents a number of questions that parents might use to assess specific programs.

REFERENCES

1. Lovaas OI. Behavioral treatment and normal educational and intellectual functioning in young autistic children. J Consult Clin Psychol 1987; 55:3–9.

2. Anderson SR, Avery DL, DiPietro EK, Edwards GL, Christian WP. Intensive home-based early intervention with autistic children. Educ Treat Child 1987; 10:352–366.

3. Birnbauer JS, Leach DJ. The Murdoch early intervention program after 2 years. Behav Change 1987; 10:63–74.

4. McEachin JJ, Smith T, Lovaas OI. Long-term outcome for children with autism who received early intensive behavioral treatment. Am J Ment Retard 1993; 97:359–372.

5. Fenske EC, Zalenski S, Krantz PJ, McClannahan LE. Age at intervention and treatment outcome for autistic children in a comprehensive intervention program. Anal Intervent Dev Disabil 1985; 5:49–58.

6. Hoyson M, Jamieson B, Strain PS. Individualized group instruction of normally developing and autistic-like children: the LEAP curriculum model. J Div Early Child 1984; 8:157–172.

7. Eikeseth S, Smith T, Jahr E, Eldevik S. Intensive behavioral treatment at school for 4- to 7-year old children with autism: a 1-year comparison controlled study. Behav Modif 2002; 49–68.

8. Rogers SJ. Empirically supported comprehensive treatments for young children with autism. J Clin Child Psychol 1998; 27(2):168–179.

9. Skinner BF. Science and Human Behavior. New York: Macmillan, 1953.

10. Lovaas OI. Behavioral treatment and normal educational and intellectual functioning in young autistic children. J Consult Clin Psychol 1987; 55:3–9.

11. Rogers SJ. Empirically supported comprehensive treatments for young children with autism. J Clin Child Psychol 1998; 27(2):168–179.

12. Heckaman K, Alber S, Hooper S, Heward W. A comparison of least to most and progressive time delay on the disruptive behavior of students with autism. J Behav Educ 1998; 8:171–202.

13. Touchette PE, Howard J. Errorless learning: reinforcement contingencies and stimulus control transfer in delayed prompting. J Appl Behav Anal 1984; 17:175–181.

14. Skinner BF. Verbal Behavior. MA: Copley, 1957.

15. Sundberg ML, Partington JW. Teaching Language to Children with Autism or Other Developmental Disabilities. Version 7.1. Pleasant Hill, CA: Behavior Analysts, Inc., 1998.

16. Partington JW, Sundberg ML. The Assessment of Basic Language and Learning Skills. Version 1.0. Pleasant Hill, CA: Behavior Analysts, Inc., 1998.

17. Sundberg ML, Michael J. The benefits of Skinner's analysis of verbal behavior for children with autism. Behav Modif 2001; 25:698–724.

18. Iwata BA, Dorsey MF, Slifer KJ, Bauman KE, Richman GS. Toward a functional analysis of self-injury. Anal Intervent Dev Disabil 1982; 2:3–20.

19. Iwata BA, Dorsey MF, Slifer KJ, Bauman KE, Richman GS. Toward a functional analysis of self-injury. Anal Intervent Dev Disabil 1982; 2:3–20.

20. Carr EG, Durand VM. The social-communicative basis of severe behavior problems in children. In: Reiss S, Bootzin RR, eds. Theoretical Issues in Behavior Therapy. New York: Academic Press, 1985:219–254.

21. Frost LA, Bondy AS. The Picture Exchange Communication System Training Manual. Cherry Hill, NJ: Pyramid Educational Consultants, 1994.

22. Charlop-Christy MH, Carpenter M, Le L, LeBlanc LA, Kellet K. Using the picture exchange communication system (pecs) with children with autism: assessment of pecs acquisition, speech, social-communicative behavior, and problem behavior. J Appl Behav Anal 2002; 35:213–231.

23. Sundberg ML, Partington JW. Teaching Language to Children with Autism or Other Developmental Disabilities. Version 7.1. Pleasant Hill, CA: Behavior Analysts, Inc., 1998.

24. Koegel LK, Koegel RL, Harrower JK, Carter CM. Pivotal response intervention. I. Overview of approach. J Assoc People Spec Handicaps 1999; 24:174–185.

25. Koegel R, O'Dell MC, Koegel LK. A natural language paradigm for teaching nonverbal autistic children. J Autism Dev Disabil 1987; 17:187–199.

26. Gray C. The New Social Story Book. Illustrated ed. Arlington, TX: Future Horizons, Inc., 2000.

27. Charlop-Christy MH, Le L, Freeman KA. A comparison of video modeling with in vivo modeling for teaching children with autism. J Autism Dev Disord 2000; 30:537–552.

28. Handleman JS, Harris SL, eds. Preschool Education Programs for Children with Autism. 2nd ed. TX: Pro-Ed, 2001.

29. Lord C, McGee JP, eds. Educating Children with Autism. Washington, DC: National Academy Press, 2001.

30. Division 12 Task Force. Training in and dissemination of empirically validated psychological treatments: report and recommendations. Clin Psychol 1995; 48:3–23.

31. Weiss MJ, Piccolo E. The Rutgers autism program. In: Handleman JS, Harris SL, eds. Preschool Education Programs for Children with Autism. Austin, TX: Pro Ed, 2001:13–27.

32. Smith T, Donahoe PA, Davis BJ. The UCLA young autism project. In: Handleman JS, Harris SL, eds. Preschool Education Programs for Children with Autism. Austin, TX: Pro Ed, 2001:29–48.

33. Romanczyk RG, Lockshin S, Matey L. The IGS Curriculum–Version 9. Vestal, NY: CBTA, 1998.

34. Romanczyk RA, Lockshin SB, Matey L. The children's unit for treatment and evaluation. In: Handleman JS, Harris SL, eds. Preschool Education Programs for Children with Autism. TX: Pro Ed, 2001:49–94.

35. Taylor J, Ekdahl M, Romanczyk RG, Miller M. Escape behavior in task situations: task versus social antecedents. J Autism Dev Disord 1994; 24:331–344.

36. Taylor J, Romanczyk RG. Generating hypotheses about the function of student problem behavior by observing teacher behavior. J Appl Behav Anal 1994; 27:251–265.

37. Rogers SJ, Hall T, Osaki D, Reaven J, Herbison J. The Denver Model: a comprehensive, integrated educational approach to young children with autism and their families. In: Handleman JS, Harris SL, eds. Preschool Education Programs for Children with Autism. Austin, TX: Pro Ed, 2001:95–133.

38. Meyer LS, Taylor BA, Levin L, Fisher JR. Alpine learning group. In: Handleman JS, Harris SL, eds. Preschool Education Programs for Children with Autism. Austin, TX: Pro Ed, 2001:135–155.

39. McGee GG, Morrier MJ, Daly T. The Walden early childhood programs. In: Handleman JS, Harris SL, eds. Preschool Education Programs for Children with Autism. Austin, TX: Pro Ed, 2001:157–190.

40. McClannahan LE, Krantz PJ. Behavior analysis and intervention for preschoolers at the Princeton child development institute. In: Handleman JS, Harris SL, eds. Preschool Education Programs for Children with Autism. Austin, TX: Pro Ed, 2001:191–213.

41. Marcus L, Schopler E, Lord C. TEACCH services for preschool children. In: Handleman JS, Harris SL, eds. Preschool Education Programs for Children with Autism. Austin, TX: Pro Ed, 2001:215–232.

42. Lord C, McGee JP, eds. Educating Children with Autism. Washington, DC: National Academy Press, 2001.

43. Harris SL, Handleman JS, Arnold MS, Gordon RF. The Douglass developmental disabilities center: two models of service delivery. In: Handleman JS, Harris SL, eds. Preschool Education Programs for Children with Autism. Austin, TX: Pro Ed, 2001:233–260.

44. Greenspan SI, Wieder S. An integrated developmental approach to interventions for young children with severe difficulties in relating and communicating. Zero to Three: National Center for Infants, Toddlers, and Families 1997; 17:5–18.

45. Greenspan SI, Wieder S. Developmental patterns and outcomes in infants and children with disorders in relating and communicating: a chart review of 200 cases of children with autistic spectrum diagnoses. J Dev Learning Disord 1997; 1:87–141.

46. Strain PS, Hoyson M. The need for longitudinal, intensive social skill intervention: LEAP follow-up outcomes for children with autism as a case in point. Topics Early Child Spec Educ 2000; 20:116–122.

47. McClannahan LE, Krantz PJ. Behavior analysis and intervention for preschoolers at the Princeton child development institute. In: Handleman JS, Harris SL, eds. Preschool Education Programs for Children with Autism. Austin, TX: Pro Ed, 2001:191–213.

48. Quill K, Gurry S, Larkin A. Daily life therapy: a Japanese model for educating children with autism. J Autism Dev Disord 1989; 19:625–635.

49. Lovaas OI. Behavioral treatment and normal educational and intellectual functioning in young autistic children. J Consult Clin Psychol 1987; 55:3–9.

50. McEachin JJ, Smith T, Lovaas OI. Long-term outcome for children with autism who received early intensive behavioral treatment. Am J Ment Retard 1993; 97:359–372.

51. Scheinkopf SJ, Siegel B. Home-based behavioral treatment of young children with autism. J Autism Dev Disabil 1998; 28:15–23.

52. Green G. Early behavioral intervention for autism: what does research tell us? In: Maurice C, ed. Behavioral Intervention for Young Children with Autism. Austin, TX: Pro-Ed, 1996:29–44.

53. Fenske EC, Zalenski S, Krantz PJ, McClannahan LE. Age at intervention and treatment outcome for autistic children in a comprehensive treatment program. Anal Intervent Dev Disabil 1985; 5:49–58.

54. Eikeseth S, Smith T, Jahr E, Eldevik S. Intensive behavioral treatment at school for 4- to 7-year old children with autism. Behav Modif 2002; 26:49–68.
55. Clinical Practice Guidelines: The Guideline Technical Report: Autism/Pervasive Developmental Disorder, Assessment and Treatment for Infants and Young Children (Age 0–3 Years). Albany: New York State Department of Health Early Intervention Program, 1999:IV–12.

9

Communication Disorders in Children with Autism: Characteristics, Assessment, Treatment

Elaine Dolgin Schneider
Pediatric Neurological Associates, White Plains, New York, U.S.A.

I. ROLE OF THE SPEECH PATHOLOGIST IN TREATING CHILDREN WITH ASD

The field of speech language pathology encompasses the diagnosis and treatment of communication disorders in a population ranging from infancy to geriatrics. A pediatric speech pathologist has extensive training in the evaluation of speech production and language development. Speech production is characterized as the way one forms the sounds of one's language (articulation), the rhythm and inflection (prosody), the fluency of the production, and the vocal quality. These qualities have a significant impact on a child's ability to communicate effectively and intelligibly.

Language is the meaningful use of words that are symbols that enable us to convey our ideas and express our needs and wants. Language development includes receptive and expressive language. Receptive language is the ability to understand the meaning of verbal language. Expressive language is the ability to use verbal behaviors.

Pragmatic language is the ability to use language in a social setting. This skill develops in infancy as children use eye gaze to interact with their caregivers.

Children instinctively use nonverbal and verbal language to regulate the behavior of others through protesting (No, don't touch) and requesting objects (i.e., I want cookie) and actions (i.e., Tie my shoe). Young children may socially interact by greeting, showing off (i.e., Did you see that red fire truck?), requesting assistance (i.e., Help me), answering questions, and posing questions to seek information. Finally, children establish joint attention, which is defined as the ability to share attention. Deficits in joint attention are considered by many researchers to be an early predictor of childhood autism (1) and are considered to be pivotal to deficits in language, play, and social development in the autism spectrum disorder (ASD) population.

A. Speech Characteristics of Children with ASD

Delay and abnormality in development of speech are very common in children with ASD. The difficulties vary and can range from the absence of speech, to repetitive use of language, to the emergence of novel and creative speech with mistakes in grammar and word meaning. Children with Asperger's syndrome (AS) may develop normal speech without any differences in grammar and vocabulary. However, closer analysis reveals subtle and, often, less than subtle differences in the use of language. These children may speak very little, speak at length about a particular subject, or use language that is repetitive, rather than conversational. They have difficulty transitioning from one event to another and have weakness in social judgment. The inability to use language to share social interaction is among the core characteristics of individuals with ASD.

Children with autism have impaired social interactions, repetitive behavior and restricted play, and differences in communication. The speech pathologist working with children with autism must be sensitive to the communication disorders associated with this disorder. These characteristics occur in children with language delays exclusive of autism; however, the severity of disorder in autism is far greater than observed in the nonautistic population.

II. MUTISM

It is reported that up to 40% of children with ASD are nonverbal, that is, make few sounds or words. Nonverbal children with ASD do not spontaneously develop gestural or other nonverbal means of conveying complex messages as nonverbal children with hearing impairment do. A nonverbal child who acquires language prior to 5 years of age has a better prognosis.

Some nonverbal children with ASD cannot communicate due to verbal apraxia. Children with verbal apraxia have difficulty coordinating and/or initiating the sequential movements for speech in the absence of weakness or paralysis of the speech musculature. Verbal dyspraxia is different from oral motor apraxia in which the coordination of the movement of the articulators is compromised for nonspeech (i.e., tongue movements) and feeding (i.e., chewing) skills. Children with verbal apraxia, without ASD, possess intact comprehension and acquire linguistic concepts consistent with their chronological age. Children with verbal apraxia tend to be quiet as babies, with limited vocal play or babbling. Depending on the severity of the apraxia, a child's imitation skills are impaired. Despite a model, children with severe verbal apraxia may not be able to imitate oral movements, vowels, consonants, or consonant-vowel combinations. If the child does possess speech, the most salient characteristic of apraxia is the inconsistent production from one attempt to another. The prosody of speech, including inflection, stress, and pitch, is often affected, particularly as the child's language skills increase. Children with ASD may have speech apraxia in addition to the pragmatic language deficits, which will hamper speech development (2).

III. ECHOLALIA

Children normally acquire language through single words. By 19–21 months of age, children will progress from single words to two-word utterances. By 24–30 months, three-word combinations are noted and grammatical morphemes (smallest units of language: i.e., plural /s/, present progressive verb ending: walking) emerge. Language is productive, creative, and increases in complexity.

Along with this "analytical mode" of language development, in the early stages of development (through 18–24 months), children learn language through imitation. The children will repeat a parent's verbalizations in chunks that are specific to the situation. This is the "gestalt" mode of learning. For example, the children may generalize the phrase "go out," previously learned from the parent to now mean "Let's go outside" or "Let's go to visit Grandma." For children who develop language normally, analytical and gestalt modes may co-occur in very early stages with rapid movements to a primarily analytical mode.

Children with ASD become masters at echoing the content of what others say, without the vocal inflection and rhythm (prosody). Children with ASD may rely on or be limited to a gestalt mode for extended periods of time (3). Children with ASD who are echoic have not progressed in their language development. Their language acquisition reflects their "gestalt" thinking process (4).

Prizant (3) described two types of echolalia. Immediate echolalia is defined as "the repetition of a word or phrase just spoken by another person." Immediate echolalia can serve a communicative purpose to initiate or maintain an interaction. When asked if the child wants a cookie, the child may request the cookie by repeating the last word produced, i.e., "cookie." Immediate echolalia may also be noninteractive and serve as an aid to process the information to facilitate understanding or to help the children move through an activity.

Delayed echolalia is defined as "echoing of a phrase after some delay or lapse of time." People who use delayed echolalia have been observed to repeat scripts from television shows, movies, or videos, or even parental reprimands (i.e., "Don't do that."). Prizant identified 14 possible functions of delayed echolalia (3). As noted in immediate echolalia, delayed echolalia can be purposeful or noninteractive. The key to understanding the purpose of delayed echolalia lies in the listener's familiarity with the child's idiosyncratic use of verbalizations and past experience with the child's language patterns.

IV. LANGUAGE DISTURBANCES

As children with ASD acquire novel language, their comprehension remains concrete and their expressive language may be limited to single words. Regulation of behavior is often achieved by naming or labeling objects as a form of request. If a child wants milk, then a child with emergent language may communicate through a single utterance: "milk." The listener has the burden of interpreting the child's intent. The young child may advance to spontaneous sentences, with frequent mistakes in grammar and vocabulary.

Children with ASD often confuse pronouns. They generally substitute "You" for "I." An individual with ASD may say, "You want train," instead of "I want the toy train." Pronoun reversal is one of the most difficult errors to correct. Children with ASD may avoid using pronouns altogether and refer to themselves by their proper name.

Semantic weakness is evident. Children communicating at the single-word level may confuse words (i.e., brush/comb), while children who are at a higher language level have difficulty understanding and using words with multiple meanings (i.e., There is a fork in the road). Pivot words (i.e., the, in, on, before, because) do not have meaning for these children and they may leave them out altogether, resulting in messages that sound telegraphic (i.e., Matthew go store).

Children with semantic and grammatical weakness often process information partially. They have a tendency to reply to one or two words in the question or direction and ignore the rest of the statement. When asked, "Bring mom the book on the chair in the kitchen," a child with processing deficits may bring a chair rather than the book.

A major characteristic of children with ASD is their literal interpretation of language. These children may respond seriously to teasing as they have little to no understanding of jokes or sarcasm. Verbal children with autism may be excessively verbose, posing the same question over and over again. They have a preoccupation with the verbal exchange rather than the content of the conversation and insensitivity to the nonverbal cues of boredom displayed by the listener. They lack role taking and have poor perception of the listener and the listener's needs.

V. NONVERBAL COMMUNICATION

Children who are acquiring language normally understand gestures, facial expressions, and bodily movements that accompany the speech of those with whom they interact. Children who immigrate to a new country will rely on nonverbal cues rather than the content of the unfamiliar language to make sense of the communicative intent. Even children with a language disorder will be able to recognize the emotions expressed by a person or understand the intent of a finger pointing into the distance.

Children with high-functioning autism or AS do not readily acknowledge or understand the nonverbal clues. Children with AS have difficulty recognizing emotions and may not be able to interpret the meaning and clues that come from facial expressions or natural gestures.

Expressively, individuals with ASD may use unconventional forms of nonverbal communication. They may grab, pull, or reach to gain desired objects. Their ability to point to a desired object is delayed, if present at all. Simple gestures that are noted in children under the age of 18 months, including nodding and shaking the head, may or may not develop in children with autism.

VI. DISORDERED PROSODY

Many children with ASD have odd intonation, characterized by monotonous or inappropriate inflection. Monotone speech is described as an utterance consisting of successive words, without change in pitch or key. It has been reported that infants who are later diagnosed with ASD often babble without inflection. Speech differences also include atypical use of loudness. While many children tend to speak too loud, there are others who communicate in barely audible speech. Their voices sound mechanical and have a robot-like quality. In addition, they may self-stimulate through vocalizations (high-frequency sounds, glottal Fry, buccal sounds).

Shriberg et al. studied children with high-functioning autism and AS. From their findings they concluded that children with ASD displayed differences in articulation and inappropriate prosody in the areas of phrasing, stress, and resonance (5).

VII. FEEDING DISORDERS

Parents of children with ASD often complain that their children are very picky eaters. These children are overly selective in their choice of foods and will not taste foods shared by other members of the family. Idiosyncratic differences in processing of tactile, auditory, olfactory, proprioceptive, and visual information are common in children with ASD and may be the basis of food selectivity. Children who are hypersensitive to touch may react negatively and emotionally when offered food. They may be unable to tolerate the food inside their mouth, where touch may trigger a tonic bite reflex or a hypersensitive gag response. These children may develop feeding aversions as a way of protecting themselves from the negative feelings. Aversions include negative responses to specific textures, tastes, smells, and temperatures of foods, and the children may avoid eating. Ahearn et al. evaluated 30 individuals with ASD or PDD-NOS who had a history of aberrant feeding patterns (6). More than half of the participants exhibited low overall levels of food acceptance, while several individuals refused all food presented.

VIII. ASSESSMENT

The Quality Standards Subcommittee of the American Academy of Neurology and the Child Neurology Society issued a report outlining the parameters for both the screening and diagnosis of ASD (7). While it is recommended that every child have a comprehensive hearing evaluation, a speech and language evaluation is recommended if babbling and gesturing have not emerged by 12 months, if there is a loss of language or social skills, if true words do not emerge by 15 months, and if two-word combinations are not observed by 24 months. The American Academy of Pediatrics (AAP) issued a technical report on the pediatrician's role in the diagnosis and management of ASD children (8). Their recommendations included the need to monitor developmental milestones, especially in the areas of speech, language, and social skills, and to elicit parental concerns.

Once the early signs of ASD have been recognized, the speech pathologist should be asked to evaluate the core deficits associated with ASD—social interaction, communication and play, and behaviors—in detail. In addition to a hearing evaluation, an oral motor speech assessment, feeding evaluation, and speech/phonological assessment should be included in the battery of tests. Rating scales and checklists such as Autism Diagnostic Interview–revised (ADI-R) (9) and the Communication and Symbolic Behavior Scales (CSBS) (10) can be incorporated into a comprehensive assessment. The former is for use in both children and adults, while the latter was specifically designed to meet the assessment needs of children with ASD. Each of these tools requires considerable training to ensure reliability.

Direct observation of social behavior, communication, and play in children suspected of having autism may be made using standardized tools such as the Autism Diagnostic Observation Schedule (ADOS) (11), the Pre-Linguistic Autism Diagnostic Observation Schedule (PL-ADOS) (12), and the ADOS-G (13). ADOS and ADOS-G are observational scales used for children and adults, while the PL-ADOS (12) serves as a downward extension of the ADOS to evaluate nonverbal young children. The ADOS-G is a semistructured assessment of social interaction, communication, play, and imaginative use of materials to evaluate individuals with ASD across their life span.

The CSBS model (10) evaluates children in seven areas of pragmatic function. It looks at a child's ability to respond with emotion and establish eye contact during interactions. It examines a child's ability to use language to regulate the behavior of others, to interact socially, and to establish joint attention. Use of natural gestures, sounds, words, and objects is evaluated, along with a child's understanding of words.

A. Background Information

Prior to an assessment, it is necessary to obtain as much background information as possible. Parents serve as the primary source of information about a child's communication, play, and behavior in the first 2 years of life. Parent recollections can be enhanced with a review of videotapes taken over the course of the 2 years. Information pertaining to use of natural gestures, social eye gaze, understanding of the spoken word, and vocalizations may be analyzed prior to an assessment.

B. Social Communication

Evaluation of a child's social use of language is central to an assessment of communication in ASD. Informal and formal tools are available to evaluate a child's conversational skills, ability to share information, and ability to understand contextual cues.

The *Test of Pragmatic Language* (TOPL) is the only evaluation devoted specifically to the assessment of language pragmatics. It is used for children 5–13 years of age (14).

The *Prutting Pragmatic Protocol* is a descriptive taxonomy of 30 pragmatic parameters (i.e., variety of speech acts, topic selection, topic introduction, topic maintenance) rated according to whether they are used "appropriately" or "inappropriately" or "not observed" (15).

The *Checklist of Communicative Function and Means* is an evaluation of a child's intent gained through a natural play setting (16). Wetherby and Prizant identified communicative functions that a child uses to interact, especially when language is limited (17). A child's earliest use of language is to regulate the behavior of others. Conventional means of protest would include shaking the head "no" or stating "no." A child may gesture his intention by pushing an object away or averting eye gaze. Nonconventional means include loud vocalizations, having tantrums, and aggressive behaviors. Social interaction is a higher communicative behavior. A child will use social interactions to call attention by stating "look." The child may seek information by asking "what's that," interact through greeting, request permission by stating "please," and show off. The most defining area of social communication is the establishment of joint attention. Children use joint attention to comment, request information, and provide information about past events.

C. Receptive and Expressive Language Testing

A number of published measures are available to evaluate the children's understanding and use of language. These evaluate either receptive and/or expressive language development, but do not rule in or rule out a diagnosis of autistic spectrum disorder. The results will give specific information as to the level of language comprehension and use that the child possesses.

Language skills are measured by tasks of increasing complexity within the receptive and expressive domains. These tests assess specific aspects of a child's understanding and use of vocabulary, grammar, and syntax. These published assessments are merely a sampling of testing available.

The *Infant/Toddler Checklist for Communication and Language Development* is a checklist designed to identify different aspects of development in children and in toddlers (15). This checklist was designed for a caregiver to complete for children between the ages of 6 and 24 months to determine whether or not a referral for a comprehensive assessment is needed.

The *Infant Toddler Language Scale* is a criterion-referenced evaluation designed to assess receptive and expressive language development, play, natural gestures, and pragmatics of children from birth through 36 months (18).

The *Reynell Developmental Language Scale (RDLS)* is a measure of a child's development in receptive and expressive language areas. The scale evaluates children from 1 to 7 years of age. It provides qualitative and quantitative information into expressive language and verbal comprehension. This test was developed to evaluate children suspected of having a language delay (19).

The *Preschool Language Scale–Fourth Edition* (PLS-4) (English and Spanish) evaluates children from birth to 6 years, 11 months of age. The PLS-4 is comprised of two subscales assessing receptive and expressive language. The assessment includes the precursors to language development, comprehension, and use of vocabulary and grammar. It assesses the child's ability to process complex sentences and communicate over successive statements (20).

The *Oral and Written Language Scales* is a standardized tool designed to evaluate children ranging from 3.0 to 21.11 years of age. This assessment, accompanied by visual cues, was designed to evaluate an individual's understanding and use of spoken language (21).

The *Expressive One-Word Picture Vocabulary Test* is a picture-naming test that evaluates a children's vocabulary on the single-word level. This evaluation was developed to assess the word retrieval skills of children aged 2.0–18.11 years (22).

D. Play

A child's cognitive, nonlinguistic abilities are often evaluated through play. The goal of the play assessment is to determine whether the child is able to use objects for truly imaginative play or is just preoccupied by unusual aspects of objects. Is the play repetitive and stereotyped?

Westby described 10 stages in the development of symbolic play abilities. The *Symbolic Play Scale* evolved from a Piagetian model (23).

Between the ages of 9 and 12 months (Stage I), the child is developing object permanence and will find a toy if it is hidden under a scarf.

Between 13 and 17 months (Stage II), the child explores a toy, operates it by pulling levers and strings, and will attempt to act upon it by pushing, pulling, turning, and pounding. The child will hand a toy to an adult if unable to operate independently.

Between 17 and 19 months (Stage III), Westby identified the emergence of pretend skills. The child may pretend to go to sleep, drink from a cup, or eat from a spoon. At this age level, true language is emerging and a marked growth occurs in the number of words that a child uses.

By 19–22 months (Stage IV), the child extends the symbolism beyond him or herself to include the caregiver or a doll. The child may feed the doll, brush the doll's hair, or put the doll in the bed.

By 24 months (Stage V), the child will represent his daily experiences through play. The child plays house and takes on roles. A true sequence of events has not emerged.

By $2\frac{1}{2}$ years (Stage VI), the child begins to represent events less frequently experienced. The child may pretend to be the doctor and take care of a sick child. The child continues to play alongside his peers; however, associative play appears.

By the age of 3 (Stage VII), the child's actions have a sequence (i.e., the doctor checks the patient, calls the ambulance, takes the patient to the hospital).

By $3\frac{1}{2}$ years (Stage VIII), the child is less dependent on realistic toys such as a dollhouse, farm, parking garage. He is more interested in using blocks for building and will use one object to represent another.

At approximately 4 years of age (Stage IX), the child is able to hypothesize about future events and *problem-solve* events he has not experienced. Dolls and puppet play becomes more elaborate and is used to resolve issues regarding "what would happen if."

By the final stage of play at age 5 (Stage X) reflects the child's ability to plan out pretend situations in advance. The child gives roles to himself and to the other children and full cooperative play emerges.

E. Articulation and Oral-Motor Skills

Difficulties with articulation or specific oral-motor difficulties should be assessed when appropriate. An oral-motor-sensory feeding assessment ought to be completed if the child is nonverbal or if the child's speech production is highly unintelligible. This evaluation ought to determine whether or not the speech difficulties are associated with a verbal dyspraxia, a motor planning speech disorder often noted in children with ASD. A number of published evaluations are available to evaluate a child's speech production on the single-word and sentence levels based on a phonological, articulation, or motor planning approaches to assessment.

IX. INTERVENTION

A. Play

Play is a free-choice activity that is self-motivated, enjoyable, process-oriented, and not literal. The materials, time, and roles of the "players" are made up by the children. Children play because they like it. They do not play for praise, food, money, or rewards.

Motor play helps the brain to develop gross and fine muscles, nerves, and brain functions.

Social play encourages learning to give and take, cooperation, and sharing. The children use play to learn to use moral reasoning and values.

Constructive play encourages children to manipulate their environment. Building cities with blocks and making castles in the sand are forms of constructive play.

Fantasy play helps the children to try out new roles, rehearse a variety of possible situations, and experience language and emotions.

Teaching a child to play games with rules is helpful in addressing turn taking, social interaction, and learning to play by the rules imposed by another. Games with rules teach children a very important concept—we all must follow rules.

B. Social Language

Children with ASD benefit from intervention that teaches specific social goals. The role of the speech pathologist is to identify the complex social behavior (i.e., conversation) and analyze the prerequisite behaviors and rules that can be memorized and practiced in a variety of settings. Several models and interventions have proven to be quite effective in addressing the social communication and language needs of young and older children with ASD.

1. SCERTS Model

The social communication, emotional regulation, and transactional support (SCERTS) model was developed by Wetherby and Prizant as a tool to enhance the communication and social emotional development in young children on the autistic spectrum (24). This model addresses the challenges and issues at each level of language development—including prelinguistic, emergent language, early language, and the more advanced language stage—through an individualized and developmental approach.

2. Social Stories

Social stories, developed by Gray and Garand, is a technique used to teach a critical component of social interactions (25). Its development was based on the understanding that children and adults with ASD are impaired in their ability to consider the perspective of others. The intention of the social stories is to help the person with ASD to learn strategies to interact in a variety of social situations. These stories can be tailored to meet the individual needs of the person for whom the story is written. The stories can be used to teach children social routines (i.e., greeting a new person), how to ask for help, and how to respond to their feelings. Social stories are considered an effective tool to teach children social skills and how to make sense of social situations.

3. Teach Me Language

Teach Me Language, by Freeman and Dake, identifies and helps to teach speech and language concepts to children on the autistic spectrum, including AS (26). This book was designed to meet the specific needs of children with ASD with ABA teaching techniques. It is most effective for children who perceive visually presented information better than orally presented information. The children must be able to communicate in some way, either verbally or through total communication.

C. Speech Production

Therapy to address speech production is dependent on the diagnosis of the speech disorder, whether the problem is due to an apraxia (motor planning disorder) or a dysarthria (speech disorder), or even a phonological disorder (linguistic basis). Many children with ASD experience motor planning speech disorders.

Traditional articulation therapy is useful for teaching a child to produce one sound at a time in isolation until he or she can master this sound. Once the child masters the sound, the therapist will increase the complexity of the word until the child can produce this sound on the sentence and conversational levels. However, this approach does not address the significant obstacles presented by a child with a motor planning disorder/apraxia or muscular weakness/dysarthria.

The preferred approach for treating children with verbal apraxia is to focus on the motor movements in sequence for the production of a meaningful word. The therapy will start with sounds already in the child's phonemic repertoire and use these sounds to increase the consistency of sound production in a variety of syllables and words. For example, a child with apraxia may have learned to produce the "o" sound; however, the child will state "apa" instead of "open." The goal of the therapy is to patiently repeat the sound in varying words and word combinations and provide the child the opportunity to practice and repractice until the new sounds are integrated.

Tactile cueing is an essential technique in working with children with motor planning disorders. PROMPT (prompts for restructuring oral muscular phonetic targets) is a cueing technique developed by Hayden (27). Using tactile-kinesthetic-proprioceptive cues, a speech pathologist using the PROMPT method would restructure the speech production output of children and adults with speech disorders. The input presented to the individual helps the individual achieve voluntary control of the motor speech system as he or she begins to integrate the motor, cognitive-linguistic, and social-emotional aspects of communication. The cues, which are applied externally to the muscles of the face and the mylohyoid muscle under the chin, nose, and jaw, help to reshape sounds on the individual (i.e., "a"), syllable (i.e., "ma"), word (i.e., mom, mommy), phrase (i.e., my mommy), and sentence levels. As the length of the word increases, the child who has an emergent speech system benefits from the hands-on cues to stimulate the articulatory movements. As the child integrates the correct sequence of movements to achieve speech sound production, the hand cues are faded.

Speech disorders due to muscular involvement are best addressed through an oral motor program. The children with a dysarthria will demonstrate weakness through the jaw, tongue, lips, cheeks, and soft palate. This weakness will affect all motor speech processes, including breathing, sound production, articulation, resonance, and the prosody (melody) of speech.

D. Feeding Issues

Feeding issues tend to have both a motor and sensory basis. As noted, children with feeding issues often have hypersensitivities and specific food preferences. A team approach is recommended, comprised of the parent, teacher, occupational therapist, and speech pathologist. A physical therapist may be part of the team in the case of children with a neuromuscular disorder.

Interventions utilize techniques to normalize sensory defensiveness and aversive responses to tactile, auditory, and olfactory stimulation. Calming music, oral stimulation of the tongue, lips, and facial region, an explanation of expectations, and graded modifications in texture and temperature can be presented as techniques to help reduce oral hypersensitivity.

E. Total Communication

A total communication approach with children with ASD would provide a range of effective and accessible means available to communicate including alternative and augmentative systems. Speech, when available, provides an effective and accessible means for children to communicate, but augmentative systems may be necessary for children who are preverbal and are experiencing difficulty in acquiring speech. These systems encourage the children to communicate without precluding the acquisition of verbalizations. Research suggests that the use of alternative communication systems actually promotes the development of more complex skills (28).

Augmentative and alternative communication (AAC) and assistive technology (AT) are used to provide new communication possibilities for the children who are nonverbal and when speech is not an effective means of communication. A wide variety of products are available, ranging from a device that has a few words to more sophisticated devices that are programmable to include an individualized vocabulary of pictures and/or written words.

The picture exchange communication system (PECS) developed by Frost and Bondy, uses drawing to help young children with severe speech disorders to communicate. PECS uses pictures to convey words and concepts (29).

Sign language is a viable intervention when working with nonverbal or apraxic/dysarthric children until language emerges. It involves introducing natural gestures along with oral language to build communication skills.

X. CONCLUSION

On November 12, 2002, Ms. Polly Morrice wrote about her struggle with autism in *The New York Times* (30). Her son, who was 11 years at the time of this op-ed article, was diagnosed with ASD and enrolled in a specialized preschool program at the age of 3. She described autism as a "window-of-opportunity disorder," which she elaborated by stating that "the earlier in a child's life you intervene to adjust the faulty neural wiring that causes it, the better the outcome." According to many clinical practice guidelines developed by experts, such as the *Clinical Practice Guideline–Autism/Pervasive Developmental Disorders: Assessment and Intervention for Young Children (Ages 0–3 years)* supported by the New York State Early Intervention Program, treatment is most effective when intensive training is provided to young children (31). Although the applied behavioral analysis program, similar to the intervention developed by Lovaas, has been endorsed by some of these guidelines, including the New York State guidelines, other models, such as Greenspan's floor time (32) may be effective if applied early and intensely. Each of these interventions encourages the integration of a speech pathology component in a comprehensive program.

REFERENCES

1. Osterling J, Dawson G. Early recognition of children with autism: a study of first birthday home videotapes. J Autism Dev Disord 1994; 24:247–257.
2. Strand E. Treatment of motor speech disorders in children. Semin Speech Lang 1995; 16:126–139.
3. Prizant BM. Language acquisition and communicative behavior in autism: toward an understanding of the "whole" of it. J Speech Hear Disord 1983; 48:296–307.
4. Grandin T. Thinking in Pictures: and other Reports from My Life with Autism. New York: Doubleday, 1995.
5. Shriberg LD, Rhea P, McSweeny JL. Speech and Prosody characteristics of adolescents and children with high-functioning autism and Asperger syndrome. J Speech Lang Hear Res 2001; 44:1097–1115.
6. Ahearn WH, Catine T, Nault K, Green G. An assessment of food acceptance in children with autism or pervasive developmental disorder—not otherwise specified. J Autism Dev Disord 2001; 3:505–511.
7. Filipek PA, et al. Practice parameter: screening and diagnosis of autism, report on the Quality Standards Subcommittee of the American Academy of Neurology and the Child Neurology Society. Neurology 2000; 55:468–479.
8. Committee on Children with Disabilities, American Academy of Pediatrics. Technical report: the pediatrician's role in the diagnosis and management of autistic spectrum disorder in children. Pediatrics 2001; 107:1–18.
9. Lord C, Rutter M, Le Couteur A. Autism diagnostic interview–revised: a revised version of a diagnostic interview for caregivers of individuals with possible pervasive developmental disorders. J Autism Dev Disord 1994; 24:659–685.

10. Wetherby AM, Prizant BM. Communication and Symbolic Behavior Scales Developmental Profile (CSBS DP). Baltimore, MD: Paul H. Brooks Publishing Co. Inc., 2002.
11. Lord C, Rutter M, Goode S, Heemsbergen J, Jordan H, Mawhood L, Schopler E. Autism diagnostic observation schedule: a standardized observation of communicative and social behavior. J Autism Dev Disord 1989; 19:185–212.
12. DiLavore PC, Lord C, Rutter M. The pre-linguistic autism diagnostic observation schedule. J Autism Dev Disord 1995; 25:355–379.
13. Lord C, Risi S, Lambrecht L, Cook EH Jr, Leventhal BL, DiLavore PC, Pickles A, Rutter M. The autism diagnostic observation schedule-generic: a standard measure of social and communication deficits associated with the spectrum of autism. J Autism Dev Disord 2000; 30:205–223.
14. Phelps-Terasaki D, Phelps-Gunn T. Test of Pragmatic Language. Austin, TX: Pro-Ed, Inc., 1992.
15. Prutting CA, Kirchner DM. A clinical appraisal of the pragmatic aspects of language. J Speech Hear Disord 1987; 52:105–119.
16. Wetherby A, Prizant B. Infant/Toddler checklist for communication and language development. Appl Symbolix, Langley, B.C., Canada: SKF Books, 1998.
17. Wetherby A, Prizant B. Profiling young children's communicative competence. In: Warren S, Reichle J, eds. Causes and Effects in Communication and Language Intervention. Baltimore, MD: Paul Brookes, 1990; 217–251.
18. Rossetti LM. Infant Toddler Language Scale. East Moline, IL: Linguisystems, Inc., 1990.
19. Reynell JK. Reynell Developmental Language Scale. Wood Dale, IL: Stoelting Co., 2001.
20. Zimmerman I, Steiner V, Evatt Pond R. Preschool Language Scale–Fourth Edition. San Antonio, TX: Psychological Corporation, 2001.
21. Carrow Woolfolk E. Oral and Written Language Scales. Circle Pines, MN: American Guidance Service, 1995.
22. Gardner M. Expressive One-Word Picture Vocabulary Test. Novato, CA: Academic Therapy Publications, 2000.
23. Westby C. Language abilities through play. Lang Speech Hear Serv Schools, 1980; XI: 154–168.
24. Wetherby A, Prizant B. SCERTS model. Presented in Conference by Wetherby and Prizant, August 2000, Providence, RI.
25. Gray C, Garand JD. Social stories: improving responses of students with autism with accurate social information. Focus Autist Behav 1993; 8:1–10.
26. Freeman S, Dake L. Teach Me Language. Langley, B.C., Canada: SKF Books, 1996/1997: 26.
27. Hayden D. The PROMPT System — Therapeutic Intervention Hierarchy, August 1994.
28. Kangas KA, Lloyd L. Early cognitive skills as prerequisites to augmentative and alternative communication use: what are we waiting for? Augment Altern Commun 1998; 4:211–221.
29. Bondy A, Frost L. The picture exchange communication system. Focus Autist Behav 1994; 9:1–19.

30. Morrice P. Few options for treating autism. New York Times, November 2002.
31. Autism/Pervasive Developmental Disorders Guideline Panel. Clinical practice guideline – autism/pervasive developmental disorders: assessment and intervention for young children (Ages 0–3 years). Clinical Practice Guideline No. 1, NYDOH. Albany: New York State Department of Health, Early Intervention Program, 1999.
32. Greenspan SI, Wider S. Developmental patterns and outcomes in infants and children with disorders in relating and communicating: a chart review of 200 cases of children with autistic spectrum diagnoses. J Dev Learning Disord 1997; 1:87–141.

10

Sensory Integration and Occupational Therapy Intervention for Autistic Spectrum Disorders

Patricia M. Stevens, Sallie Tidman, and Kari A. Glasgow
Children's Hospital, Richmond, Virginia, U.S.A.

I. INTRODUCTION

> I was destructive as a child. I drew all over the walls not once or twice, but anytime I got my hands on a pencil or crayon. I remember really "catching" it for peeing on the carpet. So the next time I had to go, instead of peeing on the carpet, I put the drape between my legs. I thought it would dry quickly and Mother wouldn't notice. Normal children use clay for modeling; I used my feces and then spread my creations all over the room. I chewed up puzzles and spit the cardboard mush out on the floor. I had a violent temper, and when thwarted, I'd throw anything handy—a museum quality vase or left-over feces. I screamed continually, responded violently to noise and yet appeared deaf on some occasions. (1)

The above quote graphically depicts the chaotic and overwhelming world of individuals with autism. The overt behaviors that occur because of this inner chaos can be daunting and overwhelming for parents, physicians, teachers, and all who come in contact with them. Occupational therapists believe that much of this behavioral chaos occurs because of a failure of individuals with autism to organize their sensory experiences, or sensory integration dysfunction (DSI). Sensory integration theory was developed over 50 years ago by a pioneering occupational therapist, A. Jean Ayres, while she was working with children with perceptual, learning, and behavioral problems of unknown etiology. She set out to examine how the brain processed sensations, not just sensations of the eyes and ears but other parts of the body as well (2). Ayers referred to sensory integration (SI) as "the organization of sensory input for use, through sensory integration, [of] the many parts of the nervous system [that] work together so that a person can interact with the environment effectively and experience appropriate satisfaction" (2). Carol Kranowitz broke down SI into four sequential steps: receiving, organizing, and using sensory information, and reacting to sensory information (3). Sensory information is picked up peripherally, and travels to the CNS for organization and planning. The reaction and execution is then carried out in the motor system. DSI occurs when sensory information is not processed, integrated, or organized properly in the brain, resulting in dysfunction of information processing, behavior, and the ability to meet the demands of the environment (3). DSI makes it hard for the child to learn from his/her experiences.

II. MAKING SENSE OF THE WORLD THROUGH THE SENSES

The five senses obtained via the sense organs of eyes, ears, mouth, hands, and nose are vision, auditory, gustatory, touch, and olfactory, respectively. These are often referred to as "far senses" because the input comes from outside one's body. SI also adds three "near senses," or hidden senses. These are tactile, vestibular, and proprioceptive. They are called hidden because the information comes from within one's body (3).

Tactile includes the sensations of touch, pressure, vibration, pain, and temperature, which we obtain through the skin all over the body. These sensations determine: Does the person like to be hugged, or shies away from a hugging, kissing relative? Does the person like to walk in the surf at the beach getting wet and sandy? Does the person have the label in the back of a shirt cut out because it is bothersome? What is the person's pain tolerance?

Vestibular is the sense that receives and responds to input from movement of the body and from changes in the head position. This information is received in the inner ear (3). Vestibular sense tells a person that he or she is moving—forward, backward, upward, or downward. It tells one how fast he or she is moving, or how slow he or she is moving. Vestibular sense tells one whether he or she is upright or upside down. It also tells one when his or her head is tilted or rotated looking at the horizon. The vestibular sense determines if a person is an amusement park thrill-ride seeker or the thought of a roller coaster makes him nauseous.

The last hidden sense is proprioception, or the internal "position sense." It tells us how the body and the body parts are positioned. This information comes from the muscles, ligaments, and joints. The brain registers when muscles are contracted or elongated; it also registers when the joints flex, extend, or when joint traction occurs (2). This sense determines if a child maintains an upright sitting posture at the table or shifts constantly, falling out of the chair.

The three basic senses, vestibular, proprioceptive, and tactile, are integral in developing a child's body perception, coordination of the two sides of the body, motor planning, activity level, attention span, and emotional stability. Along with the far senses, particularly vision and auditory, a child learns to make sense of his or her world (2). Children with autism fail to organize their sensory information. The inability to organize this information often leaves a person with autism appear highly reactive to sensory information. Temple Grandin's description of riding a spinning amusement ride is an excellent example of sensory organization:

> Frightened but dared, I bought a ticket for the ride and with trembling legs, walked up the few steps to enter the barrel. My heart in my mouth, I leaned against the side. The sound of the motor starting up sent a chill skittering down my spine. Then the "rotor" picked up speed and the motor sounded like a giant's hum. The colors of the blue sky, the white clouds, the yellow sun blended together like a spinning top. The smell of cotton candy, Karmel Corn and tacos swirled around individually until they too, combined into the carnival smell. Glued to the side of the barrel, I waited for the floor to drop out. Fear tasted bitter in my mouth and I tried to press harder against the side. With a creak on the hinges the floor opened to the ground below but now my senses were so overwhelmed with stimulation that I didn't react with anxiety or fear. I felt only the sensation of comfort and relaxation. (1)

III. PROCESS OF SENSORIMOTOR INTEGRATION

The process of sensorimotor integration includes the following elements.

A. Sensory Modulation

In a review of recent research literature, Wilbarger and Stackhouse (4) define modulation as "the intake of sensation via typical sensory processing mechanisms such that the intensity and quality of response are graded to match environmental demand and so that a range of optimal performance/adaptation is maintained." The human organism seeks to maintain a state of homeostasis, or sensory balance. Typical children can modulate their level of arousal and alertness to be able to attend to stimuli. They can regulate themselves to achieve, monitor, and change a state of attention that matches the demands of the environment. They can modulate a response in relation to the task required. They can discriminate and attend to selected stimuli (sensitization) and accommodate to the constant bombardment of stimuli in daily life (habituation). Modulation states can vary widely during a typical day in both the neurotypical and atypical child, depending on environment, stresses, and physiological needs (hunger, sleep).

Children with autistic spectrum disorder (ASD) demonstrate deficits of sensory modulation. As they function through the day, their regulation states may not match the level of intensity in a given situation. For example, the child may have completed the morning routine of waking, eating, dressing, and transitioning to school in a highly aroused state with very poor ability to focus on a visual motor activity requiring attending and inhibition of extraneous stimuli (auditory and tactile as well as emotional arousal). For this child to participate, he or she will need to modulate or bring his or her arousal state to a level of matching the environment. For the neurotypical child, this can be accomplished through following a set of routines and verbal and social cues to "settle down" and sit at a desk in the classroom. For the atypical child, the requirement to "settle down" has no context or strategy to accomplish. This child may need sensorimotor cues to ease the transition. It might well start with waking up with a deep pressure massage and followed by clothing that is less irritating to the skin. A breakfast with textures that provide proprioceptive input such as a chewy bagel and drinking through a straw may assist in regulating the arousal level. Once the child arrives at school, having a structured task involving controlled movement may again assist in regulation of activity level. The modulation problems include low registration of stimuli, hypo- and hyperresponse to stimuli, and sensory avoidance.

B. Sensory Discrimination

Sensory discrimination is the ability to differentiate between incoming stimuli based on prior experience to make meaningful adaptive responses. It provides the foundation for sorting and classifying information. It allows the individual to prioritize what information is important and what is not necessary at the moment. At the sensory level, this happens unconsciously. An easy example is all the auditory information received constantly (hums of electrical equipment, people talking, background music, etc.), and the ability to screen it all out, yet still be able to discern something unusual or important. Discrimination is necessary for both habituation and sensitization. It allows the individual to put multiple attributes to a sensory experience and integrate the information for further learning.

C. Motor Planning

Praxis, or motor planning, is the ability to conceive, organize, and execute an unfamiliar motor activity (2). It involves physically or mentally constructing the movement in a goal-directed manner. Adequate movement skills require proper postural mechanisms such as adequate muscle tone, balance, strength, and development of normal gross and fine motor skills. Motor planning itself involves ideation or generating an idea of the new movement and then executing it based on sensory information. The child with DSI will frequently demonstrate deficit in both the planning and execution of a movement.

IV. SENSORY ISSUES IN AUTISM

> A child can rarely describe his sensory experiences to others, for he has no internal baseline with which to compare them.—T. Berry Brazelton

A. Problems of Sensory Modulation

Lack of sensory modulation or inability to regulate arousal is a common observation in autism. Children with ASD are frequently in states of under- or overarousal in regard to incoming sensory input and reactivity to the demands of the environment. The various problems of sensory modulation are as follows.

1. Low Registration

The child appears to show dull affect with little interest in the external environment and requires a significant amount of stimulation to achieve an alerting response. Threshold or the amount or quality of stimulus required to have a CNS reaction is high (5).

2. Underresponsive

The child has a diminished perception of self as moving and interacting within his environment. He seeks sensations to remain alert, but has difficulty reaching an alert status because of impaired processing. He may appear to be very active and disorganized as he attempts to gain enough sensory input to organize self and respond; threshold is high.

3. Increased Registration

This results in poor ability to discriminate or select sensation to respond or process to habituate. A child demonstrates defensive behaviors to protect from incoming sensory information from the environment and may typically display "fight, fright, or flight" behaviors in response to environmental demands; threshold is low.

4. Hyperresponsive

Children with this behavior demonstrate overreaction or defensiveness to sensory input. Their motor responses are fearful, cautious, withdrawing, or aggressive and they may appear negative and angry.

B. Sensory Avoidance

The child avoids sensory input that is perceived as painful and overwhelming to the nervous system and develops routines and rituals to avoid external stimuli. Threshold is low (5).

C. Sensory Seeking

Self-stimulatory and self-injurious behaviors and constant motion fall into this category. Within the concept of threshold and habituation, the self-stimulating child may be seeking to meet the sensory need, but the arousal/threshold is not met and the behavior recurs. The child may also be seeking to extinguish unpleasant sensory or environmental stimuli by blocking them with stimuli that turn his or her attention inwardly. Extremes of seeking proprioceptive or vestibular stimulation may be observed with repeated pounding with the extremities, head banging, pushing, and seeking of deep pressure or "squeezing" (6). Temple Grandin and several others have reported relief with the "squeeze machine." Spinning and rocking are commonly seen as both alerting and calming for the child. Through the visual-vestibular connection, the child may also engage in seeking out the same sensory information through spinning toys and objects.

D. Sensory Defensiveness

This is a sensory disorder characterized by a "fight, flight, or fright" reaction to sensory stimulation most individuals would consider harmless. The nervous system does not adequately discriminate different sensory stimuli and responds in a survival mode: aggressive response, withdrawal from stimuli, rigid routines to avoid stimuli and maintain control over the environment, and other nonfunctional responses to the environment.

E. Tactile Defensiveness

This is commonly seen in DSI. The child may be irritated by clothes and may refuse to wear certain clothes. He or she may not like the texture of certain foods and may refuse to eat them. Socially the child may be seen as aggressive when he or she avoids contact with others or responds aggressively when touched unexpectedly. Self-care may be affected in terms of bathing, haircuts, and other grooming activities.

F. Auditory Defensiveness

This is an aversive reaction to sounds, common and unexpected. Sounds, such as a vacuum cleaner, a telephone ringing, or a timer on a stove, may be enough to disrupt the child, eliciting flight or withdrawal. Both sound intensity and pitch may disturb the child.

G. Visual Defensiveness

This includes hypersensitivity to light or avoidance of gaze. Busy visual environments may be overwhelming because of poor figure ground discrimination. The child may have difficulty in transitioning from indoor to outdoor because of the light sensitivity.

H. Oral Defensiveness

This child with ASD may refuse many foods because of oral defensiveness and may become more selective as he or she gets older instead of using a broad selection of foods. It may be difficult to clean the child's face after eating, creating a problem of hygiene. Olfactory defensiveness may also be present. Food selections in oral sensitivity may be based on taste and/or texture and it is important to note the taste and texture of preferred foods.

I. Gravitational Insecurity

This is a form of hyperresponsivity to vestibular sensations, particularly sensations from the otolith organs, which detect linear movement through space and the pull of gravity (2). The child may show an excessive fear to ordinary movement and is challenged by changes in head position and movement, particularly with head tilted back or up and down. The child may demonstrate intolerance to movement imposed or on an unstable surface. Movement through the environment is difficult and confusing for the child. The fear that the child feels is very real and impacts movement and balance.

J. Decreased Imitation

Children with autism have difficulty in imitating others. Imitation and development of praxis require adequate development of body awareness and kinesthetic processing. The sensory inputs from the tactile, proprioceptive, and vestibular systems all contribute to support motor skills. When the child is unable to plan a movement through imitation or receives faulty feedback from the movement he completes, his motor coordination is affected. Children with autism frequently have difficulty with initiating movements and performing goal-directed motor complex activities.

V. IMPACT OF SENSORY ISSUES

> Here's your hat, Temple... My ears felt as if they were being squashed together into one giant ear. The band of the hat pressed tightly around my head. I jerked the hat off and screamed. Screaming was the only way of telling Mother that I didn't want to wear the hat. It hurt. It smothered my hair.—Temple Grandin

Tasks of daily living can be very challenging for a child with ASD and his caregivers. Sensory processing and modulation disorder combined with language impairment make the routines of daily living a constant challenge. Frequently, the child falls into patterns of routines and unchanging rituals to self-regulate his day. By controlling the environment in this manner, the child can have an internalized set of expectations and outcomes with each activity. But when a new challenge or change in routine is introduced, the child lacks the ability to plan, compensate, or react in a meaningful manner to it.

Dressing can be a major issue for children with autism, especially as it relates to tactile processing. Abnormal reactions may relate to hypersensitivity or hyposensitivity. The hypersensitive child may refuse clothing altogether, or be very selective in terms of textures, tags, or clothing that is loosely touching the skin. The child does not become habituated to his perceived source of irritation and seeks constant relief from it. The hypersensitive child may also demonstrate a need to be covered on all extremities and body parts by layering of clothing. By layering and wrapping clothing tightly, the child is self-regulating and providing not only a protective barrier from touch, but deep pressure to inhibit irritating stimuli and calm him. The hyposensitive child requires significant amounts of stimuli for arousal and attention and seeks sensation. This child may tightly wrap clothing on his or her body and extremities or may not want to wear clothing to maximize the sensory input being received by the CNS.

Mealtimes also present significant issues in regard to sensory processing. Environmentally, the modulation required to regulate sounds, smells, and body position to stay at the table may present as a challenge. Decreased proprioceptive awareness in the hands to hold a utensil may result in finger feeding or passively waiting to be fed. The motor plan to scoop the spoon and bring it to the mouth, while maintaining the grasp, is a challenge for many of the children.

Visual as well as tactile food aversions are commonly seen. Children with autism may prefer certain food textures, may avoid foods that are multitextural (casseroles, cereal in milk, salads, or oranges, for example), may select foods that are all of similar textures (smooth, least resistive, less taste), and frequently may prefer foods that are savory and sharp over sweet (barbeque flavor, bacon, etc.).

Sensory processing and modulation impact daily routines and requirements. Transitions in arousal states begin with waking in the morning and progress throughout the day. Modulation is often on the high end of arousal and a small amount of sensory input can cause the child to react strongly and emotionally. From a sensory point of view, the child with autism seeks out the routine and ritual to decrease the amount of input and novelty the system needs to accommodate and act upon. Always walking against a wall and limiting food and clothing preferences decrease tactile input. Vestibular dysfunction is characterized by gravitational insecurity and decreased movement from place to place. The child may show extreme distress at a diaper change because of the head tilt and body movement imposed by lying the child down. Toilet training may become difficult as the child is perceiving fear of feet off the ground and the tactile and auditory sensations of the bathroom are overwhelming to the nervous system.

Rearranged furniture in a familiar room may cause an extreme reaction, as if the child has "lost" the visual motor plan of the room and is unable to recognize the room out of context. Without the ability to "reorganize" internally, the point of control becomes restoring the room to the familiar state.

Self-stimulatory and self-injurious behaviors may serve a sensory function to the child with autism (6). The behaviors frequently center on tactile, proprioceptive, and or vestibular input. The child may use these behaviors to alert and arouse or to assist with calming and blocking other, more aversive stimuli.

Children are frequently noted to engage in oral stimulation by mouthing nonfood items and hands, as well as extraoral stimulation with fabrics and light touch. Hands are frequently engaged in light touch patting and rubbing preferred textures and favorite items to hold. The self-seeking stimulation of this type often appears with the tactile defensive child, yet that is the child that who refuses touch imposed upon him or her. Once again, it appears to be an issue of controlling the sensory input. This child may also seek to rub and hug against a caregiver, but refuse reciprocation as a defensive measure. The extremes of this behavior may be seen in biting, hair pulling, and slapping. The hyporesponsive child may engage in extreme sensory-seeking behavior when in actuality, the child may be trying to produce sensation that he or she can perceive.

Proprioceptive self-stimulatory behaviors are seen in a variety of ways. Compressing and stretching the muscles over a joint gives the strong proprioceptive feedback the body is seeking to assist with muscle tone, body image, and regulation of movement effort. Flapping, jumping, slapping, and other movements that involve jarring of the joints give intense proprioceptive stimulation. Toe walking stretches the leg muscles, also giving the deep proprioceptive input. Frequently, oral behaviors such as hitting against the face, pulling against resistance with teeth, clenching teeth, and even guttural sounds are providing proprioceptive input to the child. The chewing gum industry has been aware of how people seek out this type of stimulation. The extremes of this sensation seeking may be seen in head butting and hitting against walls, biting oneself, and slapping and hitting oneself.

The focus of vestibular self-stimulation is responsively to head movement. Rocking the body, isolating head movements in linear movements, twirling, and spinning are all movements related to vestibular stimulation. The close association of visual-vestibular processing gives rise to the concept of using visual stimulation (watching spinning objects, finger flickering in the periphery) to arouse the vestibular system.

VI. ASSESSMENTS OF SENSORY ISSUES

SI issues are assessed by an occupational therapist through interviews and questionnaires, standardized tests, and formal and informal clinical observations.

A. Interviews and Questionnaires

During an evaluation the therapist will ask the caregiver about the child's difficulties to decide if the problems are sensory-related. For example, the child may have difficulty with tolerating a certain clothing fabric owing to tactile defensiveness. Interviewing the family provides the therapist with important medical history.

The Sensory Profile, developed by Dunn in 1999, is a standardized caregiver questionnaire, which assists therapists in measuring the sensory-processing abilities of children. The original profile was designed for ages 5–10. There are now, however, additional profiles available for infants, adolescents, and adults. The profile consists of 125 questions and is grouped into three categories: sensory processing, modulation, and behavioral and emotional responses. The caregiver fills in the questionnaire according to how often the behaviors occur (always, frequently, occasionally, seldom, never). The profile assists therapists in targeting the sensory processing issues affecting daily life (5).

Another questionnaire is the Sensory Integration Inventory–Revised: For Individuals with Developmental Disabilities. This questionnaire provides the same information for children and adults with developmental delays and disabilities and is based on observations of behavior patterns. It is divided into tactile, vestibular, proprioceptive, and general reactions. Information is gathered through interviewing familiar caregivers and uses clinical observations. Yes and no questions are asked and scored to provide the therapist with a profile as to the areas where there are difficulties that need to be targeted (6). Other questionnaires available include the Touch Inventory for Elementary School-aged Children (TIE) and behavior checklists for families and teachers.

B. Standardized Tests

Only a few standardized tests have been developed to test sensory integration specifically. It is important to evaluate fine motor, visual motor, and activities of daily living (ADL) skills because sensory issues affect everyday life and skills. The following section will comment on several of the available tests.

The Sensory Integration Praxis Tests (SIPT) is one of the main standardized tests used to evaluate sensory dysfunction. It contains 17 subtests, which measure tactile, vestibular, and proprioceptive sensory processing; visuomotor perception (including position in space); motor planning; and bilateral and sequencing skills. This test takes $2\frac{1}{2}$ hr to administer and score but it can be broken into sections and administered separately (7).

A sensory test for younger children is the Test of Sensory Functions in Infants (TSFI). It can be administered in 20 min. It is for ages 4–18 months and will assist with children who are at risk for developing sensory issues later. DeGangi-Berk and Berk also developed the TSI, which is the DeGangi-Berk Test of Sensory Integration, and is for children 3–5 years of age. This test requires 30 min to administer.

Testing of fine motor skills can be completed using the Peabody Developmental Motor Scales–Second Edition (PDMS-2) or the Bruninks-Oseretsky Test of Motor Proficiency, depending on the age of the child. The PDMS-2 tests children from birth to 72 months of age in gross motor (reflexes, locomotion, bilateral coordination) and fine motor skills (grasping and visual motor integration). It requires approximately an hour for administration and scoring (8). The Bruninks test is for ages 4–17, and tests gross motor and fine motor skills (response speed, bilateral coordination, upper-limb speed and dexterity, and visual motor coordination). This test requires $1\frac{1}{2}$ hours, but can be broken into sections (9).

Other tests include the Beery-Buktenica Developmental Test of Visual-Motor Integration (VMI). This test is administered quickly and can be interpreted in three components: visual motor integration, visual integration, and motor skills. The age range is 3–18 years and a short form is available that can be used with children up to 8 years (10). The Developmental Test of Visual Perception–2 (DVPT-2) is for ages 4–10 years. It measures visual perceptual skills through eight subtests (eye-hand coordination, position in space, copying, figure-ground, spatial relations, visual closure, visual-motor speed, form constancy). It can be administered in sections and the time frame can range from 30 min to 1 hr (11).

Evaluation of ADL skills is mostly completed through clinical observation and interview. Areas addressed include: grooming, dressing of the upper and lower body, and toileting. A therapist will want to know how much assistance is needed in each area and will determine if the abilities of the child are age-appropriate.

C. Clinical Observations

Clinical observations can be completed in several settings including the home, a clinic, or any other natural environment for the child. Observations include play skills and interactions with objects in the environment, muscle tone, reflex integration, and strength.

VII. INTERVENTIONS

> i want to go on with the therapy as long as planned
> and i want to go on with the music
> it is calming and smoothes my nerves
> it is a feeling of gentle peace internal warmth and a place
> free of anxiety like i never knew before.—Berger Sellin (12)

Guiding principles of sensory integration therapy include:

Controlled sensory input can be used to elicit an adaptive response.
Registration of meaningful sensory input is necessary before an adaptive response can be made.
An adaptive response contributes to the development of sensory integration.
More mature and complex patterns of behavior are composed of consolidations of more primitive behaviors.
The more inner-directed a child's activities are, the greater the potential of the activities for improving neural organization (4).

Occupational therapy intervention often involves activities that incorporate sensory activities based on proprioceptive and vestibular input. Use of suspended equipment such as swings and trapeze can provide a variety of movement experiences in the different planes of movement. Vestibular input is a strong sensory input that has potential to affect arousal states (2), as the receptors are located in the inner ear. For the child who needs intense stimulation secondary to low registration and high threshold, engaging in movement on a circular or orbital plane may assist in arousing. Conversely, moving in a linear, slow plane of movement may calm and focus the child who is operating at an increased arousal level. But not all intervention requires swings or other suspended equipment. Assisting the child to move using scooter boards, changing running speed, and movement through complex motor skills can also assist with integration of sensation.

A key concept in therapy is providing structured input to organize the nervous system. Proprioceptive input has a strong effect on modulation. Trampolines and other equipment that provide deep pressure to the joints are frequently used to provide input to promote sensory stimulation. Many of the repetitive or self-stimulatory behaviors seen in autism have a basis in proprioception-seeking behaviors. By increasing the amount and duration of varied input, the need for this type of behavior can be decreased.

To provide a program of vestibular-proprioceptive input, the program must be structured to meet the child's sensory needs and be flexible to meet the child's changing status. Occupational therapy begins with finding the child's arousal state and establishing the child's sensory responsiveness. Challenge to motor skills and modulation is ongoing and toward the goal of increasing tolerance for the changing environment and the child's ability to make an adaptive response. A "sensory diet" is frequently set up with the family. This refers to evaluating a child's day and keying into those times and activities that appear to be most disruptive for the child. Evaluating whether incorporating a sensory component into that activity would assist with completion, as well as increase the learning potential for the child, is one of the roles of the occupational therapist. As an example, a bedtime routine is frequently a challenge for families. The child may be in a state of overarousal and unable to stay in bed or sleep. The sequence of events prior to bedtime may be examined and evaluated with the parents. A typical experience may be that the child has been free-playing until bedtime. The parent tries to make the child brush his teeth, wash, change into nightclothes, and settle with a book to sleep. However, the child is not at a place where transition to sleep can be easily accomplished. Changing the routines to have a time to brush teeth (a high-arousal activity), then providing deep proprioceptive input, slow vestibular input (slow movement in a glider-rocker chair, wrapup in bath towels), and evaluating the sleep area (use of weighted blanket or sleeping bag) may assist with the transition. A sensory diet is an ongoing evaluation of the child's status and must be flexible. It requires task analysis from the therapist and the family for it to be successful.

Other interventions focus on tactile and oral processing. The defensive behaviors discussed previously are responsive to touch pressure as well as increasing discrimination. Slow exposure to tactile experience and acceptance of input is often the focus of therapy. Setting up the environment to support the child's ability to integrate sensory experience is essential for a successful experience. Oral motor and feeding issues involve motor planning. A child with ASD may not be able to plan the movements of bringing food to the mouth, chewing, and swallowing. Tactile and visual aversions to food may be present. To be successful in promoting good nutrition, the therapist requires a good understanding of the child's sensory status and needs to use a sensory model within the context of a behavioral model.

Interventions include providing the opportunity to increase body awareness and giving proprioceptive and tactile inputs for the body to recognize where it is in relation to position in space. Incorporating sensory motor stimulation in a directed manner assists in the development of motor skills, because successful motor planning requires adequate sensory processing. The therapist teaches motor planning and sequential motor skills so that the child is able to perform complex motor skills and react in a functional manner to novel motor requirements.

VIII. TIPS FOR PARENTS

Tables 1–6 were developed by occupational therapists from Children's Hospital in Richmond, Virginia to give ideas for sensory activities for children with autism. For the best results, these should be tailored to a child's individual needs by a therapist and should be incorporated into home and school routines. The tables include various supports and activities in areas such as proprioceptive, tactile, vestibular, visual, auditory, and oral-motor sensory. Proprioceptive sensory support involves using sustained moderate to deep pressure on total body or major joints for calming. Tactile sensory support includes using slow, moderate to deep skin depression for calming influence, as well as using a variety of various textured and temperature items or substances to engage a child in activities. Vestibular sensory support involves the use of slow, predictable linear movement in horizontal or vertical direction as a calming influence. Visual sensory support entails using visual input as a calming influence or to engage a child in activities. Auditory sensory supports include the use of low-volume and low-frequency rhythmic sounds as a calming influence. Finally, oral-motor sensory support can be used to calm or alert.

IX. INTEGRATING OCCUPATIONAL THERAPY AND SENSORY INTEGRATION THERAPY INTO A LARGER AUTISM PROGRAM

Integrating an occupational therapy and sensory integration therapy program into a larger autism program can take many forms. A child can receive occupational therapy services on a regular basis: weekly, twice weekly, or monthly. Or the child may receive regular weekly therapy for a few months, then carry over at

Table 1 Proprioceptive Activities

Alerting	Calming	Other
Perform large body movements, such as climbing, pushing, pulling, and crossing obstacles, before sitting down to do hand activities	Push-and-pull activities: push and pull partner on swings, push and pull large objects around house and school, push and pull while both people are sitting facing each other holding hands with arms extended, push and pull balls, hula hoops	Swaddling activities: wrap up in futon mattress like a taco, use foam mats, comforters, or futon mattresses as tunnels or people sandwiches
	Playing "Simon Says" to walk like animals (bear walk on all fours, rabbit hop), or to push floor with arms, or push feet against wall	To release energy: jumping on trampoline, bed mattress, into piles of pillows, or beanbag chairs, and bouncing on inflated balls
	Wearing a weighted vest, hat, shoes, or put weights in pants/jacket pockets, wearing heavy clothes, wearing a weighted backpack or fanny pack	
	Napping or sleeping with heavy comforters or a weighted blanket	
	Before school or during transitions provide deep pressure to joints by pushing on joints in a steady firm manner 5–10 times (shoulders, elbows, wrists, hips, knees, ankles, fingers, feet)	

Table 2 Tactile Activities

Alerting	Calming	Other
Use vibrating toys, Vibrating Bugs, or electric toothbrushes, and attach small vibrators to other objects you want the child to play with	Slow massage with deep pressure touch: can use calming scented lotions (lavender, sandalwood; to include olfactory sensory input)	Use weighted crayons, pencils, or vibrating toys to draw in resistive clay, putty, sand, Ziploc bag filled with hair-styling gel, or construction paper.
Use a loofah sponge during bathtime and include different-textured toys in bath	Use a brushing program before transitioning to new or potentially stressful activities (dressing, bathing) and then give deep pressure to joints (get instructions concerning brushing program from an occupational therapist)	Let the child play in a sandbox
Use non-see-through box with small opening to feel and find various textured objects: keys, macaroni, koosh balls, car, truck, ball, etc.	Firm hugs, avoid light touch or tickling	Finger painting with pudding, shaving cream, nontoxic paints, etc.
	At bedtime use heavy blankets, fill bed with stuffed animals, make huge pillows by sewing sheets together with foam filling	
	Use weighted lap drapes when seated for activities	

home and school, and then come back when new developmental or sensory issues arise. Regular therapy services should include a home and school carryover program and instructions should be provided to the parents and teachers. Therapy performance and goals should be shared with the medical and instructional team for optimal outcomes. Occupational therapy services with a sensory integration focus could also occur via a consultation mode with the therapist observing the child monthly in a school or home setting and provide ideas, activities, and suggestions to be incorporated into regular daily activities. For children with moderate to severe impairment, the occupational therapists should work closely

Table 3 Vestibular Activities

Alerting	Calming	Other
Circular movements on swings	Slow rocking in lap or in rocking chair Slow swinging on various suspended swings (tire swings, regular swings, wide-platform swings, net hammocks) Attach bungee cords to swings for an up-and-down movement (be careful not to excite the child with fast bouncing)	

Table 4 Visual Activities

Alerting	Calming	Other
Use carpet to teach boundaries in play For transitioning from one activity to another, use "Simon Says" or colored and laminated feet pictures as a roadmap to the next activity; or make the child carry objects or pictures that represent the next activity; picture exchange communication system is good for transitioning	Work in a cubby or a hideout area, such as ball pit or tent to decrease visual distraction Make the environment predictable and uncluttered by arranging toys in the room in a consistent way Use deep colors with low contrast Keep the space uncluttered	Use computer games with added sounds for auditory input Use Touch Window or Big Keys to direct visual attention to the computer Use grids to decrease the visual field of choice Use red to yellow shades, bright-colored lights, and black-and-white peripheral visual input

Table 5 Auditory Activities

Alerting	Calming	Other
When trying to engage in activities, include toys that make sound (music boxes, whistles, toy cars/blocks/utensils that make noises)	Use headphones with soft lyrical music Use a slow and soft voice Present activities in a room with a rug or carpet to decrease extraneous noises	Use short and simple verbal messages when giving directions Transition to new activities by reciting children's songs or by listening with headphones

Table 6 Oral-Motor Activities

Alerting	Calming	Other
Use sour, spicy, bitter, and hard or chewy-textured foods	Use sweet, warm, and smooth-textured foods Sucking activities: hard candy, imitate smacking sounds and raspberries; use straws, aquarium or therapy tubing, crazy straws to suck up liquid, pudding, Jell-O, milkshakes, etc., to promote strong sucking; introduce strong or intense citrus flavors (Cran-mixes, etc.); choose food that is about the diameter of the mouth to promote a good suck seal, sports bottles, lollipops, Popsicles Blowing activities: musical toys, whistles, party favors, visual action toys (blow and something pops up); blow out candles, blow cotton balls, blow bubbles at bathtime; blowing activities in many positions: sitting, on stomach, on back Biting, chewing, and crunching activities: crunchy food like carrots, celery, crunchy peanut butter, potato chips, chewing on therapy tubing, licorice, taffy, etc.; food textures that encourage biting and crunching (bread sticks, apples, crackers, Cheetos); use food that is heavily textured not thin and slimy (peanut butter, Cheetos, pretzels, etc.)	Before mealtime, apply deep pressure in and around the child's mouth and on the body Prepare mouth with deep pressure before toothbrushing, and use electric toothbrush if tolerated Use weighted utensils and dishes, and nonslip surfaces (place setting, Dycem mats)

with educators and speech pathologists as a team. For children with mild impairment, the therapists should work with the families to evaluate how sensory issues impact functional performance and develop strategies to assist the child in activities of daily living.

   As with most forms of intervention, the earlier the child receives therapy, the more effect it will have on learning and functional performance.

REFERENCES

1. Grandin T, Scariano MM. Emergence: Labeled Autistic. Novato, CA: Arena Press, 1986:20, 76.
2. Ayres AJ. Sensory Integration and the Child. Los Angeles, CA: Western Psychological Services, 1979:5, 14, 59–66, 69–75, 82–83, 83–88, 91–101.
3. Kranowitz CS. The Out-of-Sync Child: Recognizing and Coping with Sensory Integration Dysfunction. New York: Berkley Publishing Group, 1998:8, 40–42, 42–47, 95–101.
4. www.ot-innovations.com/jerry.html
5. Dunn W. Sensory Profile User's Manual. San Antonio, Texas: Psychological Corporation, 1999:1–5, 33–36, 35.
6. Reisman JE, Hanschu B. Sensory Integration Inventory–Revised: For Individuals with Developmental Disabilities. Hugo, MN: PDP Press, 1999:2–5, 8–9, 20–22.
7. Case-Smith J. Occupational Therapy for Children. 4th ed. St. Louis: Mosby, 2001:359.
8. Folio MR, Fewell RR. Peabody Developmental Motor Scales Examiner's Manual. 2nd ed. Austin, TX: Pro-Ed, 2000:3, 4, 10.
9. Bruininks RH. Bruininks-Oseretsky Test of Motor Proficiency Examiner's Manual. Circle Pines, MN: American Guidance Service, 1978:11, 43.
10. Beery KE. The Beery-Buktenica Developmental Test of Visual-Motor Integration: Administration Scoring and Teaching Manual. 4th ed. Parsippany, NJ: Modern Curriculum Press, 1997:21–22.
11. Hammill DD, Pearson NA, Voress JK. Developmental Test of Visual Perception Examiner's Manual. 2nd ed. Austin, TX: Pro-Ed, 1993:5.
12. Sellin B. I Don't Want to Be Inside Me Anymore: Messages from an Autistic Mind. New York: Basic Books, 1995.
13. Berk RA, DeGang GA. Test of Sensory Function in Infants (TSFI). Los Angeles, CA: Western Psychological Services, 1990:1, 7.

11

Drug Therapy (Pharmacotherapy) of Autistic Spectrum Disorders

Vidya Bhushan Gupta
New York Medical College and Columbia University, New York, New York, U.S.A.

I. INTRODUCTION

Lack of understanding of the origins of abnormal behaviors in autism has impeded the development of rational drug therapies. Treatment is further complicated by a tremendous range of syndrome expression, perhaps due to the involvement of many neurotransmitters (1). There is no specific drug to cure autism or to treat its core symptoms of poor social relatedness and communication skills deficit. Therefore, the goal of drug treatment of autism is, at present, to decrease the frequency of maladaptive behaviors, such as hyperactivity, aggression, self-abusive behavior, temper tantrums, lability of mood, irritability, social withdrawal, anxiety, repetitive compulsive behaviors, and stereotypies. Atypical behaviors should be examined for their antecedents and contexts in which they occur and treatment should be considered only if the behaviors are maladaptive, interfere with programming, or impair the quality of life. For example, if a child flaps his hands when he is overaroused, but is still responsive to programming, his behavior may not require treatment. On the contrary, if a child turns an electric switch off and on repeatedly, and throws a tantrum when removed from the switch, his behavior is maladaptive and requires treatment. If a behavior occurs to avoid a socially threatening situation or a distressing sensory stimulus, behavioral interventions should be tried before drug treatment is initiated. An embarrassing behavior that occurs in public may be considered for treatment earlier than if it occurs in private. In other words, a proper behavioral diagnosis should be made before initiating treatment. Even if a decision is made to treat a behavior, drug treatment or pharmacotherapy should not be the sole treatment, but should be part of an overall management plan that includes other therapeutic and educational interventions. Some guidelines for drug treatment of target behaviors are given in Table 1. Although, in this chapter, medications have been grouped under the predominant symptom for which they are used, they often have effects on other symptoms as well. In other words, there are no specific drugs for target symptoms in autism and hit and trial is the rule.

II. HYPERACTIVITY, IMPULSIVITY, INATTENTION, AND DISTRACTIBILITY

The underlying basis of hyperactivity, inattention, distractibility, and impulsivity may be different in autism from that in attention deficit hyperactivity disorder

Table 1 Guidelines for the Management of Maladaptive Behaviors in Autism

1. Monitor behaviors for a period of time at home and in the school.
   Observe the frequency, setting, and antecedents of behaviors.
   Record the behaviors objectively using behavior checklists.
   Rule out medical causes of abnormal behavior (those who cannot talk act out).
   Assess if behaviors impair family's quality of life and cause parental stress.
2. Decide which behaviors are maladaptive and require intervention (target behaviors).
3. Try behavioral and environmental changes; involve therapists, teachers, and parents.
4. Once it is decided to try a medication, develop a multidisciplinary management plan for target behaviors including therapeutic and pharmacological interventions.
   Choose a medication, its dose and formulation—"start low and go slow."
   Have patience and be ready for unexpected reactions, avoid polypharmacy.
   Set realistic expectations and support parents in tolerating "bad" behavior.
   Set up goals of management (the end point).
   Plan how therapeutic response and side effects will be monitored.
   Use a behavioral checklist or a global impression scale, such as CGI[a] or CGAS[b].
   Develop a follow-up plan—how often the dose will be adjusted, when the trial will be called a failure or success, how long the drug will be continued after the acceptable response has been obtained, and the game plan for drug failure.
4. Discuss the plan with the parents, inform them about the limitations of drug therapy in autism and potential side effects of the medications, and obtain their verbal or written consent.

[a]Clinical global impressions.
[b]Clinical global assessment scale (children and adolescents).

(ADHD), because the response to psychostimulants is not as robust in autism as in ADHD. DSM-IV excludes the diagnosis of ADHD if the child has autism or PDD. Some children with autism are overfocused on a particular object, activity, or stimulus. Others may be hyperactive, but work within a narrow range of interests.

A. Psychostimulants

Although psychostimulants, such as methylphenidate and dextroamphetamine, have shown modest effects in reducing overactivity (2–4), the effects on attention and distractibility are not so obvious. Side effects of psychostimulants, such as irritability, anxiety, agitation, insomnia, aggression, delusions, and worsening of social withdrawal and stereotypies, have been reported more often in individuals with autism (5). Handen et al. reported positive response in 8/13 subjects but adverse effects, such as social withdrawal and irritability, were noted at higher doses (6). Others have reported therapeutic benefits without adverse side effects (4). Stimulants are more useful in children with Asperger's syndrome and PDD-NOS than in autism, and are not so helpful in patients who persevere within a narrow range of activities (6). Theoretically stimulants have the potential to increase stereotypic behaviors.

B. α_2-Adrenergic Agonists

Clonidine, an α_2-adrenergic agonist, has a modest effect in reducing hyperactivity, overarousal, and irritability, but has little effect on the social and communication abnormalities (7,8). Fankhauser et al. reported improvement in stereotyped body movements, self-stimulation, hypervigilance, and hyperactivity with weekly clonidine patch treatment in a double-blind, placebo-crossover study, but side effects such as sedation and fatigue occurred during the first 2 weeks of clonidine treatment (7). Clonidine was modestly effective in the short-term treatment of irritability and hyperactivity in children with autism in another study (8).

C. Antipsychotics (Neuroleptics)

Although older antipsychotics (neuroleptics), such as haloperidol, were effective in treating hyperactivity and aggression (9), they resulted in significant adverse effects, particularly tardive dyskinesia (10). Newer or atypical neuroleptics, such as risperidone and olanzapine, hold more promise in reducing hyperactivity, impulsivity, perseverative behaviors, and aggression with much less risk of tardive dyskinesia. Risperidone, an HT2A and dopamine D_2 antagonist, has been studied the most frequently (11–14). Besides open-label trials (12,13), a multi-center, double-blind, placebo-controlled study has indicated that risperidone may be effective in children and adolescents in reducing temper tantrums, aggression, and self-injurious behavior (15). It may also increase socialization in some children. The major side effect of risperidone has been increased appetite causing weight gain. Olanzapine, another atypical neuroleptic, was also found beneficial in a small open-label trial in reducing the symptoms of hyperactivity, repetitive behaviors, self-injurious behaviors, and even social relatedness in individuals with autism, but it, too, causes weight gain (16,17). Ziprasidone (Geodon) improved the symptoms of aggression, irritability, and agitation without significant weight gain in an open-label study (18). Clozapine (Clozaril) showed some positive effect in two case reports in older subjects but its tendency to cause agranulocytosis limits its use in autism and PDD (19,20). Quetiapine (Seroquel) was not tolerated well in an open-label trial because it caused sedation, behavioral activation, and weight gain (21). Atypical or newer neuroleptics used in autism are described in Table 2.

Other drugs that may be potentially used to treat hyperactivity in children with autism include opiate blockers, such as naltrexone, cyclic antidepressants, and anxiolytics (5). Among the antidepressants, clomipramine (Anfranil), desipramine (22), and mirtazapine have been found to decrease hyperactivity in small samples of individuals with autism (23). Mirtazapine (Remeron), a tetracyclic drug with both serotonergic and adrenergic properties, showed modest effectiveness for treating the symptoms of hyperactivity, aggression, self-injury,

Table 2 Newer Neuroleptics Used in Autism

Name	Side effects	Dose and formulation
Risperidone (Risperdal) (11–14): blocks D_2 and 5HT2a, α_1- and α_2- adrenergic receptors; off-label in children	Weight gain, drowsiness, tardive and withdrawal dyskinesia	Starting dose: 0.25 mg twice a day, to be increased by 0.25 mg weekly Tablets: 0.25, 0.5, 1, 2, 3, 4 mg Oral solution: 1 mg/mL
Olanzapine (Zyprexa) (16,17): blocks D_1, D_2, D_4, and 5HT1, 5HT2, adrenergic, cholinergic, histaminergic receptors; off-label in children	Weight gain, drowsiness, orthostatic hypotension, dry mouth, dizziness	Starting dose: 2.5 mg once a day, to be increased by 2.5 mg weekly Tablets: 2.5, 5, 7.5, 10, 15, 20 mg Orally disintegrating tablets (Zyprexa ZYDIS): 5, 10
Ziprasidone (Geodon) (18): higher HT2 to D_2 binding; off-label in children	No weight gain, less change in blood pressure, less anticholinergic effects, and transient sedation, QT ↑	Dose: 20–80 mg twice a day Capsules: 20, 40, 60, 80 mg

irritability, anxiety, depression, and insomnia in autistic disorder and other pervasive developmental disorders. Adverse effects were minimal and included increased appetite, irritability, and transient sedation (23). Serotonin reuptake inhibitors have not been particularly helpful in reducing hyperactivity and may, in fact, may cause behavioral activation and hyperactivity (24).

Traditional anxiolytics, such as benzodiazepines, are not helpful in the treatment of hyperactivity in autism. In fact, these might cause paradoxical hyperactivity. Buspirone (BuSpar), on the other hand, has shown some promise in reducing hyperactivity (25), but the underlying basis of hyperactivity in buspirone-responsive individuals may be anxiety. Opioid receptor blocker naltrexone (ReVia) has been noted to have modest effects on hyperactivity, but it is not clear if it decreases motor activity due to its sedative effect (26–29). Its use in children below 18 years is off-label. The starting dose is 50 mg once a day. It has a low side effect profile. Levetiracetam, a nootropic medication, decreased hyperactivity in 10 autistic children in an open-label trial (30).

In summary, drug treatment of hyperactivity in autism is, at present, unsatisfactory and additional studies of drug treatment of hyperactivity in autism are needed. For a detailed review see Aman and Langworthy (5).

III. REPETITIVE, RITUALISTIC, AND STEREOTYPIC BEHAVIORS

Some children with autism have stereotypic or repetitive motor behaviors, such as body rocking and spinning, flicking hands in front of the face, twisting of hands, twirling an object, and gesticulations. They also repeat motor sequences or scripts such as lining up toys, breaking the line, and lining them up again. Some indulge in repetitive self-stimulatory behavior such as rocking, swaying, and lying on the floor. Some repetitive behaviors, such head banging and hand biting, cause injury but perpetuate themselves, perhaps because of endorphin release. Other children with autism have compulsive behaviors such as hording or tearing paper or turning the faucet on and off. The underlying basis of repetitive behaviors in autism is unclear. Unlike typical obsessive compulsive disorder (OCD), these are not due to uncontrollable and distressing obsessions, but perhaps due to inflexibility, immaturity, or cognitive limitation. They might even have some adaptive value like stress reduction, sensory stimulation, and social attention, and escape from demands (31). Therefore, repetitive behaviors should be treated only if they are maladaptive; that is, they interfere with programming, worsen the quality of life, or are potentially harmful to the child.

Serotonin reuptake inhibitors (SRIs) and atypical neuroleptics are the major drug groups that have been used to treat repetitive, ritualistic, and stereoptypic behaviors in individuals with autism.

A. Serotonin Reuptake Inhibitors

Studies of SSRIs in autism suggest that they decrease the symptoms of repetitive behaviors, anxiety, social withdrawal, and behavioral rigidity with few side effects when used in doses smaller than used in depression or OCD (32). Higher doses of these medications, on the other hand, cause disinhibition syndrome characterized by increased restlessness, activity, agitation, and aggression. SRIs are less well tolerated and are less effective in younger autistic subjects compared with autistic adolescents and adults.

1. Nonselective Serotonin Reuptake Inhibitors

Clomipramine (Anafranil). Several trials of this tricyclic, nonselective SRI have shown that it reduces stereotypy, self-injurious behavior, and repetitive behaviors and improves social interaction in individuals with autism (33–36), but often causes serious side effects (37). Although clomipramine is approved for use in children at and above the age of 10 years for OCD, children tolerate clomipramine worse than adolescents and adults. Several side effects, such as prolongation of corrected QT interval, tachycardia, constipation, rash, enuresis, increased seizure frequency, agitation, aggression, and serotonin syndrome—myoclonus, muscle rigidity, fever, chills, diaphoresis, restlessness, tremor, agitation, irritability, confusion, and coma—have been reported (38). An open-label study of clomipramine in children had to be discontinued because of side effects (39).

2. Selective Serotonin Reuptake Inhibitors (SSRIs)

Fluvoxamine (Luvox). Fluvoxamine, a selective SSRI, was found to be effective in reducing repetitive behaviors and aggression in adults with autistic disorder in a controlled trial (40). Although controlled trials of fluvoxamine have not been done in children, case reports suggest improvement in stereotypical, repetitive behaviors with fluvoxamine in children with autism (41). Fluvoxamine is approved for use in children age 8 years and older for OCD.

Fluoxetine (Prozac). Several open-label trials of fluoxetine have reported improvement in perseverative behaviors, aggression, and self-injurious behaviors, in a quarter to third of the patients with autism and PDD, but several subjects had drug-induced behavioral activation. Side effects such as hyperactivity, agitation, decreased appetite, insomnia, and hypomania have been reported with fluoxetine (42–44). Recently, DeLong et al. have reported better results with fluoxetine in a subset of children with "unusual intellectual achievement" and family history of affective disorder (45).

Paroxetine (Paxil). Paroxetine is a serotonin and norepinephrine uptake inhibitor. There are a few reports of paroxetine use in autism and results have been similar to fluoxetine with improvement in a quarter of patients with low doses but behavioral activation at higher doses (44,46).

Sertraline (Zoloft). Sertraline is a serotonin and dopamine reuptake inhibitor. A few open-label trials of sertraline in individuals with autism have shown that it decreases self-injurious behavior, aggression, and anxiety with minimal side effects (47,48).

In summary, it seems that SRIs and SSRIs are modestly effective in adolescents and adults with autism in the management of repetitive, ritualistic, and stereotypic behaviors. These are also useful in mood disorders in individuals with autism. Their role in younger children is uncertain because of less efficacy and more side effects. There is a need for further research with controlled trials, because the current information is from case reports or open-label trials in small samples of heterogeneous subjects (49). For doses and formulations, see Table 3.

IV. AGGRESSION

Aggressive behavior in children with autism is not premeditated or predatory as in conduct disorder, but impulsive, often as a reaction to frustration and fear. Children with autism may also act aggressively to seek attention or to escape

Table 3 Serotonin Reuptake Inhibitors Useful in Autism

Name	Dose and formulation
Fluvoxamine (Luvox)	50–200 mg
Approved for use in children for OCD	Tablets: 25, 50, 100 mg
Fluoxetine (Prozac)	10–80 mg
Approved for children >7 years for OCD and >8 for depression	Tablet: 10 mg, pulvule: 10, 20, 40 Solution 20 mg/5 mL
Sertraline (Zoloft)	25–200 mg
Approved for children >6 years	Tablets: 25, 50, 100 mg
Paroxetine (Paxil)	20–80 mg
Off-label in pediatrics	Tablets: 10, 20, 30, 40 mg Oral suspension: 10 mg/5 mL
Clomipramine (Anafranil)	75–200 mg
Approved for children >10 years	Tablets: 10, 25, 40 mg Capsules: 25, 50, 75 mg

unacceptable demands. Alternatively, they may encroach upon others or attack others if the latter are in their way. At the neurochemical level, aggression is, perhaps, mediated by many neurotransmitters, including various excitatory and inhibitory amino acids, long-acting steroids, serotonin, noradrenaline, and dopamine (50–53).

Because the etiology of aggressive behaviors is diverse, many medications have been used to target this symptom, including antipsychotics, SSRIs, anticonvulsants, opioid antagonists, and lithium (54,55).

A. Antipsychotics (Neuroleptics)

Increased dopaminergic activity has been postulated to be a cause of aggression in animals (56). Extrapolating from the animal data, antipsychotics that block dopaminergic receptors, such as haloperidol, have been the mainstay of treatment of aggressive behavior in psychiatry. Campbell et al. conducted several controlled drug trials of haloperidol in autism reporting beneficial effects. Combination of haloperidol with behavior treatments resulted in acquisition of imitative speech and social skills. Haloperidol also decreased fidgetiness, withdrawal, and stereotypies and improved relatedness to the examiner. However, on long-term follow-up, 34% of children developed tardive or withdrawal dyskinesias, involving the face and mouth. Most of these movements were reversible in the long run (57). The newer antipsychotics, such as risperidone and olanzapine, cause fewer side effects and are replacing haloperidol as medications of choice. Risperidone, a 5-HT2 receptor and D_2-receptor antagonist, has been found to reduce behavioral symptoms such as aggression, self-injurious repetitive movements, and hyperactivity in many studies, both controlled and uncontrolled. Adverse side effects include weight gain, sedation, and galactorrhea (58). Olanzapine was found to be comparable to haloperidol in an open-label trial (59). Quetiapine, on the other hand, was not well tolerated by children with PDD (60), and side effects of clonazepine, particularly agranulocytosis, preclude its use in autism, except as a last resort (61).

B. Serotonin Reuptake Inhibitors

Disturbed central serotonergic function has been suggested to play a role in problems with frustration tolerance and has been correlated with increased aggression in adults, hyperactive children, children with OCD, and nonhuman primates (62,63). For a detailed discussion of SRIs, see above. Citalopram has been found to be particularly useful for impulsive aggression in children and adolescents in an open-label study (64), but has not been studied in autism.

C. Anticonvulsants

Theoretically anticonvulsants may improve the behavior of individuals with autism by controlling epilepsy and underlying bipolar disorder (65). There are case reports of individuals with autism whose behavior and language and social skills improved after anticonvulsant therapy (66–68). Many of these had epileptiform discharge on EEG with or without epilepsy. It has been suggested that some children with autism may respond to anticonvulsants because of shared neuropathology, such as abnormal electric activity in the amygdale (65). According to Rapin, although epilepsy may play a minor role in a few children with regressive autism, it is uncertain if anticonvulsants can stall autistic regression (69,70).

Affective anticonvulsants, valproic acid (VPA) and carbamazepine, are used to treat aggression, irritability, and bipolar disorder in individuals with mental retardation, with or without autism. A study of VPA in the treatment of patients with intellectual disability and aggressive or self-injurious behavior found a moderate to marked improvement in 71% of subjects. In 82% of the subjects there was a significant reduction in aggression and self-injurious behavior, in 46% other psychotropic medications could be discontinued, and in 39% the dose of other (71) psychotropic medication could be reduced. Although it is difficult to diagnose bipolar disorder in individuals with autism, it is likely that aggressive and irritability in some individuals with autism may be a manifestation of underlying affective disorder. This view is strengthened by the finding of higher prevalence of affective disorders in families of individuals with autism (72). However, anticonvulsants can have serious side effects (73,74) and should be used after careful risk-benefit analysis in individuals with autism also who have epilepsy, epileptiform discharge on EEG, cyclic aggression and irritability (75).

D. Trazodone (Desyrel)

Trazodone, an antidepressant that is neither tri- nor tetracyclic, has been mentioned as treatment of aggression and violence in autistic children (76). The response rate is 25–30% and side effects, such as orthostatic hypotension and leg swelling and pain, can occur. In males it can cause priapism.

E. Lithium

Lithium maybe used in individuals who are aggressive, agitated, and overaroused, and have cycles of overarousal and withdrawal. But its side effects and the need to draw blood for levels and tests limit its use in individuals with autism.

Buspirone and beta-blockers have also been used to treat aggressive behavior in autism. These have been discussed in other sections.

V. ANXIETY

Children with autistic spectrum disorder often have symptoms of anxiety (77), particularly in unfamiliar environments, when exposed to certain environmental stimuli, when the familiar order in their environment is changed, or when their rigidity and repetitive behavior is challenged (78). Buspirone, a 5-HT1A receptor agonist, has been found to be safe and effective in controlling the symptoms of anxiety in autism in double-blind, placebo-controlled crossover study (79). It belongs to the azipirone group of medications, does not affect mental alertness as other anxiolytics do, and is not addictive. At higher doses it inhibits 5-HT 2A receptors, and decreases striatal levels of serotonin and its metabolites. Buspirone has effects on dopamine, norepinephrine, and the GABA systems as well. It takes about 2–4 weeks for its full effects, although mild effects are seen within 1 week (80). In an open-label trial buspirone resulted in marked improvement in the target symptoms of anxiety and irritability in children with autism (81). It has also been found to decrease aggression, hyperactivity, stereotypies, and self-injurious behavior (82). Others have shown mixed results (83,84). In an open-label study, there was worsening of aggression with buspirone (84). Rarely increase in agitation and aggression and involuntary movements of the mouth have also been reported (85).

VI. SELF-INJURIOUS BEHAVIOR

Children with autism, especially the low-functioning children, indulge in self-injurious behaviors, such as self-biting, self-hitting, head banging, eye poking, and skin picking. Reduced pain sensitivity, "addiction" to endorphins, and abnormalities of opioid and dopaminergic neurotransmission in the brain have been suggested as the possible causes of self-injurious behavior in autism (86).

A. Opioid Antagonists

Positive results for self-injurious behavior have been reported with naltrexone, a long-acting narcotic antagonist (87–89). Naltrexone has been reported to decrease hyperactivity, irritability, and withdrawal, and to increase verbal output and attentiveness (90–93). Despite its initial promise, several double-blind control trials have either failed to show significant effects of naltrexone on behavioral symptoms of autism or have found rather small effects, particularly on the core symptoms of social withdrawal and communication deficits (94–96). Others have argued that only those individuals who have evidence of dysregulation of the propiomelanocortin system with elevated levels of C-terminal β-endorphin and serotonin benefit from naltrexone (95,97).

Nevertheless, naltrexone has some role in the management of hyperactivity, irritability, and self-injurious behavior in autism, because of its low side effect profile. It is given in the dose of 0.5–1.0 mg/kg body weight with an average dose of 1 mg/kg/day. Side effects, such as rash, sedation, and unsteady gait, can occur (96).

B. β-Adrenergic Blockers

β-Adrenergic blockers, such as propranolol and nadolol, have been reported to decrease aggressive outbursts and self-injurious and stereotypic behavior in a few open-label studies and case reports of individuals with mental retardation and autism. Secondary improvement in attention (98–100), language, and social skills was also reported in the one study. Nadolol was reported to be better than propranolol in a case report (101).

The use of β-adrenergic blockers is limited by their side effects of hypotension, bradycardia, exacerbation of asthma, and nightmares. For a detailed review of β-adrenergic blockers in aggression see Haspel (102).

VII. SLEEP PROBLEMS IN CHILDREN WITH AUTISM

Individuals with autism often have sleep problems, such as difficulties in settling down, frequent and prolonged nighttime awakenings, night terrors, and disturbances of sleep-wake cycle (103). Sleep disturbances may be due to disturbance of the sleep-wake cycle, underlying medical conditions, anxiety, or psychosocial stress. Disturbances of nighttime sleep affect daytime behavior and also cause parental stress (104). While behavioral interventions are the mainstay of management of sleep problems, medications are sometimes necessary. Short-acting benzodiazepines, such as triazolam (Halcion) and flurazepam (Dalmane), may have a short-term role in the treatment of pediatric insomnia but are not approved for use in children in the United States. However, tachyphylaxis and risk of misuse preclude the long-term use of benzodiazepines for the treatment of insomnia in children. Alimemazine (trimeprazine), a phenothiazine, has been shown to be effective in the short-term treatment of insomnia in young children, but does not have U.S. Food and Drug Administration approval for pediatric insomnia (105). Niaprazine, a histamine H_1-receptor antagonist with sedative properties, was found to treat insomnia in an open-label study of 25 children and young people with autism and a range of severity of mental retardation (age range 2–20 years) (106). Individuals with mild-to-moderate mental retardation were selectively better responders. Newer hypnotics, such as zolpidem (Ambien), zopiclone (Imovane), and Zaleplon (Sonata), which appear better tolerated and less habit-forming than the benzodiazepines in studies of adults, may have a role when combined with psychosocial treatments for pediatric insomnia (107,108).

Melatonin, a pineal gland hormone, was found to be effective in treating insomnia in a recent uncontrolled study of 50 children and young adults with developmental disorders (age range 3–28 years) (109). The results in people with mental retardation have been mixed (110). Side effects, such as residual drowsiness the next morning, awakening in the middle of the night, and excitement after awakening and before going to bed, can occur but are usually mild. There is no consensus about dosage and the mode of administration. It is uncertain if melatonin needs to be given continuously or can be phased out after sleep pattern has improved (111). The recommended dose is 0.5–3 mg/day.

VIII. SUMMARY

Table 4 summarizes the major drug groups and their indications in autism. The number of medications that have been or are being tried for autism is too large to be discussed in this volume. Some, such as fenfluramine, have become history. It was withdrawn from the market because of side effects. Others, such as lofexidine, amantadine, cyproheptadine, famotidine, and donepezil, have been tried in individual cases, with mixed results. Unless the neurochemical basis of autism is discovered, a specific drug in unlikely to be available for autism. Until then drug therapy will remain, at best, an adjunct to behavioral and educational interventions.

Table 4 Summary of the Use of Various Drug Groups in Autism

	Repetitive behavior	Hyperactivity impulsivity	Aggression, self-injury	Anxiety/ affective symptoms
SSRI	X			
Atypical antipsychotics	X	X	X	X
Stimulants		X		
Naltrexone		X		
Clonidine		X	X	X
Lithium			X	
β-blockers			X	
Anticonvulsants			X	
Buspirone				X

Source: Adapted from Williemsen-Swinkels SHN, Buitelaar JK. The autistic spectrum: subgroups, boundaries, and treatment. Psychiatr Clin North Am 2002; 25:811–836.

REFERENCES

1. Volkmar FR. Pharmacological interventions in autism: theoretical and practical issues. J Clin Child Psychol 2001; 30:80–87.
2. Strayhorn J. More on methylphenidate in autism. J Am Acad Child Adolesc Psychiatry 1989; 28:299.
3. Strayhorn JM Jr, Rapp N, Donina W, Strain PS. Randomized trial of methylphenidate for an autistic child. J Am Acad Child Adolesc Psychiatry 1988; 27:244–247.
4. Quintana H, Birhamer B, Stedge D, Lennon S, Freed J, Bridge J, et al. Use of methylphenidate in treatment of children with autistic disorder. J Autism Dev Disord 1995; 25:283–294.
5. Aman MG, Langworthy KS. Pharmacotherapy for hyperactivity in children with autism and other pervasive developmental disorders. J Autism Dev Disord 2000; 30:451–459.
6. Handen BL, Johnson CR, Lubetsky M. Efficacy of methylphenidate among children with autism and symptoms of attention-deficit hyperactivity disorder. J Autism Dev Disord 2000; 30:245–255.
7. Fankhauser MP, Karumanchi VC, German ML, Yates A, Karumanchi SD. A double-blind, placebo-controlled study of the efficacy of transdermal clonidine in autism. J Clin Psychiatry 1992; 53:77–82.
8. Jaselskis CA, Cook EH Jr, Fletcher KE, Leventhal BL. Clonidine treatment of hyperactive and impulsive children with autistic disorder. J Clin Psychopharmacol 1992; 12:322–327.
9. Campbell M, Cueva JE. Psychopharmacology in child and adolescent psychiatry: a review of the past seven years. Part I. J Am Acad Child Adolesc Psychiatry 1995; 34:1124–1132.
10. Neuroleptic-related dyskinesias in autistic children: a prospective, longitudinal study. J Am Acad Child Adolesc Psychiatry 1997; 36:835–843.
11. McDougle CJ, Holmes JP, Carlson DC, Pelton GH, Cohen DJ, Price LH. A double-blind, placebo-controlled study of risperidone in adults with autistic disorder and other pervasive developmental disorders. Arch Gen Psychiatry 1998; 55:633–641.
12. Posey DJ, McDougle CJ. Risperidone: a potential treatment for autism. Curr Opin Invest Drugs 2002; 3:1212–1216.
13. Masi G. Open trial of risperidone in 24 young children with pervasive developmental disorders. J Am Acad Child Adolesc Psychiatry 2001; 40:1206–1214.
14. Malone RP. Risperidone treatment in children and adolescents with autism: short- and long-term safety and effectiveness. J Am Acad Child Adolesc Psychiatry 2002; 41:140–147.
15. McCracken JT, McGough J, Shah B, Cronin P, Hong D, Aman MG, Arnold LE, Lindsay R, Nash P, Holloway J, McDougle CJ, Posy D, Swiezy N, Kohn A, Scahill L, Koenig K, Volkmar F, Carroll D, Lancor A, Tierney E, Ghuman J, Gonzalez NM, Grados M, Vitiello B, Ritz L, Davies M, Robinson L, McMahon D. Risperidone in children with autism and serious behavioral problems. N Engl J Med 2002; 347:314–321.

16. Potenza MN, Holmes JP, Kanes SJ, McDougle CJ. Olanzapine treatment of children, adolescents, and adults with pervasive developmental disorders: an open-label pilot study. J Clin Psychopharmacol 1999; 19:37–44.
17. Malone RP, Cater J, Sheikh RM, Choudhury MS, Delaney MA. Olanzapine versus haloperidol in children with autistic disorder: an open pilot study. J Am Acad Child Adolesc Psychiatry 2001; 40:887–894.
18. McDougle CJ, Kem DL, Posey DJ. Case series: use of ziprasidone for maladaptive symptoms in youths with autism. J Am Acad Child Adolesc Psychiatry 2002; 41:921–927.
19. Gobbi G, Pulvirenti L. Long-term treatment with clozapine in an adult with autistic disorder accompanied by aggressive behaviour. J Psychiatry Neurosci 2001; 26:340–341.
20. Chen NC, Bedair HS, McKay B, Bowers MB Jr, Mazure C. Clozapine in the treatment of aggression in an adolescent with autistic disorder. J Clin Psychiatry 2001; 62:479–480.
21. Martin A, Koenig K, Scahill L, Bregman J. Open-label quetiapine in the treatment of children and adolescents with autistic disorder. J Child Adolesc Psychopharmacol 1999; 9:99–107.
22. Gordon CT, Rappaport JL, Hamburger SD, State RC, Manheim GB. Differential response of seven subjects with autistic disorder to clomipramine and desipramine. Am J Psychiatry 1992; 149:363–366.
23. Posey DJ, Guenin KD, Kohn AE, Swiezy NB, McDougle CJ. A naturalistic open-label study of mirtazapine in autistic and other pervasive developmental disorders. J Child Adolesc Psychopharmacol 2001; 11:267–277.
24. Fatemi SH, Realmuto GM, Khan L, Thuras P. Fluoxetine in treatment of adolescent patients with autism: a longitudinal open trial. J Autism Dev Disord 1998; 28:303–307.
25. Realmuto GM, August GJ, Garfinkel BD. Clinical effect of buspirone in autistic children. J Clin Psychopharmacol 1989; 9:122–125.
26. Campbell M, Anderson LT, Small AM, Locascio JJ, Lynch NS, Choroco MC. Naltrexone in autistic children: a double-blind and placebocontrolled trial. Psychopharmacol Bull 1990; 26:130–135.
27. Kolmen BK, Feldman HM, Handen BL, Janosky JE. Naltrexone in young autistic children: replication study and learning measures. J Am Acad Child Adolesc Psychiatry 1997; 36:1570–1578.
28. Willemsen-Swinkels SH, Buitelaar JK, van Berckelaer-Onnes IA, van Engeland H. Brief report: six months continuation treatment in naltrexone-responsive children with autism: an open-label case-control design. J Autism Dev Disord 1999; 29:167–169.
29. Willemsen-Swinkels SH, Buitelaar JK, van Engeland H. The effects of chronic naltrexone treatment in young autistic children: a double-blind placebo-controlled crossover study. Biol Psychiatry 1996; 39:1023–1031.
30. Rugino TA, Samsock TC. Levetiracetam in autistic children: an open-label study. J Dev Behav Pediatr 2002; 23:225–230.
31. Mason G. Stereotypis: a critical review. Anim Behav 1991; 41:1015–1037.

32. Awad GA. The use of selective serotonin reuptake inhibitors in young children with pervasive developmental disorders: some clinical observations. Can J Psychiatry 1996; 41:361–366.

33. Lewis MH, Bodfish JW, Powell SB, Parker DE, Golden RN. Clomipramine treatment for self-injurious behavior of individuals with mental retardation: a double-blind comparison with placebo. Am J Ment Retard 1996; 100:654–665.

34. Gordon CT, State RC, Nelson JE, Hamburger SD, Rapoport JL. A double-blind comparison of clomipramine, desipramine, and placebo in the treatment of autistic disorder. Arch Gen Psychiatry 1993; 50:441–447.

35. McDougle CJ, Kresch LE, Posey DJ. Repetitive thoughts and behavior in pervasive developmental disorders: treatment with serotonin reuptake inhibitors. J Autism Dev Disord 2000; 30:427–435.

36. Garber HJ, McGonigle JJ, Slomka GT, Monteverde E. Clomipramine treatment of stereotypic behaviors and self-injury in patients with developmental disabilities. J Am Acad Child Adoclesc Psychiatry 1992; 31:1157–1160.

37. Brodkin ES, McDogle CJ, Naylor ST, Cohen DJ, Price LH. Clomipramine in adults with pervasive developmental disorders: a prospective open-label investigation. J Child Adolesc Psychopharmacol 1997; 7:109–121.

38. Brasic JR, Barnett JY, Sheitman BB, Lafargue RT, Kowalik S, Kaplan D, et al. Behavioral effects of clomipramine on prepubertal boys with autistic disorder and severe mental retardation. CNS Spectrum 1998; 3:39–46.

39. Sanchez LE, Campbell M, Small AM, Cueva JE, Armenteros JL, Adams PB. A pilot study of clomipramine in young autistic children. J Am Acad Child Adolesc Psychiatry 1996; 35:537–544.

40. McDougle CJ, Naylor ST, Cohen DJ, Volkmar FR, Heninger GR, Proce LH. A double blind placebo controlled study of fluvoxamine in adults with autistic disorder. Arch Gen Psychiatry 1996; 53:1001–1008.

41. Kauffmann C, Vance H, Pumariega AJ, Miller B. Fluvoxamine treatment of a child with severe PDD: a single case study. Psychiatry 2001; 64:268–277.

42. Cook-EHJ, Rowlett R, Jaselskis C, Leventhal BL. Fluoxetine treatment of children and adults with autistic disorder and mental retardation. J Am Acad Child Adolesc Psychiatry 1992; 31:739–745.

43. Fatemi SH, Realmuto GM, Khan L, Thuras P. Fluoxetine in treatment of adolescent patients with autism: a longitudinal open trial. J Autism Dev Disord 1998; 28:303–307.

44. Bradford D, Bhaumik S, Naik B. Selective serotonin re-uptake inhibitors for the treatment of perseverative and maladaptive behaviours of people with intellectual disability. J Intellect Disabil Res 1998; 42(Pt 4):301–306.

45. DeLong GR, Ritch CR, Burch S. Fluoxetine response in children with autistic spectrum disorders: correlation with familial major affective disorder and intellectual achievement. Dev Med Child Neurol 2002; 44:652–659.

46. Posey DI, Litwiller M, Koburn M, McDougle CJ. Paroxetine in autism. J Am Acad Child Adolesc Psychiatry 1999; 38:111–112.

47. Steingard RJ, Zimnitzky B, DeMaso DR, Bauman ML, Bucci JP. Sertraline treatment of transition-associated anxiety and agitation in children with autistic disorder. J Child Adolesc Psychopharmacol 1997; 7:9–15.

48. Hellings JA, Kelley LA, Gabrielli WF, Kilgore E, Shah P. Sertraline response in adults with mental retardation and autistic disorder. J Clin Psychiatry 1996; 57:333–336.

49. McDougle CJ, Kresch LE; Posey DJ Compulsive behavior: Repetitive thoughts and behavior in pervasive developmental disorders: treatment with serotonin reuptake inhibitors. J Autism Dev Disord 2000; 30:427–435.

50. Lindenmayer JP. The pathophysiology of agitation. J Clin Psychiatry 2000; 61(suppl 14):5–10.

51. Eichelman B, Hartwig AC. Discussion: biological correlates of aggression. Ann NY Acad Sci 1996; 794:78–81.

52. Eichelman B. Toward a rational pharmacotherapy for aggressive and violent behavior. Hosp Commun Psychiatry 1988; 39:31–39.

53. Miczek KA, Weerts E, Haney M, Tidey J. Neurobiological mechanisms controlling aggression: preclinical developments for pharmacotherapeutic interventions. Neurosci Biobehav Rev 1994; 18:97–110.

54. Barnard L, Young AH, Pearson J, Geddes J, O'Brien G. A systematic review of the use of atypical antipsychotics in autism. J Psychopharmacol 2002; 16:93–101.

55. Kim E. The use of newer anticonvulsants in neuropsychiatric disorders. Curr Psychiatry Rep 2002; 4:331–337.

56. van Erp AM, Miczec KA. Aggressive behavior, increased accumbal dopamine, and decreased cortical serotonin in rats. J Neurosci 2000; 20:9320–9325.

57. Campbell M, Armenteros JL, Malone RP, et al. Neuroleptice-related dyskinesias in autistic children.: a prospective , longitudinal study. J Am Acad Child Adolesc Psychiatry 1997; 36:835–843.

58. Masi G, Cosenza A, Mucci M, De Vito G. Risperidone monotherapy in preschool children with pervasive developmental disorders. J Child Neurol 2001; 16:395–400.

59. Malone RP, Cater J, Sheikh RM, Choudhury MS, Delaney MA. Olanzapine versus haloperidol in children with autistic disorder: an open pilot study. J Am Acad Child Adolesc Psychiatry 2001; 40:887–894.

60. Martin A. Koenig K, Scahill L, Bregman J. Open-label quetiapine in treatment of children and adolescents with autistic disorder. J Child Adolesc Psychopharmacol 1999; 9:99–107.

61. Gobbi G, Pulvirenti L. Long-term treatment with clozapine in an adult with autistic disorder accompanied by aggressive behaviour. J Psychiatry Neurosci 2001; 26:340–341.

62. Mitsis EM, Halperin JM, Newcorn JH. Serotonin and aggression in children. Curr Psychiatry Rep 2000; 2:95–101.

63. Mehlman PT, Higley JD, Faucher I, Lilly AA, Taub DM, Vickers J, Suomi SJ, Linnoila M. Low CSF 5-HIAA concentrations and severe aggression and impaired impulse control in nonhuman primates. Am J Psychiatry 1994; 151:1485–1491.

64. Armenteros JL, Lewis JE. Citalopram treatment for impulsive aggression in children and adolescents: an open pilot study. J Am Acad Child Adolesc Psychiatry 2002; 41:522–529.

65. Di Martino A, Tuchman RF. Antiepileptic drugs: affective use in autism spectrum disorders. Pediatr Neurol 2001; 25:199–207.
66. Pilopys AV. Autism: electroencephalogram abnormalities and clinical improvement with valproic acid. Arch Pediatr Adolesc Med 1994; 148:220–222.
67. Childs JA, Blair JL. Valproic acid treatment of epilepsy in autistic twins. J Neurosci Nurs 1997; 29:244–248.
68. Bardenstein R, Chez MG, Helfand BT, Buchanan C, Zucker M. Improvement in EEG and clinical function in pervasive developmental disorder (PDD): effect of valproic acid. Neurology 1998; 50:a86.
69. Rapin I. Autistic regression and disintegrative disorder: how important the role of epilepsy? Semin Pediatr Neurol 1995; 2:278–285.
70. Tuchman RF, Rapin I. Regression in pervasive developmental disorders: seizures and epileptiform electroencephalogram correlates. Pediatrics 1997; 99:560–566.
71. Ruedrich S, Swales TP, Fossaceca C, Toliver J, Rutkowski A. Effect of divalproex sodium on aggression and self-injurious behavior in adults with intellectual disability: a retrospective review. J Intell Disabil Res 1999; 43:105–111.
72. Bolton PF, Pickles A, Murphy M, Rutter M. Autism, affective and other psychiatric disorders: patterns of familial aggregation. Psychol Med 1998; 28:385–394.
73. Calabrese JR, Goethe JW, Kayser A, Marcotte DB, Monagin JA, Kimmel SE, Brugger AM, Morris D, Fatemi SH. Adverse events in 583 valproate-treated patients. Depression 1996; 3:257–262.
74. Beran RG, Gibson RJ. Aggressive behaviour in intellectually challenged patients with epilepsy treated with lamotrigine. Epilepsia 1998; 39:280–282.
75. Hollander E, Dolgoff-Kaspar R, Cartwright C, Rawitt R, Novotny S. An open trial of divalproex sodium in autism spectrum disorders. J Clin Psychiatry 2001; 62:530–534.
76. Gedye A, Trazodone reduced aggressive and self-injurious movements in a mentally handicapped male patient with autism. J Clin Psychopharmacol 1991; 11:275–276.
77. Muris P, Steerneman P, Merckelbach H, Holdrinet I, Meesters C. Comorbid anxiety symptoms in children with pervasive developmental disorders. J Anxiety Disord 1998; 12:387–393.
78. Gillott A, Furniss F, Walter A. Anxiety in high-functioning children with autism. Autism 2001; 5:277–286.
79. McCormick LH. Treatment with buspirone in a patient with autism. Arch Fam Med 1997; 6:368–370.
80. Schweitzer E, Rickels K. Strategies for treatment of generalized anxiety disorder in the primary care setting. J Clin Psychiatry 1997; 58(suppl 3):27–31.
81. Buitelaar JK, van der Gaag RJ, van der Hoeven J. Buspirone in the management of anxiety and irritability in children with pervasive developmental disorders: results of an open label study. J Clin Psychiatry 1999; 59:56–59.
82. Ratey JJ, Sovner R, Mikkelsen E, Chmielinski HE. Buspirone therapy for maladaptive behavior and anxiety in developmentally disabled persons. J Clin Psychiatry 1989; 50:382–384.
83. Realmuto GM, August GJ, Garfinkel BD. Clinical effect of buspirone in autistic children. J Clin Psychopharmacol 1989; 9:122–125.

84. King BH, Davanzo P. Buspirone treatment of aggression and self-injury in autistic and non-autistic persons with severe mental retardation. Dev Brain Dysfunct 1996; 6:368–687.

85. Posey DJ. The pharmacotherapy of target symptoms associated with autistic disorder and other pervasive developmental disorders. Harv Rev Psychiatry 2000; 8:45–63.

86. Sandman CA. beta-Endorphin dysregulation in autistic and self-injurious behavior: a neurodevelopmental hypothesis. Synapse 1988; 2:193–199.

87. Herman BH, Hammock MK, Arthur-Smith A, et al. Naltrexone decreases self-injurious behavior. Ann Neurol 1987; 22:550–552.

88. Lienemann J, Walker F. Reversal of self-abusive behavior with naltrexone (letter to the editor). J Clin Psychopharmacol 1989; 9:448–449.

89. Sandman CA, Barron JL, Colman H. An orally administered opiate blocker, naltrexone, attenuates self-injurious behavior. Am J Ment Retard 1990; 95:93–102.

90. Willemson-Swinkels SH, Buitelaar JK, vanEngeland H. The effects of chronic naltrexone treatment in young autistic children: a double-blind placebo-controlled crossover study. Biol Psychiatry 1996; 39:1023–1031.

91. Panksepp J, Lensing P. Brief report: a synopsis of an open-trial of naltrexone treatment of autism with four children. J Autism Dev Disord 1991; 21:243–249.

92. Campbell M, Anderson LT, Small AM, Adams P, Gonzalez NM, Ernst M. Naltrexone in autistic children: behavioral symptoms and attentional learning. J Am Acad Child Adolesc Psychiatry 1993; 32:1283–1291.

93. Campbell M, Anderson LT, Small AM, Locascio JJ, Lynch NS, Choroco MC. Naltrexone in autistic children: a double-blind and placebo controlled study. Psychopharmacol Bull 1990; 26:130–135.

94. Willemson-Swinkels SHN, Buitelaar JK, Nijhof GJ, Van Engeland H. Failure of naltrexone hydrochloride to reduce self-injurious and autistic behavior in mentally retarded adults: double blind placebo-controlled studies. Arch Gen Psychiatry 1995; 52:766–773.

95. Bouvard MP, Leboyer M, Launav JM, Recasens C, Plumet MH, Waller-Perotte D, Tabuteau F, Bondoux D, Dugas M, Lensing P, et al. Low-dose naltrexone effects on plasma chemistries and clinical symptoms in autism: a double-blind, placebo-controlled study. Psychiatry Res 1995; 58:191–201.

96. Kolmen BK, Feldman HM, Handen BL, Janosky JE. Naltrexone in young autistic children: replication study and learning measures. J Am Acad Child Adolesc Psychiatry 1997; 36:1570–1578.

97. Sandman CA, Touchette P, Marion S, Lenjavi M, Chicz-Demet A. Disregulation of propiomelanocortin and contagious maladaptive behavior. Regul Pept 2002; 108:179–185.

98. Williams DT, Mehl R, Yudofsky S, Adams D, Roseman B. The effect of propranolol on uncontrolled rage outbursts in children and adolescents with organic brain dysfunction. J Am Acad Child Psychiatry 1982; 21:129–135.

99. Ratey JJ, Bemporad J, Sorgi P, Bick P, Polakoff S, O'Driscoll G, Mikkelsen E, et al. Open trial effects of beta-blockers on speech and social behaviors in 8 autistic adults. J Autism Dev Disord 1987; 17:439–446.

100. Cohen IL, Tsiouris JA, Pfadt A. Effects of long-acting propranolol on agonistic and stereotyped behaviors in a man with pervasive developmental disorder and fragile X syndrome: a double-blind, placebo-controlled study. J Clin Psychopharmacol 1991; 11:398–399.
101. Connor DF, Ozbayrak KR, Benjamin S, Ma Y, Fletcher KE. A pilot study of nadolol for overt aggression in developmentally delayed individuals. J Am Acad Child Adolesc Psychiatry 1997; 36:826–834.
102. Haspel T. Beta-blockers and the treatment of aggression. Harv Rev Psychiatry 1995; 2:274–281.
103. Richdale A. Sleep problems in autism: prevalence, cause and intervention. Dev Med Child Neurol 1999; 41:60–66.
104. Younus M, Labellarte MJ. Insomnia in children: when are hypnotics indicated? Paediatr Drugs 2002; 4:391–403.
105. Lancioni GE, O'Reilly MF, Basili G. Review of strategies for treating sleep problems in persons with severe or profound mental retardation or multiple handicaps. Am J Ment Retard 1999; 104:170–186.
106. Rossi PG, Posar A, Parmaggianni A, et al. Niaprazine in the treatment of autistic disorder. J Child Neurol 1999; 14:547–550.
107. Kripke DF. Chronic hypnotic use: deadly risks, doubtful benefit. Sleep Med Rev 2000; 4:5–20.
108. Patat A, Paty I, Hindmarch I. Pharmacodynamic profile of Zaleplon, a new non-benzodiazepine hypnotic agent. Hum Psychopharmacol 2001; 16:369–392.
109. Ishizaki A, Sugama M, Takeuchi N. Usefulness of melatonin for developmental sleep and emotional/behavior disorders: studies of melatonin trial on 50 patients with developmental disorders. No to Hattatsu 1999; 31:428–437.
110. Mendelson WB. A critical evaluation of the hypnotic efficacy of melatonin. Sleep 1997; 20:916–919.
111. Sack RL, Hughes RJ, Edgar DM, Lewy AJ. Sleep-promoting effects of melatonin: at what dose, in whom, under what conditions, and by what mechanisms? Sleep 1997; 20:908–915.

12

Complementary and Alternative Treatments for Autism

Vidya Bhushan Gupta
New York Medical College and Columbia University,
New York, New York, U.S.A.

I. INTRODUCTION

Complementary and alternative medicine (CAM) has been defined as "a broad domain of healing resources that encompasses all health systems, modalities, and practices and their accompanying theories and beliefs, other than those intrinsic to the politically dominant health system of a particular society or culture in a given historic period" (1). Although complementary and alternative treatments are not commonly prescribed by the practitioners of conventional medicine, their use has increased in the United States in the last decade (2). Owing to the lack of satisfactory treatments, CAM use is particularly common in children with developmental disabilities (3,4). About 50% of children with autism are treated with CAM (5). Parents feel a sense of autonomy when they make therapeutic decisions for their children based on their own research. Usually a significant component of this research involves the Internet, where a lot of unauthenticated and unscrupulous information exists along with useful information. The information in this chapter is not an endorsement of CAM but an acknowledgment that it is widely used by individuals with autism, and the physicians and others who take care of children with autism should know about it so that they can counsel the families judiciously (6).

II. BIOLOGICALLY BASED THERAPIES

This category includes natural and biologically based practices, interventions, and products, including the following: phytotherapy or herbalism; special diet therapies; orthomolecular medicine; and unconventional pharmacological, biological, and instrumental interventions.

A.   Dietary Manipulation

Proponents of the gastrointestinal theory of autism posit that autism occurs because of the absorption of toxic peptides from the gut and, therefore, can be treated by eliminating the source of these toxins from the diet. See Chapter 2 for details.

1.   Casein- and Gluten-Free Diet (CFGF)

According to the gut theory of autism, casein and gluten are digested incompletely in children with autism. Autism is putatively caused by the end products of this incomplete digestion—amino acid polymers with opioid characteristics, called exorphins. Removal of casein-containing foods, such as cow's milk and dairy products, and gluten- and gliadin-containing foods, such as wheat, barley, rye, and oats, from the diet is supposed to improve the behavior of children with autism by reducing exorphins. Maximum improvement after elimination can take up to 2 years. A Medline search revealed two poorly done studies of CFGF diet and both reported positive results (7,8). In one study, skin tests for food allergy were positive in many of the subjects and many had high levels of antibodies against casein in their blood (7). Proponents recommend testing the urine for toxic peptides in their personal laboratories, but recommend eliminating casein and gluten even if the levels of urinary peptide are normal (9). For a review see Ref. 10.

2.   Sugar- and Additive-Free Diet

There is no empirical evidence that sugar and food additives, such as colorings, sweeteners, and preservatives, can cause the symptoms or that eliminating them from the diet improves the behavior of children with autism. Children with autism often have preferences for particular foods and textures, but these are due to perceptual and sensorimotor reasons and do not reflect food intolerance or sensitivity.

Elimination diets increase the burden of care on the parents, exclude the child from many pleasures of life, and can cause nutritional deficiencies (11). Instead of eliminating casein and gluten from the diet of every child, a more selective approach may be taken. Take a history of food allergies, food intolerance, and gastrointestinal (GI) symptoms in every child with PDD and refer those with a history or symptoms of food allergy to an allergist and those with food intolerance and GI symptoms to a gastroenterologist. If a child has diarrhea or constipation, and is not gaining weight or height, celiac disease may be considered and tests such as total IgA, antigliadin IgA, tissue trans-glutaminase, and antiendomyseal IgA antibodies may be ordered. Elimination diets can be tried for children with positive test results.

If testing is normal, but the parents insist that symptoms become worse when the child eats a particular food, eliminate the food item from the diet for 4 weeks and then reintroduce it, logging the foods eaten and the child's behavior in a diary. This selective approach is more benign and harmless than blanket elimination of casein, gluten, gliadin, and soy products from the diet.

B. Dietary Supplementation

1. Megavitamin B_6

In 1978, Rimland et al. reported that some autistic children responded favorably to high doses of vitamin B_6 (orthomolecular treatment) (12). In a subsequent trial, Rimland observed that some children experienced increased irritability, sound sensitivity, nausea, increased excitability, increased autistic symptoms, loose stools, and upper respiratory infection when they were given large amounts of vitamin B_6 (pyridoxine), but these problems disappeared when increased amounts of magnesium were added to the diet. Subsequent trials have, therefore, used pyridoxine with magnesium. The advocates of this treatment claim that the favorable changes in behavior are not due to general sedation but represent improvement in symptoms associated with autism. Although vitamin B_6 deficiency has not been documented in individuals with autism, according to the proponents, subclinical deficiencies could be present in individuals with autism. The effects could be mediated by neurotransmitters, because vitamin B_6 is involved in the formation of dopamine and other neurotransmitters (i.e., serotonin, γ-aminobutyric acid, norepinephrine, and epinephrine) (13). Some studies have, indeed, documented a tendency toward normalization of urinary homovanillic acid levels and evoked potentials with pyridoxine and magnesium (13,14).

Sensory neuropathy, a serious side effect, has been reported with very high doses of pyridoxine in the literature at large (15), but in studies that use ≤ 1 g/kg/day of vitamin B_6, few participants reported adverse side effects and the adverse effects were relatively minor and manageable. Once magnesium was added to the megavitamin therapy, adverse effects were even less. In the trials, dose of vitamin B_6 ranged from 1 mg/kg to 30 mg/kg, and of magnesium, from

10 to 15 mg/kg/day. Megavitamin B_6 therapy may be a relatively harmless and cheap adjunct for the treatment of autism (13,14,16). For a detailed discussion see Chapter 14.

2. Other Vitamins

Supplementation with other vitamins, such as vitamin A, folic acid, vitamin E, vitamin B_1, vitamin B_{12}, and vitamin C, is also recommended by some. As long as the dose of vitamins is within the recommended dietary allowance or slightly higher, the treatment may be harmless, but megadoses of vitamins, particularly vitamin A, D, and C, can be toxic. Vitamin C in the dose of 8 g/70 kg/day in divided dose was found to decrease stereotypic behaviors in a small sample of individuals with autism spectrum disorder (ASD) and mental retardation in a double-blind, placebo-controlled study. Except for a risk of renal stones this therapy seems to be benign (17).

3. Minerals

Advocates of trace and other minerals claim that children with autism have low levels of calcium, magnesium, copper, manganese, and chromium and higher levels of lithium and mercury in their hair samples as compared to age-and-sex-matched controls. Based on this premise, children with autism are given supplements of common minerals (calcium, magnesium, copper, manganese, zinc, chromium, and cobalt), and trace minerals (vanadium, germanium, selenium, tungsten, molybdenum, and tin). Minerals, such as zinc, have important functions in brain development and function, but dietary deficiencies or metabolic abnormalities involving trace elements are rare and have not been shown to cause autism. If the supplement contains doses within or slightly beyond the recommended dietary allowance, the treatment is harmless.

4. Fatty Acids

Supplementation with long-chain fatty acids (especially omega-3 and omega-6) has been alleged to improve the symptoms of autism in a few individuals, but there is no empirical or theoretical proof of their efficacy. The proponents argue that long-chain fatty acids restore the imbalance of prostaglandins and cytokines. If the intervention consists of merely administering oils such as evening primrose oil or borage seed oil, it is innocuous, but when the proponents recommend costly analysis of fatty acids in their personal laboratories, it becomes exploitative.

5. Inositol

Inositol is a precursor in the second-messenger system of some serotonin receptors. In animal studies and human trials, it has been found to improve behavior in depression, panic disorder, and OCD, but not in schizophrenia, ADHD, or autism (18,19). According to a controlled, double-blind, crossover trial, inositol is not helpful in autism (20).

6. Dimethylglycine

Dimethylglycine, a tertiary amine, is claimed by some to be effective in about 50% of individuals with autism (21). It has antioxidant and immunomodulating effects. In one study it was found to enhance humoral and cell-mediated immunity (22). At one time it was considered to have anticonvulsant effect as well, but controlled trials have failed to demonstrate its anticonvulsant effect (23). Two placebo-controlled trials failed to demonstrate significant benefits of dimethylglycine on behavior of patients with autistic disorder (24,25). One of these studies was faulted for using a low dose of dimethylglycine. However, dimethylglycine is a reasonably priced innocuous substance with few side effects. The recommended dose is one to four 125-mg tablets for a child, and two to eight tablets for an adult. It is also available as a liquid for younger children (26).

Other nutraceuticals, such as antioxidants, α-lipoic acid, peroxynitrate, and urecholine, have also been suggested as potential treatments for autism, but do not have any empirical or theoretical support.

Although physicians should be open to the idea of using neutraceuticals, they should provide limited leadership to the families without compromising the families' autonomy. They should carefully check the neutraceuticals for harmful ingredients because under the Dietary Supplement Health and Education Act of 1994 (DSHEA), ingredients used in dietary supplements are no longer subject to the premarket safety evaluations by the Food and Drug Administration. They should be vigilant about the side effects of neutraceuticals and should caution the families about brand-name products that make tall claims, because there is nothing unique in one concoction of minerals and vitamins over another.

C. Biologicals

1. Secretin

Fortuitous improvement in language and social behavior of three patients with autism who received a single dose of porcine secretin during a GI procedure led to an interest in secretin as a treatment for autism (27). It is a 27-amino-acid polypeptide hormone released by the cells of upper intestinal tract in response to a bolus of food to stimulate bicarbonate and bile production. Although it is widely distributed in the brain, its role in the brain is unknown. Many well-done studies have failed to demonstrate therapeutic benefits of single or multiple doses of either synthetic human secretin (28–31) or porcine secretin in individuals with autism (32–34).

At present, secretin is approved for diagnostic purposes only and its use in autism is off-label. Recommended dose for autism is 2 clinical units (CU)/kg or 0.2–0.4 mg/kg body weight (35). A sensitivity test with a smaller dose is recommended before the full bolus is given. Although the proponents claim that secretin is safe, hyperactivity and a few cases of diarrhea, seizures, and apnea have been reported. Secretin is neither innocuous nor inexpensive.

2. Antiyeast Therapy

Candida albicans, a yeast, is normally found in various parts of the body, including the gut. Generally, the amount of yeast in the gut is kept under control by other microbes that compete for the same nourishment. However, exposure to antibiotics, especially repeated exposure, can destroy these microbes, resulting in an overgrowth of *C. albicans*. According to the proponents of the yeast theory of ADD and autism, when the yeast multiplies, it releases toxins, such as aldehyde, alcohol, tartaric acid, and other organic acids, which, in turn, impair the central nervous system and the immune system. Only one laboratory in the country, owned by one of the proponents of the *Candida* theory, tests the urine for the toxic metabolites of *Candida*. The promoters of this theory recommend that this test, costing about $200, be done at the initiation of therapy and then periodically. No other commercial laboratory tests for these substances and medical insurers do not reimburse the cost.

Some of the behavior problems that have been linked to an overgrowth of *C. albicans* include confusion, hyperactivity, short attention span, lethargy, irritability, and aggression. Health problems, such as headaches, stomachaches, constipation, gas pains, fatigue, and depression, have also been attributed to *Candida*. Treatment is begun with an antifungal antibiotic, nystatin. If this does not work, other antifungal antibiotics, amphotericin B, ketoconazole, fluconazole, and terbinafine are tried. All are given orally. Additionally, the gut is replenished with a rich culture of probiotic agents or good microbes such as acidophilus. Avoiding sugar and other carbohydrate-rich foods on which yeast thrives, such as fruits, prevents overgrowth of the yeast. Interestingly, the child is supposed to become ill and to show negative behaviors for a few days after receiving antifungal treatment, because the yeast is destroyed and the debris is circulated through the body until it is excreted. A child who shows such deterioration is believed to have a good prognosis.

All evidence is anecdotal, written up in well-marketed books (36). There is no empirical evidence that there is overgrowth of *Candida* in individuals with autism (37). Whereas nystatin is relatively safe with mild risk of anemia and diarrhea, the other drugs are not so benign and may cause serious side effects, such as liver function abnormalities, headache, and rash. This treatment has no scientific basis.

3. Immunomodulator Therapy

a. Intravenous γ-Globulins (IVIG). There are two contradictory reports about the efficacy of IVIG. Gupta reported improvement in 10 children with autism who had evidence of immunodeficiency with IVIG at 400 mg/kg every 4 weeks for 6 months (38). Plioplys, on the other hand, reported benefit in only one of 10 children who did not have evidence of immunodeficiency with IVIG at 154–375 mg/kg every 6 weeks (39). Doses up to 5 g/kg every other day have been suggested without any empirical evidence. IVIG is costly and carries the risk of blood-borne infections such as hepatitis and HIV. Renal dysfunction ranging from increased blood urea nitrogen and creatinine to renal failure has been reported. IVIG is contraindicated in individuals with IgA deficiency. Thus IVIG is neither innocuous nor inexpensive.

b. Pentoxifylline. Pentoxifylline is a phosphodiesterase inhibitor with immunomodulatory, hemorrheological, and serotonergic effects. Its immuno-modulatory effect includes inhibition of tumor necrosis factor-α (40). It is approved in the United States for the treatment of intermittent claudication because of its effects on blood vessels, such as vasodilatation and increased blood flow. Its effects in autism may be mediated by its immunomodulatory or serotonergic properties. Most of the reports about its benefits in autism are either anecdotal or open-label studies without comparison groups. Until a double-blind, crossover trial confirms its benefits, it cannot be recommended.

4. Detoxification Therapies

Because the increased prevalence of autism has coincided with increasing industrial pollution, there is a considerable interest in the xenobiotic theory of autism. According to this theory, autism is caused by accumulation of heavy metals such as mercury, lead, cadmium, arsenic, and antimony in the body. The proponents use unconventional commercial panels of questionable validity to measure the body burden of heavy metals in hair and urine samples and recommend chelation if the tests are positive (41). If mercury poisoning is suspected, a careful environmental history, including the frequency, amount, and types of seafood consumed, should be taken followed by measurement of mercury concentrations in blood and urine at a reliable laboratory that uses reference values in general agreement with the published values. Blood mercury is the best test for current methylmercury exposure, while a 24-h urine collection is the best indicator of recent or chronic exposure to elemental or inorganic mercury (42). Spot collections are usually adequate but must be adjusted for creatinine concentration. Provocative chelation should not be used as a primary diagnostic test (42,43). In most cases hair testing is not required and has limited utility (42). Unconventional commercial hair, urine, and other panels should not be used (44).

Although no link has been found between patients' symptoms and mercury levels in individuals without known exposure (44), proponents of this theory recommend chelating children with autism with DMSA (2,3-dimercaptosuccinic, or Succimer) and DMPS ((2,3-dimercapto-1-propanesulfonic acid) even if there is no clinical or laboratory evidence of mercury poisoning. Blood CBC, liver, and kidney panels, and a sensitivity test are a prerequisite for this treatment. Succimer is given in the dose of 10 mg/kg/day in three divided doses for a few days followed by a rest period (45). Such cycles are repeated until heavy metals are cleared from the urine.

The reports supporting this treatment are mainly anecdotal. The treatment is neither innocuous, nor inexpensive. Both DMSA and DMPS can cause adverse reactions, such as gastrointestinal (GI) symptoms, rashes, neutropenia, and elevation of liver enzymes.

The proponents of the toxic theory also recommend supporting the cytochrome 450 and sulfation system in the liver to promote metabolism of toxic chemicals, but there is little theoretical or empirical support for such treatments. Proponents recommend glutathione and its precursors, glutamine, N-acetylcysteine, glycine, α-lipoic acid. The list of substances that are mentioned, such as methylsulfonylmethane, taurine, and molybdenum, is formidable and irrational. Even probiotics, such as lactobacilli and bifidobacteria are recommended to assist with mercury detoxification (46). The theory is pseudoscience in megawords and can be intimidating for the families. The physician should assist the families in researching the harmful effects of the ingredients offered in preparations sold on the Internet or in health food stores.

5. Famotidine (Pepcid)

One double-blind, placebo-controlled study reported some behavioral improvement in 9 children with ASD with 2 mg/kg of famotidine per day in divided doses. Famotidine is a H_2 (histamine) receptor antagonist used to treat gastroesophageal reflux. H_2 receptors in the brain are supposed to mediate exploratory behavior in animals. Although more studies are needed, the treatment is benign and worth a try (47).

III. MANIPULATIVE AND BODY-BASED SYSTEMS

This category refers to systems that use manipulation and/or movement of the body, such as chiropractic medicine, massage and bodywork, and unconventional physical and occupational therapies. There is no evidence that chiropractic or craniosacral manipulation helps children with autism and it will not be discussed further. A few controversial methods that fall in this realm of CAM are presented in this chapter.

A. Deep Pressure

It has been suggested that deep lateral pressure can reduce arousal and anxiety in autism. Occupational therapists often use deep pressure to decrease anxiety level and to increase sensory awareness of their subjects, but specific advantage of contraptions such as the Grandin Hug machine or Velvasoft Deep Pressure Sensory Tops and Shorts is not proven (48,49). Medline search came up with only one pilot study that suggested reduction in tension and anxiety for children with autism who received deep pressure (50). However, the treatment is innocuous and not very costly.

B. Auditory Integration Therapy (Tomatis Method)

This treatment is based on the premise that transmission of high-frequency human voice and music to the brain through an "electronic" ear can promote neuromaturation improving attention and behavior (51). Guy Berard introduced this therapy in France as a treatment for autism. Sensitivity of a child with autism to specific sound frequencies is tested with a detailed audiogram. The child then listens to music from which troublesome sound frequencies have been eliminated, in 20 half-hour sessions over a 10–12-day period. Although the proponents claim that AIT improves attention, auditory processing, expressive language, and auditory comprehension and decreases irritability and lethargy, there is no scientific support for these claims (52). Objective electrophysiological measures such as auditory-evoked brainstem responses fail to demonstrate differences in hearing sensitivity between autistic and nonautistic children (53). It is difficult to test children with autism. The sound level produced by the equipment can be potentially harmful (54). According to Bettison, listening to music in general may improve some aspects of autism, but there is no additional benefit of manipulated music (55).

Children with autism often like music and vocal or instrumental music is commonly used in the schools for autistic children to engage them. Music may reduce their social anxiety and self-stimulatory behavior, and may even improve their social responsiveness if participation in music is made contingent on responding, but it is not certain that these behavioral changes generalize to other settings or are curative.

C. Touch and Massage Therapy

Like music, some children with autism may respond to gentle touch and massage with calming and increased attention. Some parents even claim benefits such as reduction in hyperactivity, stereotypical and off-task behavior, and better sleep. Massage is innocuous if tolerated and certainly worth a try. There is nothing esoteric about massage beyond total loving care (TLC) and if a massage therapist asks the parents for exorbitant sums of money to use a special technique or oil, beware.

Touch has also been used in an educational approach called "rapid prompt method" in which the mother or an educator repeatedly touches, prods, and urges a child with autism to write. This prompting method has been made popular by the media, but is still awaiting scientific validation.

D. Facilitated Communication

Facilitated communication (FC) involves supporting a nonverbal individual's hand to make it easier for him/her to type out words on a typewriter, computer keyboard, or other communication device (56). Several scientific studies have suggested that facilitators may unintentionally influence the communication, perhaps to the extent of actually selecting the words themselves. There are no correct responses from the subject unless the facilitator knows the response (57,58). Many controlled studies have reported negative findings, indicating that the technique is neither reliable nor valid (59,60). The families should be aware that FC has been used to obtain allegations of abuse, particularly sexual abuse, from individuals with autism against third persons, causing negative consequences for families (61). For a detailed review of FC, see Ref. 62.

IV. ALTERNATIVE MEDICAL SYSTEMS

These include medical systems that have been practiced in other parts of the world from antiquity. Each of these systems has its unique explanation of how diseases are caused and how they should be treated. Except for homeopathic doses of secretin, there are few reports of alternative medical systems for the treatment of autism.

V. LIFESTYLE CHANGES

Lifestyle changes are helpful, actually essential, in coping with and caring for a child with autism. Parents should be encouraged to join parent support groups, obtain respite services, and practice behavioral relaxation.

A. Mind-Body Medicine

Mind-body medicine involves behavioral, psychological, social, and spiritual attempts to treat the body by exerting the influence of the mind over the body. The mind is the sum total of our thoughts, feelings, and memories. Each of our thoughts, feelings, and memories is a chemical or electrical wave in the brain that has the potential of circulating through the entire body. Thus, mind and body are intricately interlinked and constantly affect each other. Mind-body treatments, such as behavioral relaxation training, yoga, and mediation, are not effective for autism per se, but can help the parents in coping with the condition of their children.

B. Art, Music, and Dance Therapy

Such therapy has been used to improve social skills of children with autism and to enable them to engage in some acceptable activity instead of a maladaptive behavior to self-stimulate themselves.

VI. SUMMARY

The number of CAM treatments that are being promoted for autism is too large to be covered in this book. Physicians should be cautious about cynically rejecting these treatments, because some may have a placebo effect. If a treatment is not harmful, even if not useful, one should not dissuade the patents from trying it. Parents feel more empowered and in control if they make therapeutic decisions about their children, right or wrong. However, if a treatment is potentially harmful, one should caution the parents without paternalistically forbidding its use. The parents should decide for themselves what is good for their child and their family. The physician can assist them in this process but should not usurp their autonomy. A few examples of CAM are given in Table 1 and a clinical approach to CAM is presented in Table 2.

Table 1   Some Examples of CAM for Autism

Biological	Diet, vitamins, minerals, secretin, detoxification
Educational	Rapid prompt method
Communication	Facilitated communication
Sensory therapies	Auditory integration therapy
Body manipulation	Touch, massage, chiropractic

Table 2 Guidelines for Professionals Who Counsel Families About CAM

1. Keep an open mind. Instead of being overcritical, support parents in their quest for a cure for their child's condition.
2. Respect the parents' autonomy in making decisions about their child. Avoid paternalism. Do not judge and treat the parents adversely if the parents choose to try CAM along with conventional medicine.
3. Stay informed about CAM and be willing to provide guidance and assistance to the family in obtaining and reviewing information when the family is considering controversial or unproven treatments.
4. Discuss CAM options with the parents when a treatment plan is being developed. State whatever is known about a CAM, including its side effects, objectively and neutrally.
5. Discuss with the parents how to decide if CAM is based on hearsay or credible scientific research performed by a number of researchers working independently. Word of mouth, multisyllabic words, testimonials, and sponsored programs that make tall claims for a product are red flags. Counsel the parents about the importance of blinded controlled research with a comparison group. Newspapers and radio or TV talk shows cannot achieve the rigor of science. Tell the parents about reputed sources of information such as Medline Plus, the National Institute of Mental Health, the MIND Institute of the University of California, EBSCO, and ERIC.
6. Support the parents in choosing a reliable practitioner of CAM and a reliable product if they decide to try CAM. Help them develop some objective criteria to assess the efficacy of the CAM. Encourage them to use conventional treatments as well when CAM is being tried. Check for drug interactions.
7. Ensure that the treatments are not harmful to the child's health and safety.
8. Check for fraud. Check the National Health Fraud Unit, the FDA, the National Center for Complementary and Alternative Medicine (NCCAM) at *www.nccam.nih.gov*, the Federal Drug Administration (FDA) at *www.fda.gov*, and Alternative Medicine Alert, a monthly newsletter published by the American Health Consultants, to find out if the claims of the alternative provider are extravagant and fraudulent. If it is an herb, check the webpage of the Duke Center for Integrative Medicine at *www.dukehealth.org/ int_med* for its efficacy and toxicity. The Federal Trade Commission has a free consumer alert about fraudulent health advertising on the Internet, called "Virtual Treatments Can Be Real-World Deceptions." It can be obtained by writing to the Federal Trade Commission, Consumer Response Center, 600 Pennsylvania Ave., N.W., Washington, DC 20580, or by calling 877-FTC-HELP. Another useful site is *www.quackwatch.com.*
9. Check that the treatments are cost-effective and that the family's financial and emotional resources are not compromised by the use of these treatments. Check the cost of the treatment and suggest to the parents that they check with the insurance company to see if it will pay for the treatment.
10. When in doubt, acknowledge ignorance and be willing to refer for consultation.
11. Do not take away hope. Even if the positive effect of a CAM is a placebo effect, let the parents savor it, and positively acknowledge it.
12. Suggest that parents read the FDA Guide to Choosing Medical Treatments at *www.stopgettingsick.com.*

REFERENCES

1. Panel of Definition and Description, CAM Research Methodology Conference, April 1995. Defining and describing complementary and alternative medicine. Altern Ther Health Med 1997; 3:49–57.
2. Eisenberg DM, Davis RB, Ettner SL, et al. Trends in alternative medicine use in the United States, 1990–1997: results of a follow-up national survey. JAMA 1998; 280:1569–1575.
3. Chan E, Rappaport LA, Kemper KJ. Complementary and alternative therapies in childhood attention and hyperactivity problems. J Dev Behav Pediatr 2003; 24:4–8.
4. Pitetti R, Singh S, Hornyak D, Garcia SE, Herr S. Complementary and alternative medicine use in children. Pediatr Emerg Care 2001; 17:165–169.
5. Nickel RE. Controversial therapies for young children with developmental disabilities. Infants Young Child 1996; 8:29–40.
6. American Academy of Pediatrics. Counseling families who choose complementary and alternative medicine for their child with chronic illness or disability. Committee on Children with Disabilities. Pediatrics 2001; 107:598–601.
7. Lucarelli S, Frediani T, Zingoni AM, Ferruzzi F, Giardini O, Quintieri F, Barbato M, D'Eufemia P, Cardi E. Food allergy and infantile autism. Panminerva Med 1995; 37:137–141.
8. Knivsberg AM, Reichelt KL, Hoien T, Nodland M. A randomised, controlled study of dietary intervention in autistic syndromes. Nutr Neurosci 2002; 5:251–261.
9. Reichelt KL, Hole K, Hamberger A, Saelid G, Edminson PD, Braestrup CB, Lingjaerde O, Ledaal P, Orbeck H. Biologically active peptide-containing fractions in schizophrenia and childhood autism. Adv Biochem Psychopharmacol 1981; 28:627–643.
10. Shattock P and Whiteley P. The Sunderland Protocol: A Logical Sequence of Biomedical Interventions for the Treatment of Autism and Related Disorders. Sunderland, UK: Autism Research Unit, University of Sunderland, 2000.
11. Arvola T, Holmberg-Marttila D. Benefits and risks of elimination diets. Ann Med 1999; 31:293–298.
12. Rimland B, Callaway E, Dreyfus P. The effect of high doses of vitamin B_6 on autistic children: a double-blind crossover study. Am J Psychiatry 1978; 135:472–475.
13. Pfeiffer S, Norton J, Nelson L, Shott S. Efficacy of vitamin B_6 and magnesium in the treatment of autism: a methodology review and summary of outcomes. J Autism Dev Disord 1995; 25:481–493.
14. Martineau J, Barthelemy C, Garreau B, LeLord G. Vitamin B_6, magnesium, and combined B_6-Mg: therapeutic effects in childhood autism. Biol Psychiatry 1985; 20:467–478.
15. Haslam R. Is there a role for megavitamin therapy in the treatment of attention deficit hyperactivity disorder? Adv Neurol 1992; 58:303–310.
16. Rimland B, Callaway E, Dreyfus P. The effect of high doses of vitamin B_6 on autistic children: a double-blind crossover study. Am J Psychiatry 1978; 135:472–475.
17. Dolske MC, Spollen, J, McKay S, et al. A preliminary trial of ascorbic acid as supplemental therapy for autism. Prog Neuropsychopharmacol Biol Psychiatry 1993; 17:765–774.

18. Einat H, Belmaker RH. The effects of inositol treatment in animal models of psychiatric disorders. J Affect Disord 2001; 62:113–121.
19. Levine J. Controlled trials of inositol in psychiatry. Eur Neuropsychopharmacol 1997; 7:147–155.
20. Levine J, Aviram A, Holan A, Ring A, Barak Y, Belmaker RH. Inositol treatment of autism. J Neural Transm 1997; 104:307–310.
21. http://www.autism.com/ari/editorials/dmg.1html, accessed on 2.23.03.
22. Graber CD, Goust JM, Glassman AD, Kendall R, Loadholt CB. Immunomodulating properties of dimethylglycine in humans. J Infect Dis 1981; 143:101–105.
23. Gascon G, Patterson B, Yearwood K, Slotnick H. *N,N*-Dimethylglycine and epilepsy. Epilepsia 1989; 30:90–93.
24. Kern JK, Miller VS, Cauller PL, Kendall PR, Mehta PJ, Dodd M. Effectiveness of *N,N*-dimethylglycine in autism and pervasive developmental disorder. J Child Neurol 2001; 16:169–173.
25. Bolman WM, Richmond JA. A double-blind placebo-controlled, crossover pilot trial of low dose Dimethylglycine in patients with autistic disorder. J Autism Dev Disord 1999; 29:191–194.
26. http://www.autism.org/dmg.html, accessed on 2.23.03.
27. Horvath K, Stefanatos G, Sokolski KN, Wachtel R, Nabors L, Tildon JT. Improved social and language skills after secretin administration in patients with autistic spectrum disorders. J Assoc Acad Minor Phys 1998; 9:9–15.
28. Sandler AD, Sutton KA, DeWeese J, Girardi MA, Sheppard V, Bodfish JW. Lack of benefit of a single dose of synthetic human secretin in the treatment of autism and pervasive developmental disorder. N Engl J Med 1999; 341:1801–1806.
29. Carey T, Ratliff-Schaub K, Funk J, Weinle C, Myers M, Jenks J. Double-blind placebo-controlled trial of secretin: effects on aberrant behavior in children with autism. J Autism Dev Disord 2002; 32:161–167.
30. Molloy CA, Manning-Courtney P, Swayne S, Bean J, Brown JM, Murray DS, Kinsman AM, Brasington M, Ulrich CD 2nd. Lack of benefit of intravenous synthetic human secretin in the treatment of autism. J Autism Dev Disord 2002; 32:545–551.
31. Sponheim E, Oftedal G, Helverschou SB. Multiple doses of secretin in the treatment of autism: a controlled study. Acta Paediatr 2002; 91:540–545.
32. Owley T, Steele E, Corsello C, Risi S, McKaig K, Lord C, Leventhal BL, Cook Jr EH. Double-blind, placebo-controlled trial of secretin for the treatment of autistic disorder. MedGenMed 1999; Oct 6:E2.
33. Owley T, McMahon W, Cook EH, Laulhere T, South M, Mays LZ, Shernoff ES, Lainhart J, Modahl CB, Corsello C, Ozonoff S, Risi S, Lord C, Leventhal BL, Filipek PA. Multisite, double-blind, placebo-controlled trial of porcine secretin in autism. J Am Acad Child Adolesc Psychiatry 2001; 40:1293–1299.
34. Corbett B, Khan K, Czapansky-Beilman D, Brady N, Dropik P, Goldman DZ, Delaney K, Sharp H, Muller I, Shapiro E, Ziegler R. A double-blind, placebo-controlled crossover study investigating the effect of porcine secretin in children with autism. Clin Pediatr (Phila) 2001; 40:327–331.
35. http://www.autism.com/ari/secretin2.html, accessed on 2.26.03.

36. Crook WG. The Yeast Connection Handbook. Jackson, TN: Professional Books/ Future Health, Inc., 1996.

37. Horvath K, Papadimitriou JC, Rabsztyn A, et al. Gastrointestinal abnormalities in children with autistic disorder. J Pediatr 1999; 135:559–563.

38. Gupta S. Treatment of children with autism with intravenous immunoglobulin. J Child Neurol 1999; 14:203–205.

39. Plioplys AV. Intravenous immunoglobulin treatment of children with autism. J Child Neurol 1998; 13:79–82.

40. Gupta S. Immunological treatments for autism. J Autism Dev Disord 2000; 30:475–479.

41. Seidel S, Kreutzer R, Smith D, McNeel S, Gilliss D. Assessment of commercial laboratories performing hair testing. JAMA 2001; 285:67–72.

42. Agency for Toxic Substance and Disease Registry. Mercury toxicity. Am Fam Physician 1992; 46:1731–1741.

43. Forman J, Moline J, Cernichiari E, et al. A cluster of pediatric metallic mercury exposure cases treated with meso-2,3-dimercaptosuccinic acid (DMSA). Environ Health Perspect 2000; 108:575–577.

44. Kales SN, Goldman RH. Mercury exposure: current concepts, controversies, and a clinic's experience. J Occup Environ Med 2002; 44:143–154.

45. Laidler JR. DAN! Mercury Detoxification Consensus Group. Position Paper. San Diego, CA: Autism Research Institute, 2001.

46. Kidd PM. Autism, an extreme challenge to integrative medicine. Part II. Medical management. Altern Med Rev 2002; 7:472–499.

47. Lindsay LA, Tsiouris JA, Cohen IL, Shindledecker R, DeCresce R. Famotidine treatment of children with autistic spectrum disorders: pilot research using single subject research design. J Neural Transm 2001; 108:593–611.

48. Zissermann L. The effects of deep pressure on self-stimulating behaviors in a child with autism and other disabilities. Am J Occup Ther 1992; 46:547–551.

49. Krauss KE. The effects of deep pressure touch on anxiety. Am J Occup Ther 1987; 41:366–373.

50. Edelson SM, Edelson MG, Kerr DC, Grandin T. Behavioral and physiological effects of deep pressure on children with autism: a pilot study evaluating the efficacy of Grandin's Hug Machine. Am J Occup Ther 1999; 53:145–152.

51. Thompson BM. An historical commentary on the physiological effects of music: Tomatis, Mozart and neurophysiology. Integr Physiol Behav Sci 2000; 35:174–188.

52. Committee on Children with Disabilities, American Academy of Pediatrics. Auditory integration training and facilitated communication for autism (RE9752). Pediatrics 1998; 102:431–433.

53. Gravel JS. Auditory integrative training: placing the burden of proof. Am J Speech Lang Pathol 1994; 3:25–29.

54. Rankovic CM, Rabinowitz WM, Lof GL. Maximum output intensity of the Audiokinetron. Am J Speech Lang Pathol 1996; 5:68–72.

55. Bettison S,. Long-term effects of auditory training on children with autism. J Autism Dev Disord 1996; 26:361–367.

56. Jacobson JW, Mulick JA, Schwartz AA. A history of facilitated communication: science, pseudoscience, and antiscience. Am Psychol 1995; 50:750–765.

57. Smith MD, Haas PJ, Belcher RG. Facilitated communication: the effects of facilitator knowledge and level of assistance on output. J Autism Dev Disord 1994; 24:357–367.
58. Cardinal DA, Hanson D, Wakeham J. Investigation of authorship in facilitated communication. Ment Retard 1996; 34:231–242.
59. Eberlin M, McConnachie G, Ibel S, Volpe L. Facilitated communication: a failure to replicate the phenomenon. J Autism Dev Disord 1993; 23:507–530.
60. Regal RA, Rooney JR, Wandas T. Facilitated communication: an experimental evaluation. J Autism Dev Disord 1994; 24:345–355.
61. Konstantareas MM. Allegations of sexual abuse by nonverbal autistic people via facilitated communication: testing of validity. Child Abuse Negl 1998; 22:1027–1041.
62. Mostert MP. Facilitated communication since 1995: a review of published studies. J Autism Dev Disord 2001; 31:287–313.

13

Planning Education Programs for Students with Autism Spectrum Disorder

Catherine Trapani
*Marcus Institute and Emory University, Atlanta,
Georgia, U.S.A.*

I. INTRODUCTION

Twenty years ago, autism was considered to be a rare, hard-to-diagnose disorder that was far from newsworthy. Students with autism did not typically receive an education in public schools, or if they did, they were combined in self-contained classes with students with severe retardation. The salient features of the disorder include delays in language, social competence, and presence of stereotypic and persevative behaviors. These characteristics are evidenced in children before the age of 3. Currently, the number of children diagnosed with autism spectrum disorder (ASD) is 1/500 (1). As a result of the availability of assessment measures such as the Autism Diagnostic Interview Schedule–Revised (2) the diagnosis can be made reliably by the age of 2 (3), and ASD is a "hot topic" in the popular and scientific press. In 1990, autism became an educational classification in the revision of Individuals with Disabilities Education Act (IDEA) (4); thus entitling students with ASD to a free appropriate education designed to meet their needs.

Despite the increasing student body and the increasing knowledge base, no single effective "appropriate" curriculum has been isolated, and controversies rage among professional and parent groups about methods of intervention [i.e., applied behavior analysis (ABA), treatment and education of autistic and related communication-handicapped children (TEACCH), floor time]. Additionally, the amount of intervention time that should be provided (20–40 hr/week) is widely debated. Therefore, the provision of "appropriate" treatment and education for students with ASD is highly charged involving multiple disciplines and the realms of litigation and public policy.

In addition to the controversy in identifying appropriate interventions there exists the daunting mission of accessing educational and intervention services. Despite the fact that IDEA is a federal law, there is a lack of parity nationwide (between and within the states) on what constitutes an "appropriate" education for any student falling within the realm of special education (5), but this is especially true with respect to children with ASD. The operational definition of the word appropriate has itself been the topic of litigation (6), and rightly so. The language in IDEA is broad and vague making parents and schools vulnerable to the very problems the law was designed to solve. On one hand, all schools are required to provide appropriate (but not optimal) education. On the other hand, it is difficult for parents to understand why students in some states have access to ABA or TEAACH through public education (because they are deemed appropriate), while the same services in other states are deemed to be optimal and beyond what is expected of the schools. This disparity is emotionally charged and has contributed to the rapid and significant increase in litigation regarding students with ASD (7).

The litigious climate that has been created between parents and schools regarding the design and delivery of services is difficult at best. The onus of responsibility is on the parent to prove that the services provided by the school are inappropriate (8). Although the outcomes of litigation nationwide have been mixed (9), typically, the courts defer to the schools to select the methodology to be used in the individual education program (IEP) (10). Ironically, in some cases, the money involved in settling a case that has been ruled in favor of the parents could have provided "state of the art" services for a number of children (11). (For an extensive review of the special education law see Ref. 12.)

Clinicians know that the level of sophistication that parents possess regarding their rights to a free appropriate public education (FAPE) or how to approach their insurance provider is as diverse as the spectrum of autism. Some parents are well apprised of their rights and access information about the latest interventions. Others have no idea of what they should be asking during IEP meetings or how to be evaluating their children's progress from one year to the next. Clearly, all parents of children with ASD want what is appropriate for their children and realize that the stakes are high. The literature documents that receiving early intervention can circumvent many of the difficulties associated with the disorder possibly resulting in successful placement in regular education within the public schools (13). Other parents, whose children experience less success from early intervention, continue to advocate for the receipt of interventions that may assist in decreasing aberrant behaviors and increasing even a modicum of independence. They realize that gains in appropriate behavior and self-help skills will translate directly into quality-of-life issues long after the public schools are responsible for their children.

ABA has produced the largest number of controlled studies using single subject-designs documenting the efficacy of the approach (14). Additionally, the Surgeon General has noted that ABA is the most effective means of teaching children with ASD (15). Nonetheless, case studies and some empirical research have documented the positive effects of other approaches. In 2000, the National Research Council formed a committee to empirically review the research in education and public policy and to create a framework for evaluating the scientific evidence regarding features and outcomes of educational interventions (16).

The search for an effective curriculum addressing the needs of students with ASD continues, but guidance for parents, teachers, and clinicians is needed until a perfect intervention is identified. In reviewing all of the treatment paradigms, Lord and McGee (16) isolated priorities for intervention receiving consensus from all. The efficacy of the different approaches to intervention will not be reviewed in this chapter. Rather, the chapter will focus on reviewing the critical elements of instruction as identified by the National Research Council. These elements should be considered in the design of an IEP for students with autism: behavioral interventions, communication, play skills, social skills; and acquisition of cognitive and functional academic skills. For a comprehensive and critical review of the extant literature refer to the National Research Council publication Educating Children with Autism (16,17).

II. BEHAVIORAL INTERVENTIONS

Behavior problems are prevalent among persons with autism. In early childhood tantrums and disruptive behavior are displayed, whereas adolescents and young adults often exhibit aggressive, stereotypic, and self-injurious behaviors (18). Often parents, teachers, and other caregivers inadvertently enable children to manipulate their environment by displaying inappropriate behaviors, thus reinforcing and maintaining them. Persistent problem behaviors may, over time, interfere with participating in school, developing functional skills, and engaging in community activities. Additionally, placement options for young adults are often dictated by the presence of aberrant behavior (19). Once established, problem behaviors require direct intensive intervention before they are diminished. Consequently, behavioral intervention is optimal in early childhood to circumvent escalation of behaviors and is essential in older students to diminish aggression, disruption, and self-injury (20).

During the 1960s learning theorists utilizing behavioral principles produced positive gains in behavioral and educational intervention in students with autism (21,22). Over the course of 30 years, behavioral interventions have been effective in addressing a wide array of problem behaviors.

A recent critical review of the literature utilizing behavioral interventions, documented that more than half of the studies reported an 80–90% reduction in problem behaviors of students with disabilities (23). The efficacy of ABA has also been recognized by the 1997 amendment of the IDEA (24). Functional behavior assessment and a behavior intervention plan are now required in the IEPs for students with disabilities who have comorbid problem behaviors (25). Although this mandate is promising for children with ASD who exhibit problem behaviors, it is challenging for school systems that do not have the expertise or economic resources to conduct functional assessments. To meet the requirements of IDEA in a viable manner, rating scales and interviews have been utilized. Although such measures are user-friendly and inexpensive, their reliability and validity are dubious. Thus, experimental functional analysis is the assessment method that is considered to be best practice (26). Studies have documented the relationship between the precision of assessment and the success of the intervention (27). This issue is especially relevant for students who have complex severe behaviors that present a danger to themselves or others.

The purpose of functional analysis is to isolate the function of behaviors exhibited and to identify the extent to which the outcome or consequence of the behavior predicts its probability. Functional analysis differs from other assessments (e.g., interviews, standardized tests) in that the variables believed to affect behavior are systematically manipulated (28). The antecedents and consequences associated with the problem behavior are isolated during various assessment conditions (i.e., attention, toy play, demand, or alone conditions) and observed in a controlled setting. The child randomly encounters one of the four conditions in a series of 15-min sessions presented in random order. Documentation of the occurrence of high rates of a target behavior during an assessment condition is indicative of the function of the behavior (29). This is a critical process as a behavioral intervention cannot be successfully designed and implemented without identifying the specific function of the behavior (30).

When target behaviors are isolated and their functions identified, behavioral strategies can be employed to reduce the incidence of problem behaviors. For treatment to be effective, further assessment to identify reinforcers that are highly preferred (31,32) and punishers that are least preferred (33) is conducted. Fisher et al. (34) documented that the forced-choice assessment (e.g., stimuli were presented in pairs and the student was instructed to choose one of the pair) was most effective in predicting stimuli that would serve as a powerful reinforcer. Likewise, Fisher et al. (34) employed a strategy for assessing effective punishers. The punisher that produced the greatest reduction in target behaviors is selected for inclusion in the treatment protocol (34).

Currently, many schools employ positive behavior interventions that do not utilize punishers. However, some behaviors may require the inclusion of a punisher in an intervention to rapidly produce behavior change (35).

A. Issues for Planning Educational Goals

Children with limited communication skills and/or poor social development are at risk for developing problem behaviors. If aberrant behaviors develop, trained professionals should conduct functional assessments to ensure the safety of the child and the reliability of the results (36). Parents should inquire about the credentials of professionals conducting functional assessments and interventions.

The information obtained from the functional analysis should direct the design of the behavioral intervention and be reflected in the behavior intervention plan contained within the IEP (37). Sometimes, behaviors can be so challenging to parents and teachers that it is easier to give in to them than to persist in demanding compliance or appropriate behavior. Although this is understandable, it is essential that the rewards received for engaging in problem behavior are minimal. Once problem behaviors are maintained over time, they are exceedingly difficult to change. To minimize the need to engage in aberrant behavior, children should be given ways to control their environment by making choices and receiving reinforcers for appropriate behaviors (38). For behavioral interventions to be effective over time, parents and schools must work collaboratively in collecting data on target behaviors and in implementing the behavioral protocol. The systematic use of reinforcers and consequences across settings is essential to maintaining the positive effects of intervention.

III. LANGUAGE AND COMMUNICATION

Consistent with the variability present within the continuum of ASD, the population displays a wide array of language and communication deficits. Some children's language skills display idiosyncratic language or echolalia (39). Individuals who do acquire complex language encounter difficulties similar to those of their counterparts with learning disabilities, regarding conversational turn taking, shifting language levels to fit the situation and skills of their conversation partner, and following the social protocols of pragmatic language (40). Similarly, nonverbal language skills are also problematic for children with ASD (41).

Problems in joint attention and use of symbols have been isolated as core deficits in communication in this population (42). Joint attention refers to problems in coordinating attention between people and objects. It relates to skills in orienting and attending to a social partner, shifting gaze, sharing affect and experience, and following the gaze and point of another person. Symbol use refers to learning conventional or shared meanings for symbols including gestures and words. Many individuals with ASD are limited in learning symbols and in using conventional gestures such as showing, waving, pointing, and head nodding (43). These are target skills for intervention (44). A relationship seems to exist between competence in communication and behavior and overall level of outcome. Thus, language is a critical area for intervention (45).

A. Intervention

Language and communication skill interventions have utilized developmental and behavioral approaches. Although behavioral approaches to intervention are more widely represented in the research, it is one area of intervention where the two paradigms intertwine. Interventions have centered on developing functional communication, as well as verbal and nonverbal communication (46).

1. Functional Communication Training

This intervention is used when the results of a functional analysis indicate that problem behaviors such as aggression, tantrums, and self-injury are maintained because they enable individuals to manipulate the environment by gaining access to attention or escaping demands (47). Utilizing the elements of functional analysis described in the previous section, individuals are taught communication skills that provide access to the desired reinforcer (i.e., a break from work, attention, change in setting). Studies of functional communication training have culminated in robust findings in the ability to reduce problem behaviors (48). However, the efficacy of functional communication training is not limited to reducing problem behaviors, but includes teaching new methods (e.g., card exchange) of communicating requests for attention, preferred activities, and reinforcers. Functional communication can enable students to fully participate in community settings (49).

2. Verbal Communication

A vast literature documents the effects of speech and language intervention for children with autism. Most of these studies have utilized discrete trial training or more contemporary approaches of applied behavior analysis to develop verbal language skills, which have ranged from developing single-word vocabulary to describing objects and pictures and responding to questions. Perhaps the most widely known techniques are the discrete trial training protocols addressing labeling and naming skills designed by Lovaas. Limitations of discrete trial training are failure to develop spontaneous use of language and to establish generalization in natural contexts (50).

Recent discrete trial training approaches have successfully taught responses to "wh" questions and elicited descriptions of objects and pictures (51) and comprehension of prepositions (52). Other contemporary approaches include, but are not limited to, incidental teaching (53) and pivotal response training (54). Incidental teaching techniques utilize naturally occurring adult-child interactions to teach the language skills and incorporated behavioral techniques such as prompting, imitating, and requesting (55). Pivotal response training centers on initiation of communication that is considered to be a pivotal behavior. Child-initiated communication will be a catalyst for responses from others, thus providing reinforcers for communication and facilitate the development of language skills (56). It has been documented that self-initiated communications have been taught to children with autism who possessed poor spontaneous communication (57).

3. Nonverbal Communication

The use of augmentative and alternative communication systems enables persons with severe communication disorders to compensate for their disabilities by supporting existent speech or developing nonspeech symbol systems such as sign language, visual symbols displayed on communication boards, and voice output devices. The goal of these systems is to empower individuals to independently communicate their wants and needs (58).

Sign language has been used with many special education populations. It is widely documented that total communication (use of both sign language and oral speech) is an effective method of teaching receptive and expressive vocabulary to individuals with autism (59). Signing does not hinder the development of speech, but research findings suggest that it may enhance the use of speech. Acquiring skills in signing is especially important for students with limited communication who may never acquire speech (60).

It is essential to provide independent functional communication systems to students with autism. Visual symbols have been used successfully to facilitate compliance, initiate communication, and minimize dependence on verbal cues (61). Nonetheless, the efficacy of a system of visual symbols that is most widely used in public schools (the picture exchange communication system) is not empirically documented (62).

B. Issues for Planning Educational Goals

Language and communication are essential to facilitate independence and to circumvent the development of problem behaviors. Therefore, parents and professionals must be meticulous in designing language assessments and intervention. Comprehensive assessments of receptive, expressive, and pragmatic language skills are an essential first step in understanding the nature and scope of language deficits and in implementing intervention (63). Teaching sign language is helpful in providing students with a means to communicate as is functional communication training. Photographic activity schedules and augmentative communication devices should be probed. The efficacy of the intervention must be carefully evaluated so that critical time is not lost; "based on the available research with this population, progress on language and communication goals should be evident within 2 to 3 months, or different approaches should be considered." Progress should be evaluated using data collection methods consistent with single-subject design (64).

It may be helpful for parents and professional to collaborate in formulating a plan that would determine which language interventions will be implemented, the length of the trial for the intervention approach, and the next step in isolating an effective treatment. Similarly, language intervention and data collection should be implemented across home and school settings (65).

IV. PLAY SKILLS

Play presents a vast array of opportunities to assist children in developing essential skills. Appropriate play skills provide children the ability to interact with others and formulate friendships that are critical to social development throughout life. A vast literature addresses the play skills in children with autism. Skills deficits range from lack of organized, independent, cooperative play to engaging in repetitive, deviant, or aimless play (66). Studies have indicated that deficits in these areas of play are more problematic for children with ASD than for mentally retarded or normal children (67). Students experience increasing levels of difficulty playing with others as they progress in school if they have not developed the cooperative and rule-governed play skills needed for participation in group play. Functional and symbolic play have been identified in the literature as two skill deficits that are critical to the development of viable play skills (68).

Functional play involves using objects appropriately during play activities in a manner that is consistent with their function. Young autistic children show less appropriate functional play in unstructured situations (69). Symbolic play refers to the ability to substitute one object with another (i.e., using a play needle as a microphone). Difficulties in developing functional and symbolic play may be indicative of other related developmental delays. For example, researchers have identified a relationship between delayed receptive and expressive language skill deficits and functional and symbolic play skills (70). Delays in related skills impact on the ability to develop and demonstrate play skills; therefore, it is essential that those collateral skills (i.e., language, cognition, social skills, and motor skills) be assessed. Selecting play activities that are consistent with a child's level of development may facilitate learning (71). Therefore, intervention should focus on addressing the needs of the child rather than on engaging in age-appropriate activities demonstrated by same-age peers (72).

A. Play Skill Interventions

Interventions can provide opportunities to engage in developmentally appropriate play while at the same time moving children forward to higher developmental stages (i.e., zone of proximal distance) (73). Initially, adults can mediate play activities and model the appropriate varied use of toys and other playthings. Adult and child-directed play can provide exemplars to children with ASD about purposeful play that has a logical beginning and end. Such activities may have the added benefit of improving language, cognition, and social interaction (74).

In addition to teaching isolated play skills, other skills have been enhanced by including the ability to make social initiations using script-training photo and written activity schedules (75). Issues about the motivation to play have been addressed using choice making in pivotal response training (76). Additionally, integrated playgroups have created environments in which to play and provide opportunities for guided and peer-mediated intervention (77).

B. Issues for Planning Educational Goals

Engaging in developmentally appropriate play can be a catalyst for positive gains developmentally. Scheduling numerous daily structured play periods and incorporating adult and child-directed play activities is critical. Children with ASD need direct instruction and guided practice in selecting preferred playthings, using toys purposefully, and transitioning appropriately from playtime to other activities. When these skills have been obtained, children should participate in organized playgroups. Play buddies or playgroups should be carefully selected on the basis of children's skills, needs, interests, and ages. It is essential that children encounter pleasure and success from such experiences (78).

Play should be incorporated in interventions that address other critical domains such as language, social competence, and acquisition of basic academic skills. These activities can be utilized in both the school and home settings (79). Therefore, developing play skills, utilizing play across the curriculum, and planning for generalization of skills across settings should be goals included in IEPs.

The skills that are afforded by playing are foundations for abilities needed later in life, such as recreation and leisure time activity. The ability to organize free time constructively and engage in solitary or group play activities without assistance has critical ramifications regarding placement in postsecondary settings and quality of life. These issues affect all individuals with ASD, but are especially pertinent for those with moderate to severe difficulties. Recreational and leisure time skills enable individuals to access group home placements or have greater options for admission to more restricted residential settings. Likewise, these skills foster inclusion in family activities over the course of a lifetime. The importance of this cannot be underestimated. Individuals who do not initiate activities or possess interests require constant supervision and programming. Such persons are considered to be "high maintenance" and are extremely vulnerable to abuse and neglect.

V. SOCIAL SKILLS

The general literature in social competence suggests that the use of prosocial behaviors may contribute to the social adjustment of individuals and influence their interpersonal relationships. Positive as well as negative social behavior tends to be reciprocal (80). For example, observations of nursery school children's social behavior have revealed that positive social behaviors, including giving attention and affection, expressing approval and personal acceptance, and giving objects to another, are related to peer acceptance. Conversely, negative social behaviors, including noncompliance, interference, and attack, relate to rejection by others (81). Socially competent individuals posses the components of social behaviors (i.e., facial expressions, gestures, greetings), monitor those behaviors through a system of rules, and utilize these skills to obtain desired goals (82).

There are critical social skills that appear to foster friendship such as demonstrating sensitivity to the needs and feelings of others, expressing warmth and affection, and sharing goals and activities. Moreover, attitudes that precipitate friendship include finding people to be sources of satisfaction and enjoying the exchange of affection (83). Obtaining and using the skills required for reciprocal social exchanges and making friends are challenges experienced by individuals on the autism spectrum (84).

Deficits in social competence were included in the first descriptions of autism (85) and remain salient features of the disorder. Children evidence delayed or aberrant social behavior beginning in early childhood (86). Compared to same-age peers, children with autism exhibit more sterotypies and self-injurious behaviors and spend more time engaged in meaningless activity (87). Research findings suggest that social interaction is not reinforcing to many students diagnosed with ASD (88). Proximity to peers is avoided or the quality of interactions is lacking when these students do engage with others (89). This is an issue of concern as reciprocal peer exchanges are salient to the development of social relationships (90).

People with autism have difficulty talking to others (91) and coordinating joint attention (92). At higher skill levels interpreting nonverbal language (93) and comprehending humor are difficult for students with ASD (94). Additionally, demonstrating the capacity to extend beyond self is problematic in this population. A section of the Autism Diagnostic Interview Schedule–Revised (ADI-R) (95) focusing on the assessment of social development and play investigates the ability to offer comfort, among other behaviors needed to formulate relationships. Developing empathy is important, as it is a core requirement for establishing social relationships with others (96). Analyzing the parent responses in ADI-Rs can assist in formulating and sequencing appropriate goals for social development.

A. Intervention

Bandura's work in social learning theory (97) posited that specific identifiable skills form the basis for socially competent behaviors and that interpersonal difficulties may arise as a function of a faulty and/or incomplete behavioral repertoire (98).

Interventions have focused predominantly on developing social skills in young children with ASD using a variety of techniques. Social skills training has addressed initiating social exchanges (99) using picture schedules to initiate social exchanges (100) and prompting reciprocal interaction through incidental teaching (101). Other studies aimed at improving social interactions have used social scripts (102), and substantiated the power of peer-mediated interventions (103). Social behaviors have been increased by using peers in pivotal response training (104) and involving children in integrated play groups (105).

While there are numerous models for social skills training, no one model fits all needs. Social skills training models share common elements: social skills change to correspond to the social setting (106); verbal and nonverbal learned responses guide interpersonal skills (107); social competence is dependent upon the receipt of reinforcers (108); and models are designed with assumption that skills can be taught (109).

B. Issues for Parents and Professionals in Setting Educational Goals

Social skills should be assessed to determine skill deficits and identify target skills for intervention. Social skills training conducted by a school psychologist, speech and language therapist, or social worker should be incorporated into the IEPs (110). The goals of social skills training should reflect the child's cognitive ability and communication skills. Children need to receive direct instruction in this area, as they will not develop or model socially skilled behaviors merely from being in proximity to typically developing peers. Skill acquisition should be monitored so that a different intervention can be utilized if indicated. Although children with ASD may initially appear to prefer being alone, the most powerful intervention and reinforcer for using prosocial behavior comes from the natural environment. Children should have opportunities to practice the skills they are learning in settings such as the classroom, the community, and the home (111). Children should participate in playgroups, friendship groups, or groups that focus on their special interests.

VI. ACQUISITION OF BASIC SKILLS

Some students with ASD possess abilities that enable participation in a traditional academic curriculum, while others experience cognitive delays that compromise participation in a functional curriculum. Irrespective of ability level, generalizing what has been learned across materials, settings, and times is challenging. To teach toward generalization, a curriculum should plan for practicing skills in natural settings with naturally occurring reinforcers from multiple sources such as parents, teachers, and peers (112).

Consistent with other special education populations, comprehensive assessment must drive the design of the "what, how, and where" of educational programming. Consideration of issues presented in previous sections of the chapter must be reflected in the selection of the curriculum and the design of an instructional schedule. Similarly, other attributes affecting learning, such as attention, impulsivity, motivation, and cue dependence, must also be considered (113). Irrespective of the level of ability, the goal of an educational program should be to assist students in developing independence and obtaining quality of life to the greatest extent possible (114).

The infinite number of interventions aimed at improving outcomes for students with ASD is overwhelming leaving parents and professionals vulnerable to the latest fads in treatment. After completing a comprehensive critical review of instructional treatment programs for students with autism, the state of New York concluded that instruction utilizing ABA was the only one that had empirical merit and substance (115).

Although the term "ABA" is frequently used, many parents and professionals are uncertain about what ABA really is and its approach to intervention. Green (116) provides a succinct explanation in the following passage from her article on behavior analytic instruction.

> Behavior analytic instruction begins with a comprehensive assessment of each learner's current skills and needs, accomplished by observing the learner directly in a variety of situations and recording what she or he does and does not do. Every skill that is selected for instruction (often called a target) is defined in clear, observable terms and broken down into its component parts. Each component response is taught by presenting or arranging one or more specific antecedent stimuli, such as cues or instructions from another person, and/or items of interest to the learner. (116)

ABA relies on data collection so that educational and behavioral interventions can be formulated systematically. Thus, individual assessment is directly correlated with individual design and evaluation of goals, objectives, and overall curricula (117).

A. Intervention

Olley notes that the emphasis of the literature is on the method rather than the content of instruction (118). Consequently, it is easy to select a strategy of "how" to teach, but often difficult to isolate and sequence "what" should be taught. Appropriate educational programs for students with ASD require utilizing the technology of instruction in designing errorless learning and structuring environments that facilitate learning (119).

1. Instructional Techniques

In ABA, the instructional unit is the learning trial, which is defined as a structured opportunity for a response, in the presence of an antecedent, followed by a consequence (SRS) (120). Instructional methodologies address the manner in which lessons are organized and delivered and responses are evoked. Instruction can be organized in massed, spaced, and collective teaching trials. Massed trials elicit the same response from students in rapid succession. Spaced trials require students to complete a task with intervening intervals of time. Collective trials are presented sequentially to students in group instructional settings (121).

The demonstration of learning can be solicited by employing systematic antecedent and response-prompting strategies. Response prompting includes strategies such as time delay and least-to-most prompts. Time delay techniques present prompts and fade them in incremental time segments between the direction and the response. The system of least-to-most prompts utilizes a prompting hierarchy. Following the instructional cue, response prompts of gradually increasing levels of assistance are provided until the student demonstrates the correct response (122). The use of preference and reinforcer assessments (as described earlier) can assist in motivating students to learn and empowering them with choices (123).

2. Learning Environments

Students with ASD rely on external organizers embedded within the environment to anticipate tasks and expectations for performance. Thus, organizing the setting, the timing, and the sequencing of tasks and presenting materials that motivate the child to learn are essential. Dedicated space for specific learning tasks should be defined within the classroom (124). Ideally, student schedules should be organized by referring to the student assessment. Tasks that are difficult should be presented at optimal times for learning for the individual (125). Similarly, preferred activities can be used as reinforcers alternating the presentation of them with difficult, less preferred lessons.

The use of visual supports represents best practice for many students with ASD (126). Visual activity schedules using photographs or symbols provide students with advanced organizers for the daily schedule (127). Picture schedules can assist students in anticipating transitions, and in comprehending the demands of activities and social interactions (128). Recent work by Stromer et al. successfully incorporates computer technology in constructing activity schedules. Computerized activity schedules enable students to independently execute the visual and auditory prompts embedded in the program. This area has promising implications for individuals with ASD who are cue dependent (129).

B. Issues for Planning Educational Goals

Parents and professionals are desperate for solutions to the problems experienced by children with ASD. Often, interventions that are not empirically based are utilized at significant emotional and financial cost (130). To date, a cure for autism has not been identified. It is critical to investigate interventions before implementing them (131). Children are entitled to participate in a learning program that is designed to meet the needs of learners with ASD and taught by professionals who understand the disorder. Parents should refer to the guidelines of the National Research Council (132), in advocating for appropriate educational programs for their children. The recommendations regarding instructional time include instruction for a minimum of 25 hr weekly, sustained over the course of the entire calendar year. Programming should include low student/teacher ratios and family components such as parent training (132). Children should not aimlessly proceed through their years in school without making progress in IEP goals.

VII. SUMMARY

Across the nation parents with children challenged by ASD seek the services of professionals who are knowledgeable and empathic to their needs. This quest is as frustrating as the deficits that their children present, often depleting the emotional and financial resources of the family. At this time there are vast numbers of children in need of appropriate, effective intervention. Many interventions are available that produce positive outcomes. It is important for parents and professionals to be vigilant about obtaining assessments and interventions that address skills identified as priority areas of development as discussed in this chapter. It is equally important to investigate the efficacy of those interventions so that critical time is not wasted in fruitless endeavors. Behavioral and educational gains should be well documented and changes should be made in instructional strategies if progress is not demonstrated within a reasonable time. Developing self-help and leisure time activities are also critical skills for students with ASD. Obtaining assistance in securing appropriate service and developing these skills will potentially optimize future placements and enhance the quality of life for students with ASD and their families (132).

REFERENCES

1. Filipek PA, Accaerdo PJ, Ashwal MD, Baranek GT, Cook EH, Dawson G, Gordon B, Gravel JS, Johnson CP, Kallen RJ, Levy SE, Minshew NJ, Ozonoff S, Prizant, BM, Rapin R, Rogers SJ, Stone WL, Teplin SW, Tuchman RF, Volkmar FR. Practice parameter: screening and diagnosis of autism. Neurology 2000; 55:468–479.
2. Lord C, Rutter M, LeCouteur A. The Autism Diagnostic Interview Schedule Revised. J Autism Dev Disord 1994; 24(5):659–685.
3. Lord C, Storoschuk S, Rutter M, Pickles, A. Using the ADI-R to diagnose autism in preschool children. Infant Mental Health J 1993; 14(3):234–252.
4. Individuals with Disabilities Education Act (IDEA), 20 U.S.C.A. 1400-1485, originally the Education of All Handicapped Children Act (EAHCA, signed on Nov. 29, 1975 by President Ford, amended in 1978 and 1986 and incorporated into a new law in 1990.
5. Trapani C. Transition Goals for Adolescents with Learning Disabilities. Boston: Little, Brown, 1990.
6. Free Appropriate Education (FAPE) Board of Education (Hendrick Hudson Central School District v. Rowley, 458 U.S. 176 (1982).

7. Mandlawitz MR. The impact of the legal system on educational programming for young children with autism spectrum disorder. J Autism Dev Disord 2002; 32(5):495–505.

8. Turnbull HR, Wilcox BL, Stowe MJ. A brief overview of special education law with focus on autism. J Autism Dev Disord 2002; 32(5):479–493.

9. Zirkel PA. The autism case law: administrative and judicial rulings. Focus Autism Other Dev Disord 2002; 17(2):84–93.

10. Katsiyannis A, Reid R. Autism and section 504: rights and responsibilities. Focus Autism Other Dev Disord 1999; 14(2):66–72.

11. T.H. v Board of Education of Palatine Community Consol. Sch. District, No. 98 C. 4633, 98 C 4632 (N.D. Illinois 1999).

12. Herr S. Special education law and children with reading and other disabilities. J Law Educ 1999; 28(3):337–389.

13. Krantz PJ, McClannahan LE. Strategies for integration: Building repertoires that support transitions to public schools. In: Ghezzi PM, Williams WL, Carr JE, eds. Autism: Behavior Analytic Perspectives. Reno, NV: Context Press, 1999:221–231.

14. Lord C, McGee JP, eds. Educating children with autism. National Research Council. Washington, DC: National Academy Press, 2001.

15. U.S. Department of Health and Human Services. Mental Health: A Report of the Surgeon General. Rockville, MD: USDHHS, 1999.

16. Lord C, McGee JP, eds. Educating Children with Autism. National Research Council, Washington, DC: National Academy Press, 2001.

17. Lord C, McGee JP, eds. Educating Children with Autism. National Research Council, Washington, DC: National Academy Press, 2001.

18. Horner RH, Carr EG, Strain PS, Todd AW, Reed HK. Problem behavior interventions for young children with autism: a research synthesis. Focus Autism Other Dev Disord 2002; 16:205–214.

19. Horner RH, Diemer SM, Brazeau KC. Educational support for students with severe problem behaviors in Oregon: a descriptive analysis from the 1987–88 school year. J Assoc Persons Severe Handicaps 1992; 17:154–169.

20. Horner RH, Carr EG, Strain PS, Todd AW, Reed HK. Problem behavior interventions for young children with autism: a research synthesis. Focus Autism Other Dev Disord 2002; 16:205–214.

21. Risley TR, Wolf M. Establishing functional speech in echolalic children. Behav Res Ther 1967; 5:73–88.

22. Lovaas OI, Simmons JQ. Manipulation of self-destruction in three retarded children. J Appl Behav Anal 1969; 2:143–157.

23. Horner RH, Carr EG, Strain PS, Todd AW, Reed HK. Problem behavior interventions for young children with autism: a research synthesis. Focus Autism Other Dev Disord 2002; 16:205–214.

24. Individuals with Disabilities Education Act (IDEA), 20 U.S.C.A. 1400-1485, originally the Education of All Handicapped Children Act (EAHCA, signed on Nov. 29, 1975 by President Ford, amended in 1978 and 1986 and incorporated into a new law in 1990.

25. Dunlop G, Kern L, Worchester J. ABA and academic instruction. Focus Autism Other Dev Disord 2001; 16:129–136.
26. Iwata B, Vollmer T, Zarcone JR. The experimental (functional) analysis of behavior disorders: methodology, applications and limitations. In: Repp AC, Singh NN, eds. Perspectives on the Use of Nonaversive and Aversive Interventions for Persons with Developmental Disabilities. Sycamore, IL: Sycamore 1990:301–330.
27. Didden R, Duker PC, Korzilius H. Meta-analytic study on treatment effectiveness for problem behaviors with individuals who have mental retardation. Am J Ment Retard 1997; 101:387–399.
28. Fisher WW, Piazza CC, Alterson CJ, Kuhn DE. Interresponse relations among aberrant behaviors displayed by persons with autism and developmental disabilities. In: Ghezzi PM, Williams WL, Carr JE, eds. Autism: Behavior Analytic Perspectives. Reno, NV: Context Press, 1999:113–135.
29. Neef NA, Iwata BA. Current research on functional analysis methodologies: an introduction. J Appl Behav Anal 1994; 27:211–214.
30. Fisher WW, Piazza CC, Alterson CJ, Kuhn DE. Interresponse relations among aberrant behaviors displayed by persons with autism and developmental disabilities. In: Ghezzi PM, Williams WL, Carr JE, eds. Autism: Behavior Analytic Perspectives. Reno, NV: Context Press, 1999:113–135.
31. Iwata BA, Dorsey MF, Slifer KJ, Bauman KE, Richman GS. Toward a functional analysis of self-injury. Anal Intervent Dev Disord 1982; 2:3–20.
32. Fisher WW, Piazza CC, Bowman LG, Hagopian LP, Owens JC, Slevin I. A comparison of two approaches for identifying reinforcers for persons with severe and profound disabilities. J Appl Behav Anal 1992; 25:491–498.
33. Pace GM, Ivancic MT, Edwards GL, Iwata B, Page TJ. Assessment of stimulus preference and reinforcer value with profoundly retarded individuals. J Appl Behav Anal 1985; 18:249–255.
34. Fisher WW, Piazza CC, Bowman LG, Kurtz PF, Sherer MR, Lachman SR. A preliminary evaluation of empirically derived consequences for the treatment of pica. J Appl Behav Anal 1994; 27:447–457.
35. Pfiffner LJ, O'Leary SG. The efficacy of all-positive management as a function of the prior use of negative consequences. J Appl Behav Anal 1987; 20:265–271.
36. Lord C, McGee JP, eds. Educating Children with Autism. National Research Council, Washington, DC: National Academy Press, 2001:37.
37. Scotti JR, Ujcich KJ, Weigle KL, Holland CM, Kirk KS. Intervention with challenging behavior of persons with developmental disabilities: a review of current research practices. J Assoc Persons Severe Handicaps 1996; 21:123–134.
38. Fisher WW, Piazza CC, Bowman LG, Hagopian LP, Owens JC, Slevin I. A comparison of two approaches for identifying reinforcers for persons with severe and profound disabilities. J Appl Behav Anal 1992; 25:491–498.
39. Lord C, Paul R. Language and communication in autism. In: Cohen D, Volkmar F, eds. Handbook of Autism and Pervasive Developmental Disorders. New York: John Wiley & Sons, 1997:195–225.
40. Tager Flusberg H. Brief Report: Current theory and research on language and communication in autism. J Autism Dev Disord 1996; 26:169–178.

41. Lord C, Paul R. Language and communication in autism. In: Cohen D, Volkmar F, eds. Handbook of Autism and Pervasive Developmental Disorders. New York: John Wiley & Sons, 1997:195–225.
42. Sigman M, Ruskin E. Continuity and change in the social competence of children with autism, down syndrome and developmental delays. Monogr Soc Res Child Dev 1999; 64(1):114.
43. Stone W, Ousley O, Yoder P, Hogan K, Hepburn S. Nonverbal communication in 2- and 3-year old children with autism. J Autism Dev Disord 1997; 27:677–696.
44. Mundy P, Crowson M. Joint attention and early social communication: implications for research on intervention with autism. J Autism Dev Disord 1997; 27:653–676.
45. Garfin D, Lord C. Communication as a social problem in autism. In: Schopler E, Mesibov G, eds. Social Behavior in Autism. New York: Plenum Press, 1986:237–261.
46. Lord C, McGee JP, eds. Educating Children with Autism. National Research Council. Washington, DC: National Academy Press, 2001.
47. Fisher WW, Thompson R, Kuhn D. Establishing discrimination control of responding using functional and alternative reinforcers. J Appl Behav Anal 1998; 31:543–560.
48. Horner RH, Carr EG, Strain PS, Todd AW, Reed HK. Problem behavior interventions for young children with autism: a research synthesis. Focus Autism Other Dev Disord 2002; 16:205–214.
49. Goldstein H. Communication intervention for children with autism: a review of treatment efficacy. J Autism Dev Disord 2002; 32:373–396.
50. Lovaas OI, Koegel R, Simmons JQ, Stevens-Long J. Some generalization and follow-up measures on autistic children in behavior therapy. J Appl Behav Anal 1973; 6:131–166.
51. Krantz PJ, Zalewski L, Hall E, Fenski E, McClannahan L. Teaching complex language skills to autistic children. Anal Intervent Dev Disord 1981; 1:259–297.
52. Egel AL, Shafer MS, Neef NA. Receptive acquisition and generalization of prepositional responding in autistic children: a comparison of two procedures. Anal Intervent Dev Disord 1984; 4:285–298.
53. Hart BM, Risley TR. Incidental teaching of language in preschool. J Appl Behav Anal 1975; 8:411–420.
54. Koegel LK, Koegel RL, Carter CM. Pivotal responses and the natural language treatment paradigm. Semin Speech Lang 1998; 19:355–372.
55. Hart BM, Risley TR. Incidental teaching of language in preschool. J Appl Behav Anal 1975; 8:411–420.
56. Koegel L. Communication and language intervention. In: Koegel R, Koegel L, eds. Teaching Children with Autism. Baltimore, MD: Paul H. Brookes Publishing, 1995:17–32.
57. Charlop M, Trasowech J. Increasing autistic children's daily spontaneous speech. J Appl Behav Anal 1991; 24:379–386.
58. Beukelman D, Mirenda P. Augmentative and Alternative Communication: Management of Severe Communication Disorders in Children and Adults 2d ed. Baltimore, MD: Paul H. Brookes, 1998.

59. Goldstein H. Communication intervention for children with autism: a review of treatment efficacy. J Autism Dev Disord 2002; 32:373–396.

60. Yoder PJ, Layton TL. Speech following sign language training in autistic children with minimal verbal language. J Autism Dev Disord 1988; 18:217–230.

61. Mirenda P, Santigrossi J. A prompt-free strategy to teach pictorial communication system use. Augment Altern Commun 1985; 5:3–13.

62. Goldstein H. Communication intervention for children with autism: a review of treatment efficacy. J Autism Dev Disord 2002; 32:373–396.

63. Ogeltree BT, Oren T. Application of ABA principles to general communication instruction. Focus Autism Other Dev Disord 2001; 16(2):102–109.

64. Lord C, McGee JP, eds. Educating Children with Autism. National Research Council, Washington, DC: National Academy Press, 2001.

65. Lord C, McGee JP, eds. Educating Children with Autism. National Research Council, Washington, DC: National Academy Press, 2001.

66. Volkmar FR, Cohen DJ, Paul R. An evaluation of DSM III criteria for infantile autism. J Am Acad Child Psychiatry 1986; 25:190–197.

67. Sigman M, Ungerer JA. Cognitive and language skills in autistic, mentally retarded and normal children. Dev Psych 1986b; 20:293–302.

68. Lord C, McGee JP, eds. Educating Children with Autism. National Research Council, Washington, DC: National Academy Press, 2001.

69. Terpstra JE, Higgins K, Pierce T. Can I play? Classroom-based interventions for teaching play skills to children with autism. Focus Autism Other Dev Disord 2002; 17(2):119–126.

70. Mundy PM, Ungerer J, Sherman T. Nonverbal communication and play correlates of language development in autistic children. J Autism Dev Disord 1987; 17:349–364.

71. Lifter K, Sulzer-Azaroff B, Anderson, S, Cowdry GE. Teaching play activities to preschool children with disabilities: the importance of development considerations. J Early Intervent 1993; 17(2):139–159.

72. Sayeed Z, Guerin E. Early Years Play. London: David Fulton Publishers, 2000:73–84.

73. Vygotsky LS. Mind in Society: The Development of Higher Psychological Processes. Cambridge, MA: Harvard University Press, 1978.

74. Kruzynski AK, Lalinec C, Zelazo PR, Reid C, Thompson S. Impact of treatment on play and mother-child interaction. Poster: International Society for Studies in Behavioral Development Conference. Quebec City, Canada, Aug. 12–16, 1996.

75. Krantz P, McClannahan L. Social interaction skills for children with autism: a script fading procedure for beginning readers. J Appl Behav Anal 1988; 31:191–202.

76. Koegel RL, O'Dell MC, Koegel LK. A natural language teaching paradigm for nonverbal autistic children. J Autism Dev Disord 1987; 17:187–200.

77. Wolfberg PJ, Sculer AL. Integrated play groups: promoting the social and cognitive dimensions of play in children with autism. J Autism Dev Disord 1993; 23:467–489.

78. Lord C, McGee JP, eds. Educating children with autism. National Research Council, Washington, DC: National Academy Press, 2001.

79. Lord C. Early social development in autism. In: Schopler E, Van Bourgondien ME, Bristol MM, eds. Preschool Issues in Autism. New York: Plenum Press, 1993:61– 94.
80. Staub EL. The Development of Prosocial Behavior in Children. Morristown, NJ: General Learning Press, 1975.
81. Hartup WW, Glazer JA, Charlesworth R. Peer reinforcement and sociometric status. Child Dev 1967; 38:1017–1024.
82. Trower P. Toward a generative model of social skills: a critique and synthesis. In: Curran JP, Monti PM, eds. Social skills training. New York: Plenum Press, 1982:339–427.
83. Herbert M. Social skills training with children. In: Hollin CR, Trower P, eds. Handbook of Social Skills Training. Vol. 1. New York: Pergamon Press, 1986:11– 32.
84. Rutter M, Mahwood L, Howlin P. Language delay and social development. In: Fletcher P, Hale D, eds. Specific Speech and Language Disorders in Children. London: Whurr, 1992.
85. Kanner L. Autistic disturbances of affective contact. Nerv Child 1943; 2:217–250.
86. Sigman M, Ruskin E. Continuity and change in the social competence of children with autism, down syndrome and developmental delays. Monogr Soc Res Child Dev 1999; 64(1):1–113.
87. Lord C. Early social development in autism. In: Schopler E, Van Bourgondien ME, Bristol MM, eds. Preschool Issues in Autism. New York: Plenum Press, 1993:61– 94.
88. McConnell SR. Interventions to facilitate social interaction for young children with autism: review of available research and recommendations for educational intervention and future research. J Autism Dev Disord 2002; 32(5):351–372.
89. McGee GG, Feldman RS, Morrier MJ. Benchmarks of social treatment for children with autism. J Autism Dev Disord 1997; 27:353–364.
90. Dunn J, McGuire S. Sibling and peer relationships in childhood. J Child Psychol Psychiatry 1992; 33:67–105.
91. McGee GG, Feldman RS, Morrier MJ. Benchmarks of social treatment for children with autism. J Autism Dev Disord 1997; 27:353–364.
92. McArthur D, Adamson LB. Joint attention in preverbal children: autism and developmental language disorder. J Autism Dev Disord 1996; 26:481–496.
93. Celani G, Battachi MW, Arcidiacono L. The understanding of emotional meaning of facial expressions in people with autism. J Autism Dev Disord 1999; 29:57–66.
94. St James PJ, Tager Flusberg H. An observational study of humor in autism and Down syndrome. J Autism Dev Disord 1994; 24:603–617.
95. Lord C, Rutter M, LeCouteur. The Autism Diagnostic Interview Revised. Western Psych, 1999.
96. Herbert M. Social skills training with children. In: Hollin CR, Trower P, eds. Handbook of Social Skills Training. Vol. 1. New York: Pergamon Press, 1986:11– 32.
97. Bandura A. Social Learning Theory. Englewood Cliffs, NJ: Prentice-Hall, 1977.

98. Hops H. Children's social competence and skill: current research practices and future directions. Behav Ther 1983; 14:3–18.

99. Taylor B, Leven L. Teaching a student with autism to make verbal initiations: effects of a tactile prompt. J Appl Behav Anal 1998; 31:651–654.

100. Krantz PJ, MacDuff MT, McClannahan LE. Programming participation in family activities for children with autism: parents' use of photographic activity schedules. J Appl Behav Anal 1993; 26:137–138.

101. McGee GC, Almeida MC, Sulzer-Azaroff B, Feldman RS. Prompting reciprocal interaction via peer incidental teaching. J Appl Behav Anal 1992; 25:117–126.

102. Krantz PJ, McClannahan LE. Social interaction skills with children with autism: a script-fading procedure for beginning readers. J Appl Behav Anal 1998; 31:191–202.

103. Odom SL, Strain PS. Peer-mediated approaches to promoting children's interaction: a review. Am J Orthopsychiatry 1984; 54:544–557.

104. Pierce K, Schreibman L. Multiple peer use of pivotal response training social behaviors in children with autism: effects of peer-implemented pivotal response training. J Appl Behav Anal 1997; 30:157–160.

105. Wolfberg PJ, Sculer AL. Integrated play groups: promoting the social and cognitive dimensions of play in children with autism. J Autism Dev Disord 1993; 23:467–489.

106. Rinn RC, Markley A. Modification of skill deficits in children. In: Bellack AS, Hersen M, eds. Research and Practice in Social Skills Training. New York: Plenum Press, 1981:107–129.

107. Trower P. Skills training for adolescents' social problems: a viable alternative. J Adolesc 1978; 1:319–329.

108. Asher SR, Oden SL, Gottman JH. Children's friendships in school settings. In: Katz LG, ed. Current Topics in Early Childhood Education. Norwood, NJ: Ablex, 1977; 1:33–57.

109. Gresham F. Social skills training with handicapped children: a review. Rev Educ Res 1981; 51:139–176.

110. McConnell SR. Interventions to facilitate social interaction for young children with autism: review of available research and recommendations for educational intervention and future research. J Autism Dev Disord 2002; 32(5):351–372.

111. Odom SL, Strain PS. Peer-mediated approaches to promoting children's interaction: a review. Am J Orthopsychiatry 1984; 54:544–557.

112. Matson J. Behavioral treatment of autistic persons: a review of research from 1980 to the present. Res Dev Disord 1996; 17(6):433–465.

113. Trapani C. Psychoeducational assessment of children and adolescents with attention deficit hyperactivity disorder. In: Accardo PJ, Blondis TA, Whitman BY, Stein MA, eds. Attention Deficits and Hyperactivity in Children and Adults. 2d ed. New York: Marcel Dekker, Inc., 2000:197–214.

114. Lord C, McGee JP, eds. Educating Children with Autism. National Research Council. Washington, DC: National Academy Press, 2001.

115. Department of Health. Clinical Practice Guideline: The Guideline Technical Report—Autism/Pervasive Developmental Disorders Assessment and Intervention. Albany: Early Intervention Program, New York State Department of Health, 1999.

116. Green G. Behavior analytic instruction for learners with autism: advances in stimulus control technology. Focus Autism Dev Disord 2001; 16(2):72–85.

117. Deno SL. Curriculum-based measurement and special education services: a fundamental and direct relationship. In: Shinn MR, ed. Curriculum-Based Measurement: Assessing Special Children. New York: Guilford Press, 1989:1–17.

118. Olley JG. Curriculum for students with autism. School Psychol Rev 1999; 28(4):595–607.

119. Heflin LJ, Alberto PA. Establishing a behavioral context for learning for students with autism. Focus Autism Other Dev Disord 2001; 16(2):93–101.

120. Green G. Behavior analytic instruction for learners with autism: advances in stimulus control technology. Focus Autism Other Dev Disord 2001; 16(2):72–85.

121. Green G. Behavior analytic instruction for learners with autism: advances in stimulus control technology. Focus Autism Other Dev Disord 2001; 16(2):72–85.

122. Wolery M, Ault, Doyle P. Teaching Students with Moderate to Severe Disabilities. New York: Longman, 1992.

123. Dunlap G, Kern L, Worchester J. ABA and academic instruction. Focus Autism Other Dev Disord 2001; 16(2):129–136.

124. Stainback W, Stainback S, Froyen L. Structuring the classroom to prevent disruptive behavior. Teach Ex Child 1987; 16:12–16.

125. Egel AL, Shafer MS, Neef NA. Receptive acquisition and generalization of prepositional responding in autistic children: a comparison of two procedures. Anal Intervent Dev Disord 1984; 4:285–298.

126. Prizant BM, Rubin E. Contemporary issues in interventions for autism spectrum disorders: a commentary. J Assoc Person Sev Hand 1999; 24:199–208.

127. MacDuff GS, Krantz PJ, McClannahan LE. Teaching children with autism to use photographic activity schedules: maintenance and generalization of complex response chains. J Appl Behav Anal 1993; 26:89–95.

128. McLannahan LE, Krantz PJ. Activity Schedules for Children with Autism: Teaching Independent Behavior. Bethesda, MD: Woodbine House, 1999.

129. Stromer R, Kinney EM, Taylor BA, Kimball JW. Activity schedules, computer technology and teaching children with autism spectrum disorders. Behav Mod (accepted 2002).

130. Simpson RL, Myles BS. Facilitated communication and children and youth with disabilities: an enigma in search of a perspective. Focus Excep Child 1995; 27:1–16.

131. Simpson RL. ABA and students with autism spectrum disorders: issues and considerations for effective practice. Focus Autism Other Dev Disord 2001; 16(2):68–71.

132. Lord C, McGee JP, eds. Educating Children with Autism. National Research Council. Washington, DC: National Academy Press, 2001.

14

Science as a Candle in the Dark: Evidence-Based Approach to Evaluating Interventions

Charlene Butler
Seattle School District, Seattle, Washington, U.S.A.

I. INTRODUCTION

> At the heart of science is an essential balance between two seemingly contradictory attitudes—an openness to new ideas, no matter how bizarre or counterintuitive, and the most ruthlessly skeptical scrutiny of all ideas, old and new. This is how deep truths are winnowed from deep nonsense. The collective enterprise of creative thinking and skeptical thinking, working together, keeps the field on track.
> Carl Sagan, *The Demon-Haunted World: Science as a Candle in the Dark* (1996)

The judicious mix of these two modes of thought is crucial to the success of science in the pursuit of truth. Good scientists do both. They churn up many new ideas and winnow the wheat from the chaff by critical experiment and analysis to try to distinguish the promising ideas from the worthless ones.

Earlier chapters of this book have demonstrated that treatment of autism, like diagnosing it and understanding its cause(s), is still in flux. With a sense of urgency created by a growing prevalence of autism, the health care and educational communities have risen to the task of creative thinking and continue to produce a plethora of new and appealing ideas about interventions that may benefit children with autism.

Treatment for autism remains a particular challenge because it is still a phenomenological diagnosis, that is, a diagnosis based on the symptoms of a disorder—the social and language impairments and stereotypical patterns of behavior. This is in contrast to an etiological diagnosis, which is based on the causes of a condition. An etiological diagnosis is superior to a phenomenological diagnosis because knowing what has gone wrong can lead to more specific and effective treatment. Unfortunately, the causes, or etiologies, of autism are still unknown; therefore, interventions have been somewhat hit or miss—and controversial. Many quasi-scientific interventions are being promoted for autism through the Internet and print and broadcast media without an objective analysis of their efficacy. The multidisciplinary nature of some interventions makes it difficult for professionals to assess the evidence from other disciplines. Despite a logical façade and popular usage, many interventions for autism have not been found to be efficacious under scientific scrutiny. It was this growing realization in medicine that created the new movement in medicine called evidence-based medicine.

The practice of evidence-based care requires individual practitioners to use interventions whose efficacy has been proved scientifically rather than interventions based on clinical intuition. New tools are, therefore, needed to help busy practitioners to view and scientifically scrutinize evidence. It is the purpose of this chapter to demonstrate a new tool, called evidence-based reports, developed by the American Academy for Cerebral Palsy and Developmental Medicine (AACPDM), for skeptical thinking that can be applied to old, new, and yet-to-be-offered interventions.

II. TOOL FOR CRITICAL APPRAISAL OF INTERVENTIONS

Evidence reports aggregate disparate data produced by a multidisciplinary field to produce an evidence table after a systematic review process. The objective of the AACPDM evidence reports is to provide the current state of evidence about various interventions for the management of developmental disabilities. These reports can be read on its online Database of Evidence Reports. It is possible for anyone to create an evidence report by following a step-by-step process outlined in the online Methodology for Developing Evidence Tables and Reviewing Treatment Outcome Research (1).

An evidence table conveniently summarizes research findings and makes it easy to identify current "best evidence" to inform individual recommendations and choices. Best evidence is represented by a study (or studies) in an evidence table that most closely approximates the client characteristics of interest to the clinician, that used a therapeutic regime most like the one the clinician is considering and can provide, that investigated outcomes of greatest concern to this client, and that provided the most convincing or valid results.

The AACPDM adopted a two-part framework for its evidence table that uses: (1) a dimensions-of-disablement classification within which to gather and interpret disparate research data in a meaningful way, and (2) a levels-of-evidence classification that puts the quality of all available evidence in a meaningful perspective.

A. Dimensions-of-Disablement Classification: What Kind of Evidence Is There?

Dimensions-of-disablement is a concept and a classification system developed by the World Health Organization (2) that facilitates the description, measurement, and management of rehabilitation outcomes and minimizes the barriers between medical and social models of rehabilitation. Central to the concept is the idea that the consequences of a medical condition occur in and are mediated at four different reference levels of human experience: impairment of body functions, impairment of body structures, activity limitations and participation restriction, and environmental factors. Just as the disablement of autism can be described according to the different dimensions in which it manifests, interventions and outcomes can also be categorized by this classification.

1. Impairment of Body Structures

The Autism Tissue Program, a brain tissue donation program for the study of brain tissue, may help to discover impairments of body *structures* that, in turn, may lead to appropriate intervention in that dimension. Gene therapy may be an example of an intervention with potential to alter body structures.

2. Impairment of Body Function

Neuroleptic drugs or megavitamins represent intervention in this dimension because the intervention is expected to improve brain function, and, in turn, social behavior, by altering the concentration of neurotransmitters such as dopamine and serotonin. Expected treatment effects of sensory integration therapy also target impairment of function, in this case, of impaired sensations and response to them. Similarly, speech and language therapy to stimulate more normal language development intervenes at this level.

3. Activity Limitations and Participation Restriction

Specific pragmatic language training to improve social interactions, on the other hand, targets the activity/participation dimension. The use of systematically developed "social stories" to increase understanding and handling of specific social situations also attempts to intervene at this level.

4. Environmental Factors

Influencing social policies, reducing architectural barriers, and making low-cost drugs available represent interventions in this dimension. Parent counseling or training to enhance their parenting or coping skills improves the microenvironment of the child and belongs in this dimension.

B. Levels of Evidence Classification: How Good Is the Evidence?

The actual effectiveness of an intervention can only be established through empirical research, i.e., direct observation and comparison of outcomes under systematic and controlled conditions. The purpose of research is to tease out attribution. In other words, it seeks to establish the extent to which any change observed to occur in the presence of an intervention can be attributed to the intervention rather than to some other factor present during a research study. For example, it is possible that an observed change could be attributed to natural history; that is, people with the medical condition of interest are known to get better over time. The change may be attributable to normal variation in symptoms, including periods of complete remission. Greater improvement observed in a treated group may be attributed to the fact that the treated group contained fewer severely involved individuals than the control group. There may be any number of differences between the treated and control circumstances of a study that can account for change observed in the presence of an intervention. These "threats to internal validity" must be systematically controlled for there to be confidence that an observed outcome can be attributed to the intervention.

AACPDM evidence reports classify evidence into levels-of-evidence based on (1) a hierarchy of research designs that range from the greatest to least according to ability to reduce bias and error combined with (2) a means of assessing the thoroughness with which the particular research study was conducted including use of statistical calculations or other determinants of probability. The five levels of evidence reflect the methodological strength of a study. Stronger levels of evidence (Levels I and II) suggest that there are fewer sources of error present in the study design so that greater confidence can be placed in the results. The weakest level of evidence (Level V) can only hint at a possible connection between an intervention and an outcome because it is not evidence derived from research but from theory or simple description of an outcome that was observed with exposure to, or subsequent to, an intervention.

The conduct of the study serves as a second gauge to a study's rigor, since even a Level I study can contain flaws that decrease confidence in its results. Given the opportunities possible under the research design, the strength of the evidence depends on the extent to which possible threats to validity within that design were *actually* controlled. The AACPDM assessment of the conduct of the study results in a rating of strong, moderate, or weak.

C. Internal Versus External Validity

Unlike some others, the AACPDM classification is confined to gauging only the internal validity of a study. Internal validity is the ability of a study to demonstrate that the intervention—and not other factors in that study—was responsible for the observed outcomes. External validity is the confidence with which a finding might be expected to be true for others outside the study. As yet, the bodies of evidence in developmental disabilities are neither robust nor comprehensive enough to allow confident generalization to groups of people-at-large. Therefore, external validity is not reflected in the Academy level of evidence. Instead, whether a finding can be expected to generalize is believed to be more appropriately determined by individual users of the evidence reports who will focus on only the specific aspects of similarity between a patient of interest and the people who have been studied (e.g., their age, severity and type of autistic behaviors, secondary medical conditions, circumstances of treatment).

D. Group Results Versus Uniformity of Effect Results

In a trial that compares one group with another, not all the participants will respond in the same way. In a positive trial, not all will have benefited from therapy; in a negative trial, there may have been a subgroup, but too small to be reliably detected, who actually benefited. Some studies report only how the group as a whole fared, i.e., the averaged effect in the experimental group compared to the averaged effect in the control. Other studies report only the uniformity of effect within the treated group, i.e., how many of the participants improved, were unchanged, or were worse. Some studies report both. The AACPDM summary of results and evidence tables accommodate both types of these important results.

III. USING AACPDM EVIDENCE REPORTS TO EXAMINE TREATMENT OPTIONS IN AUTISM

Autism has a history of theories and treatments proposed in multiple disciplines. This is a strength in the sense that new knowledge and approaches continually press us to reconsider assumptions and strategies. On the other hand, in the absence of a coherent focus based on widely accepted theory, general clinical support, and systematic medical research, such a diversity of approaches can also be divisive.

The numerous intervention options this situation has generated can be mind-boggling to the initiate. The Autism Society of America (ASA) (3) has attempted to organize the various approaches. This listing does not imply endorsement, efficacy, or even general acceptance by the field, by the ASA, or by this author. It represents the kind of information that parents may have when they consult health care and education professionals.

To demonstrate the AACPDM evidence report strategy as a useful tool for sorting the wheat from the chaff, three interventions have been chosen from the ASA list and one from the Cure Autism Now website. Evidence reports will be developed and, in one case, only a critically appraised topic is possible. This exercise will reveal the surprising lack of scientific evidence in place to support even the most accepted, noncontroversial intervention (TEACCH). It will then describe the body of evidence for a well-established but still controversial intervention (sensory integration therapy) as well as a less widely used, even more controversial intervention (megavitamin B_6 therapy). Finally, it will demonstrate how the popular press/media "buzz" about an intervention can create the appearance of much evidence when there is essentially none, scientific or otherwise (rapid-prompt method).

All four of these interventions are based on theoretical assumptions that the inappropriate behaviors observed in autism are related to a dysfunctional nervous system that is typified by cognitive and sensory-processing problems. In TEACCH, integration and organization of sensory inputs for learning is *externally* applied to the child through a highly structured, visually based teaching method. In the newly proposed rapid-prompt method, the intervention is also external to the child, but there is no attempt to integrate simultaneous sensory inputs. Rather, the lack of sensory integration is recognized, but focus is placed on using the child's primary learning channel while ignoring other channels, on giving sufficient time for a child to switch from one sensory channel to another when necessary to do so, and on providing constant verbal prompting for children. On the other hand, sensory integration and megavitamin B_6 therapies are attempts to *internally* correct sensory processing. In sensory integration therapy, the nervous system is thought to permanently change with better ability to modulate, organize, and integrate through increasingly appropriate responses to therapeutically designed somatosensory and vestibular activities. Likewise, megavitamin B_6 therapy is expected to alter brain neurochemistry and, thereby, correct faulty sensory processing. All four interventions attempt to intervene in the dimension of impairment of body function but at different reference levels: vitamin B_6 attempts to alter function at the cellular level (neurotransmitters), sensory integration attempts to alter function at the organ system level (the central nervous system), and TEACCH and rapid-prompt methods attempt to alter emotional, social, and language function (developmental domains).

Searches for studies about each intervention were conducted as follows. Electronic searches on MEDLINE and Clinical Trials.gov were conducted via PubMed; on ERIC, via AskERIC; and on CINAHL, via ERLWebSPIRS. Further trials were sought through examination of references in studies and in review publications. Full text of English-language publications that were available through the extensive University of Washington health sciences and other library collections were examined. In addition to, or in the absence of, professionally peer-reviewed publications, a search on the Internet was conducted, with particular attention given to the websites of Cure Autism Now, ASA, and Autism Research Institute.

A. Evidence for Effects of TEACCH (Structured Teaching) for Individuals Diagnosed with Autism

1. What Is TEACCH?

Treatment and education of autistic and related communication-handicapped children (TEACCH) has had a most profound and long-lasting impact on the treatment and education of children with autism (4,5). It started as a research project that fundamentally changed thinking about autism and grew into a comprehensive program of services for children and their families in the state of North Carolina, and of research and professional training. This system of clinics, classrooms, training programs, social outreach, and materials research and development is funded by the state but administered by Division TEACCH, Department of Psychiatry, University of North Carolina School of Medicine. TEACCH has been endorsed by a number of groups over the years including the National Society for Autistic Children (1972), American Psychological Association (1986), and the American Psychiatric Association (1972). It is recognized nationally as a center of excellence in autism.

TEACCH began in 1966 with Eric Schopler, whose NIMH-funded Child Research Project tested the assumption that parental pathology caused autism. Autism was considered an emotional problem—a withdrawal from pathological parenting. Current thinking was that children needed to be under psychiatric care in psychodynamic play therapy, be removed from their parents to residential treatment, and be educated in classrooms established on the assumption that children's emotional learning problems would improve through freedom and unstructured self-expression. Schopler found that autism was not caused by parental pathology but by some form of brain abnormality and that parents of children with autism were no more or less pathological than the general population. Autism was not a form of social withdrawal but a developmental disability characterized by impairment in relationships and communication skills from the beginning of life and by repetitive preoccupations and movements.

In the ensuing years, Division TEACCH became foremost in the field, publishing over 50 books, chapters, and articles to promote its precepts, and editing the *Journal of Autism and Developmental Disorders* to keep up-to-date on other work in the field. One of its main ongoing contributions has been the diagnostic instruments and many special curricula developed by its research unit in collaboration with its clinical units with subsequent field trials in TEACCH classrooms and centers before publication. The curricula include social skills, communication skills, preschool programs, teacher training, family training, behavior management, prevocational training, job advocacy and placement, and family advocacy (6,7). The concepts introduced by TEACCH that were so novel at its inception have become "best practice," and often standard practice, in special education, and even mandated by law. Individualized education plans (IEPs), for example, are now required by federal law and are based on individualized assessment with parents as integral members of IEP teams.

More recently, a new principle has evolved at Division TEACCH. This posits that people with autism should be understood and worked with, not in the context of "normalization," but in the context of a "culture of autism" (7). This holds that people with autism are part of a distinctive group with common characteristics that are different from, but not necessarily inferior to "normal" people. Indeed, the differences between people with autism and others may sometimes favor people with autism. Their relative strengths in visual skills, recognizing details, and memory, among other areas, may become the basis of successful adult functioning, if properly promoted and nurtured. Therefore, the goal for helping people with autism is not to make them more normal but to cultivate and emphasize their strengths and interests. This is in direct contrast to most programs for developmental disabilities; they emphasize remediation of deficits with exclusive focus on that goal. Moreover, capitalizing on individual's interests, however unusual they may seem to the outside observer, increases motivation of people with autism for engagement and learning. Focus on strengths and interests can enhance efforts to work positively and productively with people with autism, rather than coercing and forcing them in directions that do not interest them and that they may not comprehend.

TEACCH was, initially, an approach to management of autism characterized by a new interpretation of autism that vindicated families, established the need for structured teaching for children, established a multifaceted professional-parent relationship, and provided an organizational structure with collaborative policies that provided service and support to families across multiple aspects of life and across the life span. The professional-parent relationship included two-way trainer/trainee interaction, mutual emotional support, shared community advocacy, collaborative staff selection, and working together in classrooms and other settings.

The TEACCH approach today is characterized by understanding and managing autism in the context of a "culture of autism," developing appropriate structures, promoting independent work skills, emphasizing strengths and interests, and fostering communication, social, and leisure outlets. Of continued importance in the TEACCH model is that these aspects of management are implemented on a systems level (i.e., applied across age groups and agencies) (7).

Since its inception, TEACCH has also been regarded as a more discrete intervention—a structured teaching program (1) with special emphasis on training social skills and communication, (2) through a visual, nonverbal restructuring of the teaching environment, (3) individualized to each child's developmental levels, (4) in which parents are regarded as critical agents of change and are trained to be active collaborators and teachers. This specific method of instruction is known as structured teaching. The method involves teaching children with autism to use visual schedules and visual work systems that are individualized to the developmental level of the child. These can be extended and graduated as development occurs.

2. How Is Structured Teaching Purported to Work?

Visually clear organizational components are expected to help people with autism cognitively organize and manage themselves for learning. A fundamental assumption is that a child who understands what is expected will be able to work independently on satisfying tasks that are within her/his capabilities. This child will be less likely to engage in aggressive or self-injurious behavior than a disorganized, anxious, agitated child who lacks a meaningful organizational framework in which to understand productive activity.

Management of behavior problems within structured teaching is based on the assumption that all inappropriate behaviors result from the cognitive and sensory-processing problems that typify autism. For example, agitation (i.e., screaming without apparent cause) and aggression (i.e., pushing someone, running away) may result from noxious hypersensitivity to sounds that the child may attribute to people in the surroundings. It may be due to excessive frustration experienced when the child needs to negotiate himself or herself out of an upsetting situation—but has severe communication limitations. TEACCH intervention responds to aggressive behaviors or behaviors that interfere with learning by examining deficit areas associated with autism, then developing skill training (i.e., training to become more functionally communicative or develop frustration management skills), and environmental manipulation to reduce or remove obstacles that are too great for the person with autism (8). If the behavior, e.g., finger tapping, does not interfere with the child's learning, this behavior is accepted in the belief that this will advance the accomplishment of educational objectives.

Most people will need special classrooms (or social or job settings) for part or all of the time where their physical environment, curriculum, and personnel can be structured to support individual needs. Some higher-functioning children need less structure and can work effectively and benefit from regular educational or other programs.

3.   What Studies Have Been Done?

Electronic search for outcome studies using TEACCH with individuals diagnosed with autism yielded only four citations: three studies and one report listing publications by TEACCH through 1991. References in these publications led to an additional eight citations. Three provided only background information, one was a review of earlier work, and four were studies. Of the seven studies located, one was excluded because only 51% of the participants had autism with no data given for the autism subgroup. Six studies met the inclusion criteria and are summarized in Tables 1 and 2. Table 3 is the evidence table.

4.   How Much and What Kind of Evidence Is There?

Impairment of Body Function. Social-emotional development and language development are the primary developmental domains that are impaired in autism. Therefore, it is surprising that developmental status in only the cognitive, motor, and perceptual domains has been measured. However, developmental domains do influence one another. In 12 of 13 measures, exposure to TEACCH resulted in improved developmental scores. The thirteenth measure showed the TEACCH group to have slightly worse eye-hand coordination than the control group.

What about the impact on autistic behaviors that are expected to improve with the behavioral supports provided by TEACCH intervention? Unexpectedly, this has been measured or reported anecdotally only five times. The impact of structured teaching was positive with reductions in problem behaviors in all five results; however, only one measure was statistically significant, three were not statistically evaluated, and two were not statistically significant.

Activity Limitations and Participation Restrictions. Is more meaningful activity and participation in family, school, and community life displayed as the result of TEACCH? Out of three results about whether children were more engaged with their environment (all positive), only one result was statistically significant, one was not, and one was not statistically evaluated.

Table 1 Summary of Studies About TEACCH (Structured Teaching): Interventions and Participants

Study	Intervention	Duration	Sample population	Age	N
1971 Schopler (9)	Structured vs. unstructured treatment sessions	8 wk	Autistic children within psychotic range by Creak criteria; social maturity quotient 29–86; 4 boys, 1 girl; all social classes	4–8 yr	5 (acted as own controls)
1978 Marcus (10)	Parent training for and delivery of structured teaching/behavior management	2 mo	Mothers of autistic children (psychosis rating range 4–6 on Psychotic Rating Scale; IQ range 12–89; all social classes; 9 boys, 1 girl)	33–69 mo	10
1980 Short (11)	Parent training for and delivery of structured teaching/behavior management	3 mo	Psychotic (autistic) children		Not known
1982 Schopler (12)	TEACCH system of programs vs. no community support	Not reported	Moderate to severely autistic older adolescents	≥17 yr	115 in TEACCH series
1993 Cox (8)	Structured teaching	2 wk	Males with moderate to severe autism, moderate mental retardation, severe temper tantrums and dangerous aggressive attacks	16 and 19 yr	2

Table 1 *Continued*

Study	Intervention	Duration	Sample population	Age	N
1997 Panerai (13)	Structured teaching	12 mo	Autistic children and adolescents with severe and profound mental retardation, stereotyped movement and behaviors, aggressiveness and self-injury; not able to work independent of adult supervision; inadequate communication (gestures, crying, vocalizations)	7–18 yr	18
1998 Ozonoff (14)	Parent training for and delivery of structured teaching in home program vs. no treatment	8–12 wk	9 Boys, 2 girls with autism, most with mental retardation; 2-parent family; 21 Caucasian American, 1 Hispanic American; in day preschools (15 in special autism programs; 7 in noncategorical public preschools)	2–6 yr	11 treated plus 11 control

Table 2 Summary of Studies About TEACCH (Structured Teaching): Methods, Outcomes, Measures, and Results

Study and research design	Outcome of interest	Dim. of disability	Measure	Result	Clin. imp.	Statistics	LOE
1971 Schopler: crossover trial (ABAB design)	Attending in meaningful activity	A&P	Observation/time sample	+	Yes	$p = <.10$ ns	II-S
		—		—	—	—	—
	Affective behavior	A&P	Observation/time sample	+	Yes	$p = <.10$ ns	II-S
	Bizarre behavior	IBF	Observation/time sample	+	Yes	$p = <.10$ ns	II-S
	Relating to people	A&P	Observation/time sample	+	Yes	$p = <.10$ ns	II-S
	Using meaningful language	A&P	Observation/time sample	+	Yes	$p = >.10$ ns	II-S
1978 Marcus (10): before and after case series	Child compliance behavior (staying on task)	A&P	Video observation	+	Yes	$p = <.005$	IV-S
		—		—	—	—	—
	Maternal teaching effectiveness	EF	Structure Rating Scale	+	Yes	$p < .005$	IV-S
1980 Short (11): before and after case series	Autistic behavior	IBF	Video: direct behavior	+			IV-W
	Parent involvement	EF	Video: direct behavior	+			IV-W
1982 Schopler (12): cohort study with retrospective control group	Family and community participation (residence)	A&P	Rates of institutionalization	+	Yes		III-W
1993 Cox (8): case reports	Aggressive behavior	IBF	Observation	+	Yes		V

Table 2 *Continued*

Study and research design	Outcome of interest	Dim. of disability	Measure	Result	Clin. imp.	Statistics	LOE
1997 Panerai (13): before and after case series	Adaptive development	IBF	Vineland	+	Yes	$p < .01$	IV-S
	Perceptual development	IBF	PEP-R subscale score	+		$p < .05$	IV-S
	Gross motor development	IBF	PEP-R subscale score	+		$p < .05$	IV-S
	Fine motor development	IBF	PEP-R subscale score	+		$p < .05$	IV-S
	Cognitive development	IBF	PEP-R subscale score	+	Yes	$p < .05$	IV-S
	Stereotypical behaviors	IBF	Structured observations	+	Yes	$p < .01$	IV-S
	Aggressive behavior	IBF	Structured observations	+	Yes	ns	IV-S
	Behavior problems	IBF	Anecdote	+	Yes		V
	Attending and working	A&P	Anecdote	+	Yes		V
	Cooperating and working	A&P	Anecdote	+	Yes		V
	Communication: frequency and variety	A&P	Anecdote	+	Yes		V
1998 Ozonoff (14): cohort study with prospective control group	Overall development	IBF	PEP-R total score	+	$p < .05$		II-S
	Eye-hand coordination dev.	IBF	PEP-R subscale score	−	—		II-S
	Cognitive verbal dev.	IBF	PEP-R subscale score	+	$p < .15$		II-S
	Perceptual development	IBF	PEP-R subscale score	+	$p < .15$		II-S
	Imitation development	IBF	PEP-R subscale score	+	$p < .05$		II-S
	Gross motor development	IBF	PEP-R subscale score	+	$p < .05$		II-S
	Fine motor development	IBF	PEP-R subscale score	+	$p < .01$		IL-S
	Cognitive development	IBF	PEP-R subscale score	+	$p < .01$		II-S

These 30 results reflect comparisons of two groups, the same group under two conditions, status of a group before and after TEACCH structured teaching, or simply describe a group without any comparison.

LOE, level of evidence; IBF, impairment of body function; A&P, activity and participation; EF, environmental factors; +, improved; −, worse; ns, not statistically significant; Vineland, Vineland Adaptive Behavior Scales-Survey Form (communication, socialization and self-help care); PEP-R, PsychoEducational Profile, Revised.

Table 3 Evidence Table: Outcomes of TEACCH (Structured Teaching)

Outcomes by dimensions of disability	Improved result (statistically significant)	Improved result (not statistically evaluated)	Unchanged or ns ($p = > .05$) result	Worse result (statistically significant)
Impairment of body structures				
Impairment of body functions	••••• ••• •	•••	••	•
Developmental status (cognitive, motor, perceptual domains)	II-S (14,14,14,14,14,14) IV-S (13,13,13,13,13) IV-S (13)			II-S (14)
Behavior (autistic, bizarre, aggressive, problem)	IV-S (13)	IV-W (11) V (8,13)	II-S (9) V (13)	
Activity and participation				
Engaging in work and play activities (on-task, attending)	IV-S (10)	V (13)	II-S (9)	
Engaging with people (affective, relating, complying, cooperating)		V (13)	II-S (9,9)	
Using language/communicating		V (13)	II-S (9)	
Family and community participation (living at home)		III-W (12)		
Environmental factors				
Parent influence on child (effective teaching/involvement)	IV-S (10)	IV-W (11)		

The dots reflect 30 results from Table 4. Each dot is elucidated by its level of evidence (coded I–V for type of research design + S, M, or W for strong, moderate, or weak control to threats to validity in conducting the study) followed by the citation number for the study that produced this result.

There were also three results, positive, about engaging with other people, but two were not statistically significant and the other was only an anecdotal report.

Did TEACCH intervention produce more meaningful use of language? There were three, positive, results about increased communication, but, again, two were not statistically significant and the other was anecdotal.

Finally, one measure of participation limitation showed that even older adolescents who were moderately to severely autistic were able to remain living at home when supported by the TEACCH support system of structured teaching at home and school plus training of and collaboration with parents. This result was not statistically evaluated.

Environmental Factors. Parent influence on the child improved (with statistical significance) in two measures that explored effect of structured teaching training for parents. Parents became more effective in teaching their own children and being involved with them.

5. How Good Is This Evidence?

This is an astonishingly weak body of evidence considering that Division TEACCH has been the leader in autism theory and practice for over 30 years and contains a university research unit that has published and taught professionals and parents so extensively.

Levels of Evidence. The level of evidence derived from these studies is Level II and III (one study each), Level IV (three studies), and Level V. In addition, 6 of the 30 results are anecdotal and, consequently, reflect Level V evidence.

Consistency of Results. While all the raw scores and anecdotal reports, except one, were consistently positive in support of TEACCH, there were only 30 results of which only 15 demonstrated statistical significance.

Extent to Which Population Has Been Sampled. Only 41 children (and 11 control children) have ever been studied in five studies between 1971 and 1998. Rates of institutionalization reported in the sixth study reflect residential data for an additional 115 children.

6. Are There Subgroups for Whom TEACCH May Be More Effective?

None of these studies reported uniformity of effect, that is, how many children were better, worse, or unchanged after exposure. Factors that may account for differing response to structured teaching were minimally explored in three studies with no identification of subgroups on the basis of chronological age, social age, socioeconomic status, severity of autism, and length of time in treatment. Correlation with chronological age was inconsistent. One study (10) found that younger children improved more than older children with mothers trained to use TEACCH, but two others (9,14) found no correlation between age and improvement. There was a tendency for children of lower socioeconomic status to improve more when maternal teaching effectiveness and child compliance were measured (10). Severity of autism correlated with improvement in one of the studies (14) in that mildly autistic children who had higher initial cognitive and language abilities benefited most, but in another study (9) more severely involved adolescents were able to be managed at home (versus being institutionalized) as often as were less severely involved adolescents. Social age and length of time in treatment did not correlate with improvement (9).

B. Evidence for the Effects of Sensory Integration Therapy for Individuals Diagnosed with Autism

1. What Is Sensory Integration Therapy?

A 1999 survey of occupational therapists showed that 99% of the 72 respondents relied on sensory integration (SI) theory to inform their practice and provide the therapy techniques they used with 2- to 12-year-old-children with autism (15). The theoretical framework for SI therapy (16), based on the work of Jean Ayres beginning in the early 1970s, holds that there is a natural human drive toward purposeful somatosensory activity with its concomitant sensory input. The neurophysiology of autism greatly reduces the capacity for this normal engagement with the environment. Lacking the capacity for more complex interaction as well as lacking normal somatosensory processing, the autistic person's drive toward action and sensory input is expressed, instead, in nonproductive, stereotyped actions. Improving the person's somatosensory processing and capacity to register, orient to, and interact purposefully with the environment will theoretically result in improved interactions and reduce the need for autistic patterns of self-stimulation. The need for constant external reinforcement will fade accordingly. Permanent changes in central nervous system functioning are theorized to occur if the therapeutic process occurs early in life while the system is still plastic.

SI therapy has been used in a number of pediatric populations. Meta-analyses (17) of studies have shown effect sizes to vary from low to moderately high depending on the populations studied, recency of the studies, and specific parameters measured. Outcomes in psychoeducational and motor categories were stronger than in other areas, at least for SI studies compared to no treatment conditions; however, effects appeared to be equivocal when compared with alternative treatments. However, autism is not a population that was represented in these meta-analyses.

Clinical observations of children with autism and reports from Temple Grandin (18) and Tito Mukhopadhyay (19), two individuals with autism who have been able to write about their sensory experiences, lend credence to the theory that autism involves a dysfunctional nervous system that does not adequately modulate incoming sensory stimulation. Tactile defensiveness, "nerve attacks," anxiety, screaming, and tantrums may be overreactive responses to incoming sensory stimuli by an overaroused nervous system. Stereotyped and self-stimulatory behaviors may be attempts to calm one's overly aroused nervous system. The child may withdraw from the environment and people in it to block out an onslaught of incoming stimulation. Alternatively, a child's nervous system may be underreactive to the extent that normal levels of sensory input fail to register. Hyperactivity, stereotyped behavior, self-stimulation, and even self-mutilation may reflect attempts of an underaroused nervous system to compensate for the experience of physiological sensory deprivation. In such cases, spontaneous abnormal motility (stereotyped behaviors) may be a way of intensifying kinesthetic feedback.

2. How Is SI Therapy Purported to Work?

Disruptions in SI functions are treated by providing controlled, therapeutically designed, meaningful sensory experiences (vestibular, kinesthetic, deep pressure, and tactile stimuli) to which a child responds with adaptive motor actions. Through this meaningful sensory input and appropriate active response to it, the abnormal neurochemistry is corrected, and new neural circuits form to repair the damaged nervous system (20).

3. What Studies Have Been Done?

Searching electronic databases and examining references in reviews and general background articles yielded 25 citations. Upon examination, 11 articles provided general information or were review articles and two (21,22) were studies not relevant to this report. Twelve citations proved to be research studies in which SI therapies were used for individuals with autism. Two (23,24) were not retrievable for direct examination but were thoroughly reported in review articles and were, therefore, included.

Variation of treatment implementation in studies has made it difficult to establish equivalence of SI therapy for determining efficacy. Baranek (25) classified the SI therapy that has been used in published studies as follows.

SI-Classical Therapy. SI therapy is classically a one-on-one intervention model in a clinic environment that uses specialized equipment, specifically suspended swings. Treatment plans are designed individually to provide a just-right challenge to the child and engage that child in developmentally appropriate play interactions. Therapy is guided by the child's meaningful play, not by adult-determined cognitive-behavioral strategies or repetitive drills. Treatment goals center on improving sensory processing to either (1) develop better sensory modulation as related to attention and behavioral control, or (2) integrate sensory information to form better perceptual schemas and practice abilities as a precursor for academic skills, social interactions, or more independent functioning. The therapy is carried out in 1-hour sessions by an SI-trained occupational therapist, 1–3 times per week, usually for several months. Home/ school programs are often provided concurrent with the direct intervention.

SI-Based Approaches. These are interventions that deviate from classic SI techniques in one or more criteria. (1) Somatosensory (e.g., brushing) and vestibular activities are provided, but suspended equipment is not used. (2) Treatment is more adult-structured or passively applied rather than being child-directed play. (3) Treatment is more cognitively focused. Structured perceptual-motor training approaches, sensory summation approaches (i.e., Sensory Diet), and cognitive-behavioral approaches (i.e., Alert program) are examples. In Sensory Diet therapy, the child is provided with a home and/or school program of sensory-based activities aimed at fulfilling the child's sensory needs. In the Alert program a child (usually with higher functioning level and verbal abilities) is given additional cognitive strategies to assist with his/her arousal modulation. These models often utilize a direct intervention (one-on-one or group) plus consultation/collaboration with caregivers who carry out home and school programs.

Sensory Stimulation Techniques. These interventions use techniques (i.e., touch pressure, vestibular stimulation) that vary but involve the passive provision of some type of sensory stimulation in a prescribed regime. They may be used in isolation or be incorporated in a broader SI-based program. The assumptions vary but most are based on neurophysiological principles stipulating that a given sensory experience provides facilitatory or inhibitory influences on the nervous system that change arousal modulation and behavior. For example, the commonly used technique of "touch pressure" to provide a calming effect may be applied via therapeutic touch (e.g., massage, joint compression) or an apparatus (e.g., Hug Machine, pressure garments, or weighted garments). Vestibular stimulation, another technique, applied in different ways may be used to modulate arousal, facilitate postural tone, and increase vocalizations.

Four of the 12 studies matched Baranek's criteria (25) for classic SI therapy (16,26–28). Three studies matched the criteria for SI-based approaches (23,24,

29). (Two used structured sensorimotor interventions based on SI principles and one used Sensory Diet. No studies of specific perceptual-motor treatments or Alert program in which the children had autism were found.) Five studies were found in which sensory stimulation techniques were the intervention (30–34). One of these reviewed effects of vestibular stimulation (30) and the others investigated effects of somatosensory stimulation (i.e., some type of touch or deep pressure). These 12 studies are summarized in Tables 4 and 5, Parts A and B. Table 6 is the evidence table in Parts A and B.

4. How Much and What Kind of Evidence Is There?

Impairment of Body Function. Given that impaired sensory processing and modulation is the primary problem in autism according to SI theory and practice, it was surprising that outcomes about processing and modulation have been measured only four times in two studies. While all four of these showed improvement, only two measures were statistically significant, one was not, and one was not statistically evaluated.

Autistic behaviors that are presumed to arise from sensory dysfunction have been measured 19 times in seven studies with 17 positive results and two unchanged results. However, only four of the positive results were statistically significant, and 10 were not statistically evaluated. Five of the six measures of anxiety (physiological and behavioral) in one study (34) were not statistically significant.

One measure (29), not statistically evaluated, documented notable improvement in physical posture after SI therapy.

Activity Limitations and Participation Restrictions. Was there an increase in meaningful activity and participation in family, school, and community life? Twenty-three results suggest there was. Greater engagement in productive activity was measured five times. However, only two of these results were statistically significant; two were not; one was not statistically evaluated.

One measure of self-help activity (toileting) was positive but not evaluated statistically.

There were six measures about engagement with other people, two of which showed statistically significant improvement with SI therapy. Another positive measure was not statistically significant, and three were not subjected to statistical evaluation.

What about communicating? These results were much weaker, including three that showed the control group demonstrating greater improvement. Only two of nine measures were positive but without statistical significance.

Finally, two anecdotes reported improvements in family and community participation. After SI therapy, the single participant in one study (29) was able to accompany family in the car safely and take advantage of community dental care rather than requiring expensive, specialty dental care necessary before.

Environmental Factors. An anecdotal report (29) for the same child indicated that caregiving in general was made easier as a result of SI therapy.

5. How Good Is This Evidence?

Levels of Evidence. Three studies used relatively strong research designs, which produced half of the outcomes shown in Part A of Table 6. Twenty results represent Level I evidence; 6, Level II; 5, Level III; 6, Level IV; and 11, Level V. Part B results that illuminate how many of group did better represent Level IV (nine results) and Level V (one result) evidence. Although the conduct of the two Level I studies was also strong and one Level IV study was moderate, there can be little confidence in the validity of the evidence from the others because it derived from poorly conducted studies that employed weak designs.

Consistency of Results. Forty-one of the 48 group-average results and all 10 of the uniformity-of-effect results were positive. All 24 results about impaired function were consistently positive.

Extent to Which Population Has Been Sampled. The greatest weakness in this body of evidence is that only 75 people have ever been studied. Evidence is available from only 12 studies, 6 of which contained only a single individual. Only four studies contained 10 or more participants.

6. Are There Subgroups for Whom SI Therapy May Be More Effective?

The uniformity-of-effect data in Part B of Table 6 shows that all individuals did not respond equally to SI therapy. Six of 10 studied by Ayres and Tickle (26), all five studied by Case-Smith and Bryan (27), and both studied by Linderman and Stewart (28) showed improvement on some, but not all, measures.

Three studies investigated factors that may be associated with better outcomes. Ayres and Tickle (26) and Edelson et al. (34) analyzed variables that correlated with better and poorer responses to therapy. Ayres and Tickle found that their good responders were those who, though few, initially presented with normal reactions to sensory input. Of those with abnormal reactions, the ones who initially showed tactile defensiveness ($p < .05$) had the best outcomes. Good responders also were those who initially tended to react to touch pressure ($p < .10$), vibration ($p < .10$), and movement ($p < .10$). Reaction to air puff, pain, joint traction, insecurity in gravitational forces, postrotary nystagmus, watching spinning stripes, bell and white noise sound, odor, and taste (flavor) did

Table 4 Summary of Studies About Sensory Integration Therapy: Interventions and Participants

Study	Intervention	Duration	Sample population	Age	N
1980 Ayres (26)	SI-Classic: 50 min, 2×/wk	1 yr	Autism: 2 mild, 5 moderate, 3 severe; 2 deaf; 1 partially sighted; 6 ethnic groups; in special education programs	3–13 yr	10
1983 Ayres (16)	SI-Classic: 2×/wk	2 yr	Severe autism, partially-sighted, deaf, female	11.5 yr	1
1999 Case-Smith (27)	SI-Classic: 30 min/?+school consultation	10 wk	Autism, mental retardation; 2 bilateral hearing impairment; 1 bipolar disorder; in half-day special needs preschool; detailed behavioral description of each child	4–5 yr	5
1999 Linderman (28)	SI-Classic: 1 hr/wk in clinic	7, 11 wk	Autism, tactile hypersensitivity 2; vestibular hyposensitivity 1	3 yr	2
1983 Reilly[a] (23)	SI-based therapy/vestibular treatment vs. tabletop activities (2× 30-min sessions of each)	3 wk	Autism	6–11 yr	18 (own controls)
1999 Larrington (29)	SI-based therapy/oral motor stim., sensory stim. + school and home program	2 yr	Severe mental retardation/autism, male; increasingly destructive and self-abusive; normal hearing and sight, no speech, some sign language and receptive language	15	1

Study	Intervention	Duration	Characteristics	Age	
1999 Stagnitti[b] (24)	SI-based therapy/sensory diet (brushing, joint compression, etc.) 3–5×/day + home program	2 wk, 2×, 5 mo apart	Sensory defensiveness, possible autism	5 yr	1
1988 Ray (30)	SS techniques/self-initiated vestibular activity (15 min 2×/wk) + daily SI therapy	4 wk	Autism, male, dyspraxia, dysarthric speech, low muscle tone, sluggish activity level, normal hearing, sleep problems, delayed cognitive, motor and social development, better receptive language, actively seeks vestibular stimulation	9 yr	1
1990 McClure (31)	SS techniques. Part 1: daily elastic pressure wraps (elbow splints); baths: vestibular inputs. Part 2: elastic wraps, arms or legs vs. no wraps, 4 sessions	Part 1: 53 days Part 2: 15 days	Autism; mental retardation; male; severe aggression, self-injury, stimulatory behaviors; in psychiatric unit	13 yr	1
1991 Zissermann (32)	SS techniques/pressure garments worn only during measurement. Part 1: Gloves (5–30-min/sessions). Part 2: Jobst vest (9–30-min sessions)	Part 1: 2 mo Part 2: 18 wk	Autism; female; severe developmental delay, possible seizures; self-stimulation; non-ambulator; in special education class for students with multiple disabilities	8 yr	1

Table 4 *Continued*

Study	Intervention	Duration	Sample population	Age	N
1997 Field (33)	SS techniques/touch therapy vs. placebo/1:1 quiet play held in lap (each 15 min 2×/wk)	4 wk	Autism diagnosed DSM-IIIR, in half-day special preschool, 12 boys, middle socioeconomic status	4.5 yr mean	11/11
1999 Edelson (34)	SS techniques/touch pressure (Hug Machine) vs. placebo (no pressure) 2×20 min/wk	6 wk	Autism; 9 boys; meaningful communication 6, nonverbal or echolalic 6	4–13 yr	5/7

[a]Data extracted from review papers (25,35,36).
[b]Data extracted from review (25).

Table 5 Summary of Studies About Sensory Integration Therapy: Methods, Outcomes, Measures, and Results

Part A. Average-of-Group Results: Experimental versus control groups, same group under experimental versus control conditions, before versus after status of treated group, or description of posttreatment only

Study and research design	Outcome of interest	Dim. of disability	Measure	Result	Clin. imp.	Statistics	LOE
1983 Ayres (16): prospective case study	Self-stimulatory behaviors	IBF	Time samples	+[a]	Yes		V
1983 Reilly (23):	Variety of speech	A&P	SVB of ASIEP[b]	—		Sign.	II[c]
single subject alternating treatments ABAB design	Mean length of utterance	A&P	SBV of ASIEP[b]	—		Sign.	II[c]
	Autistic speech	A&P	SVB of ASIEP[b]	—		Sign.	II[c]
	Speech function	A&P	SVB of ASIEP[b]			ns	II[c]
	Articulation	A&P	SVB of ASIEP[b]			ns	II[c]
	Rate of vocalizations	A&P	SVB of ASIEP[b]			ns	II[c]
1999 Larrington (29): single-subject AB design	Physical posture	IBF	Photographs	+	Yes		IV-W
	Destructive behavior	IBF	Home/school charts/notes	+	Yes		IV-W
	Engaging/playing	A&P	Home/school charts/notes	+	Yes		IV-W
	Toileting	A&P	Home/school charts/notes	+	Yes		IV-W
	Family activity participant	A&P	Parent report/anecdote	+	Yes		V
	Going to dentist	A&P	Parent report/anecdote	+	Yes		V
	Easier caregiving	EF	Group home/family anecdote	+	Yes		V
1999 Stagnitti (24):	Tactile tolerance	IBF	Anecdote	+[d]	Yes		V
	Affect	A&P	Anecdote	+[d]	Yes		V

Table 5 *Continued*

Study and research design	Outcome of interest	Dim. of disability	Measure	Result	Clin. imp.	Statistics	LOE
descriptive case report	Activity level	IBF	Anecdote	+[d]	Yes		V
	Temper tantrums	IBF	Anecdote	+[d]	Yes		V
1988 Ray (30) single-subject ABA design	Vocalizing	A&P	Avg. % of time (audiotapes)	+	Yes		III-W
	Spontaneous vocabulary	A&P	New word count (audiotapes)	+	Yes		III-W
1990 McClure (31): Part 1: descriptive case report; Part 2:	Part 1: Long term	—	Part 1.	—	—		—
	Self-stimulation	IBF	Clinical notes	+	Yes		V
	Self-injury	IBF	Clinical notes	+	Yes		V
	Interaction	A&P	Clinical notes	+	Yes		V
	Part 2: Short term	—	Part 2.	—	—		—
	Self-stimulation	IBF	Observation: % of time	+[e]	Yes		III-W
	Self-injury	IBF	Observation: % of time	+[e]	Yes		III-W
	Interaction	A&P	Observation: % of time	+[e]	Yes		III-W
1991	Part 1:	—	Part 1.	—	—		—
Zissermann (32): single-subject ABA design	Self-stimulation	IBF	Observation/frequency count	+	Yes		IV-M
	Part 2:	—	Part 2.	—	—		—
	Self-stimulation	IBF	Observation/frequency count	+	Yes		IV-M
1997 Field (33): randomized controlled trial	Orienting to sounds	IBF	Classroom observation	+		$p < .05$	I-S
	Stereotypic behaviors	IBF	Classroom observation	+		$p < .01$	I-S
	Touch aversion	IBF	Classroom observation	+		ns	I-S
	Off-task behavior	A&P	Classroom observation	+		ns	I-S
	Sensory responses	IBF	ABC (sensory score)	+		$p < .05$	I-S

Relating	A&P	ABC (relating score)	+		$p < .05$	I-S
Object use	A&P	ABC (object use score)	+		ns	I-S
Language	A&P	ABC (language score)	+		ns	I-S
Social skills	A&P	ABC (social skills score)	+		ns	I-S
Autistic behavior	IBF	ABC (total score)	+		$p < .05$	I-S
Attention	A&P	ESCS (joint attention score)	+		$p < .05$	I-S
Behavior regulation	IBF	ESCS (regulation score)	+		$p < .01$	I-S
Social behavior	A&P	ESCS (social beh. score)	+		$p < .05$	I-S
Initiating behavior	A&P	ESCS (init. beh. score)	+		$p < .01$	I-S
1999 Edelson (34): randomized controlled trial	IBF	Tension Scale[f]	+	Yes	$p < .01$	I-S
	IBF	Anxiety Scale[f]	+	Yes	$p < .10$	I-S
	IBF	Restlessness/Hyperactivity Sc[f]	+	Yes	$p < .10$	I-S
	IBF	Galvanic skin response-min	U	—	ns	I-S
	IBF	Galvanic skin response-max	U	—	ns	I-S
	IBF	Galvanic skin response-range	+	—	$p < 10$ ns	I-S

LOE, level of evidence; IBF, impairment of body function; A&P, activity and participation; EF, environmental factors; +, improved; —, worse; U, unchanged; ns, not statistically significant.

[a]Effective at 20 weeks, then deteriorated during subseqent 26 weeks while in body case following scoliosis surgery and after subsequent menarch.

[b]Sample of Vocal Behavior of the Autism Screening Instrument for Educational Planning.

[c]Inadequate information to rate conduct of study.

[d]Improvement faded by 5 months posttreatment but 6- and 9-month assessments showed "sensory defensiveness cured."

[e]Carryover also present; ABC, Autism Behavior Checklist; ESCS, Early Social Communication Scales.

[f]Based on items from Conners Patent Rating Scale.

Table 5 *Continued*

Part B. Uniformity-of-Effect-Within-a-Treated-Group Results

Study and research design	Dim.	Outcome of interest	Measure	Improved result	Worse result	Unchanged result	LOE
1980 Ayres (26): single-subject ABA design; pre and post measures	IBF	Behavior (language, awareness of environment, purposeful activities, self-stimulation, social and emotional behavior)	Observations (qualitative and different for each participant)	6/10[a]			IV-W
1999 Case-Smith (27): single-subject ABA design: 3 wk baseline, 10 week treatment	A&P	Mastery play	Engagement check/videotapes	3/5*			IV[b]
	A&P	Nonengagement	Engagement check/videotapes	4/5*			IV[b]
	A&P	Interactions	Engagement check/videotapes	1/5*			IV[b]
1999 Linderman (28): single-subject ABA design: 2 wk baseline, 7 or 11 wk treatment	A&P	Social interaction	FBA for CSID[c]	2/2[*d]		—	IV-W
	A&P	Response to affection	FBA for CSID[c]	1/1[*d]		—	IV-W
	A&P	Response to movement	FBA for CSID[c]	1/1[*d]		—	IV-W
	A&P	Approach new activities	FBA for CSID[c]	1/1[*d]		0/1	IV-W
	A&P	Functional communication	FBA for CSID[c]	—			
	IBF	Disruptive behaviors	Anecdote	2/2			V

*Indicates a statistically significant ($p < .05$) result.

[a]All improved but 6 were rated as good responders and 4 as poor responders.

[b]Inadequate information to rate conduct of study.

[c]Modified Functional Behavior Assessment for Children with Sensory Integrative Dysfunction.

[d]Visual analysis of trend, slope, level, and serial dependency calculations.

not predict the good responders. Edelson et al. found that their best responders were those who presented with higher anxiety levels compared with those with lower levels.

Ayres and Mailloux (16) reported a tendency for regression in adolescent years associated with the onset of puberty. The authors offered this as possible support for the success of SI therapy being based, at least in part, "on the capacity to enter into the neurobiological development of the child during the early critical period for maturation of sensory integrative mechanisms."

7. Have Any Medical Complications Been Documented?

None were reported in the only study that tracked unintentional side effects (34).

C. Evidence of the Effects of Megavitamin B_6 in Children Diagnosed with Autism

Linus Pauling's orthomolecular hypothesis appeared in 1968, proposing that some forms of mental illness and disease are related to biochemical errors in the body. In the early 1970s, Rimland (37), an advocate of megavitamin therapy, reported that some autistic children responded favorably to high doses of vitamin B_6. In a subsequent trial of megavitamin B_6, Rimland (38) observed that some children experienced increased irritability, sound sensitivity, and enuresis when vitamin B_6 was given in large amounts, but these problems disappeared when increased amounts of magnesium were added to dietary intake. Otherwise, there was no evidence that massive doses of vitamin B_6 had been harmful. Studies that followed, therefore, used pyridoxine or vitamin B_6 supplemented with magnesium.

1. How Does Megavitamin B_6 Therapy Purport to Work?

The proposed mechanism of action for megavitamin B_6 is that a disturbance in dopaminergic systems causes faulty central nervous system functioning that is responsible for autistic behaviors. Vitamin B_6 is involved in the formation of dopamine and other neurotransmitters (i.e., serotonin, aminobutyric acid, norepinehrine, and epinephrine) (39). Although vitamin B_6 deficiency has not been documented in individuals with autism (40), subclinical deficiencies might be present, and vitamin therapy is believed to be a means of compensating for such errors.

Table 6 Evidence Table: Outcomes of Sensory Integration Therapy

Part A. Average-of-Group Results. Experimental vs. control groups, same group under experimental vs. control conditions, before vs. after status of treated group, or posttreatment-only description

Outcomes by dimensions of disability	Improved result (statistically significant)	Improved (but not statistically evaluated)	Unchanged or ns ($p = < .05$) results	Worse result (statistically significant)
Impairment of body structures				
Impairment of body functions				
Sensory response (tactile tolerance, aversion, defensiveness, orienting to sound)	• • • • • I-S (33,33)	• • • • • • • • • • V (24)	• • • • • I-S (33)	
Behavior (self-stimulation, destructive, tantrums, restlessness, activity level, self-injury, anxiety, stereotypic, behavior regulation)	I-S (33,33,33,34)	III-W (31,31) IV-W (29) IV-M (32,32) V (16,24,24,31,31)	I-S (34,34,34,34)	
Physical posture		IV-W (29)		
Activity and participation				
Engaging in work/play activities (off-task, using objects, attending, initiating)	• • • • I-S (33,33)	• • • • • • • IV-W (29)	• • • • • • I-S (33,33)	• •
Self-care (toileting)		IV-W (29)		
Engaging with people (relating, socialization, affect)	I-S (33,33)	IV-W (29) III-W (31) V (24,31)	I-S (33)	

Using language/
  communicating (various
  aspects of speech)   III-W (30,30)   I-S (33) IIᵃ (23,23,23)   IIᵃ (23,23,23)

Family/community
  participation (going to
  dentist; riding family car)   V (29,29)

Environmental factors

Caregiving   • V (29)

ᵃInadequate information to rate conduct of study.

Part B. Uniformity-of-Effect-Within-a-Treated-Group Results

Outcomes by dimensions of disability	Improved result	Worse result	Unchanged result
Impairment of body function			
Behavior (general, disruptive)	•• 6/10 IV-W (26) 2/2 V (28)		
Activity and participation			
Engaging in activities	•••••• 3/5 IV (27)* 4/5 IV (27)* 1/1 IV-W (28)*		
Engaging and communicating with people	2/2 IV-W (28)* 1/1 IV-W (28,28,28)* 1/5 IV (27)*		

*Indicates a statistically significant ($p < .05$) result.

2.   What Studies Have Been Done?

Electronic searching was completed on January 3, 2003 and yielded 15 citations of interest. One citation was a letter to an editor about a 1995 review (39) of megavitamin B_6. Bernard Rimland, of the Autism Research Institute, in his letter criticized the authors for failing to include some of the published reports. Despite his assertion that there were 18 studies and despite attempting to secure those citations directly from the Autism Research Institute, only nine discrete studies of megavitamin B_6 in which the participants had autism could be determined.

On examination of the initial 15 citations, two publications (39,41) were excluded because each was a review article rather than a study, and another (40) was an article containing only general information. Of the research studies, one trial was excluded because it used a low dose of vitamin B_6 that documented no treatment effect at low dosage (42). Four were found to be multiple publications of a study and were, therefore, excluded (43–46).

Two additional trials (39,41) were identified through the review articles. Although these trials were published only in French (47,48), there was sufficiently thorough description of the trials between the two English reviews to include them in this evidence report. Nine studies met the inclusion criteria: (1) large doses of vitamin B_6 in (2) individuals with autism only or a subgroup with autism for which separate data are given, and (3) only one publication of a study included. Tables 7 and 8 summarize the studies. Table 9 summarizes medical complications that have been reported, and Table 10 is the evidence table. Some studies reported results that compared the average of the group's results whereas one reported results according to the uniformity of the effect within the treated group (i.e., how many were better, worse, unchanged after treatment). This requires that the summary-of-results table and the evidence table be presented in two parts; Part A contains comparisons of the average of a group's results and Part B contains uniformity of effect results.

3.   How Much and What Kind of Evidence Is There?

Impairment of Body Function. Table 7 (Part A) shows 15 results that provide evidence about whether dopamine metabolism, hypothesized to regulate central nervous system functioning, responded to megavitamin B_6 therapy. Nine studies used urinary homovanillic acid (uHVA), a metabolite of dopamine (39), as a biochemical measure of dopamine neurotransmission, evoked potentials (EP) as an electrophysiological measure of dopamine neurotransmission, or both.

Children with autism did appear to have higher levels of uHVA than did healthy children based on evidence from an index group of 11 healthy children in one study (50). What happened to those high uHVA levels in individuals with autism? That was measured nine times (Table 10). Eight measures found more normal uHVA levels with megavitamin B_6-magesium; two were statistically significant, two not statistically evaluated, and four were not statistically significant. One result showed no effect on uHVA levels (52).

Evoked potentials provide an electrophysiological measure of the brain's ability to process external sensory stimuli (39). Auditory and visual-evoked potentials involve catecholamine metabolism, a system that includes the neurotransmitter dopamine. Only two of four results confirmed more normal evoked potentials when scores were averaged across occipital (O) and central (C) sites. There were lower amplitudes, shorter latency periods, and greater variability in individuals with autism compared to an index group of healthy children. Given that averaging scores may obscure a treatment effect, the most recent study calculated results for the occipital (O) and central (C) sites separately. They found a statistically significant positive effect at the O site but no treatment effect at the C site.

Did autistic behaviors diminish? Autistic behaviors were measured 13 times in seven studies (42,48–51,53,54). Although improvement was noted in each result with 5 of the 13 measures reporting moderate to marked clinical improvement (see Table 8), Table 10 shows that 8 of these 13 measures did not attain statistical significance and two were not evaluated statistically.

4. How Good Is This Evidence?

Levels of Evidence. The majority of the studies produced Level I or Level II evidence for 20 outcomes. There is Level III and IV evidence for the other 11 outcomes. In addition to using relatively strong research designs, the conduct of most studies was moderate to strong in controlling threats to validity of the results.

Consistency of Results. The 31 group-average results were not consistent. Half showed improvement in dopamine metabolism and fewer than half confirmed improvement in autistic behaviors. This may be explained in part by the uniformity of results, which showed that although behavior improved in some participants, it did not in the majority, and this positive effect for the responders would be obscured when the results for a group were averaged.

Extent to Which Population Has Been Sampled. The greatest weakness in this body of evidence is the extremely limited number of people who have ever been studied. Evidence is available from only nine studies in which the exact number of individuals who have been studied is clouded. There are 26 participants from two studies (49,54) who are clearly drawn from separate pools of participants. The rest, drawn from a pool studied in France, almost certainly reflect the repeat use of the same participants in more than one study. These seven studies were done by a French group that included Martineau (first author for four studies in this evidence report), Barthelemy, Jonas, and Lelord (each first author for one study). One study (50) is known to have used participants in another study (45). Given the time frame and place in which these studies were conducted and the participant number in some of the publications, it is highly likely that there were overlaps of participants between some or all of the studies published by the French group. Thus, the total number of individuals from whom evidence is available is almost certainly much fewer than the apparent 182 and may be as few as 86 people shown in six of the studies (45,49,14).

5. Are There Subgroups for Whom Megadoses of B_6 May Be More Effective?

In a 1989 publication (53), Martineau et al. stated that, based on their experience, approximately 15% of participants respond to B_6-magnesium treatment and 30% have mild positive effects. The only data that can be gleaned from this body of evidence, however, is from one open trial (45) (Table 10, Part B) that reported 15 of 44 participants, or 34%, to be responders. When a group of responders and nonresponders from this open trial were subsequently studied in a double-blind, placebo-controlled trial, positive effects for B_6-magnesium were documented in 12, or 57%, of the 21 participants.

Only one study (50) has attempted to identify the relationships between various factors that may illuminate who the responders are. Potential variables were examined but no relationships were discovered between uHVA and degree of autism, Rimland scale, service scale, associated deficit, language development, motor deficits, length of hospitalization, agitation, age of onset, and drug treatment.

6. Have Any Medical Complications Been Documented?

A serious side effect of very high doses of pyridoxine (i.e., sensory neuropathy) has been reported in the literature at large (41). In these studies of individuals with autism who took ≤ 1 g/kg/day of vitamin B_6, however, only three studies (Table 9) reported adverse side effects and these were said to be manageable or relatively minor. Once magnesium was added to the megavitamin therapy, adverse effects were fewer still.

IV. CRITICALLY APPRAISED TOPIC

In the absence of any scientific publications, a topic can be critically appraised. The best evidence for the rapid-prompt method, for example, describes the nature and extent of the media, popular press, or Internet reports about an intervention and what it is purported to accomplish in which dimensions of disability.

Table 7 Summary of Studies About Megavitamin B$_6$: Interventions and Participants

Study	Daily megavitamin treatment	Comparison treatment	Duration	Population	N^a	Age
1978 Rimland (49)	2.4 mg/kg to 94.3 mg/kg B$_6$ (mode 6 mg/kg)	3 Phases of no treatment and 1 phase of placebo	Variable	12 Boys, 4 girls with autistic symptoms from earlier megavitamin/cluster analysis study who were B$_6$-responsive and relapsed on withdrawal; 6 had score indicating definite presence of autism; living at home	16	4–19 yr
1980 Barthelemy (47)^a	30 mg/kg B$_6$ + 10 mg/kg Mg	Placebo phase	14 da	Autism diagnosed with DSM criteria	37	

Table 7 *Continued*

Study	Daily megavitamin treatment	Comparison treatment	Duration	Population	N^a	Age
1981 Lelord (45)	30 mg/kg B_6 + 10–15 mg/kg Mg	Part 1: 2 phases of no treatment	Variable 4 wk	Part 1: 26 boys, 18 girls with autistic symptoms: social withdrawal, stereotypies, tantrums, hypersensitivity to stimuli, aggressive toward self and others, disordered eating and sleeping behavior; 28 in long-term institutional care; 7 severe MR; 33 no speech. Heterogenous group: 16 most clearly resembled Kanner's original description of autism, 28 had other development/neurological disorders with autistic signs (11 mild signs, 9 moderate, 8 severe)	44	3.5–16 yr (mean age 9.3 yr)
		Part 2: placebo phase		Part 2: 13 responders (hospitalized in child psychiatric service) and 8 nonresponders from Part 1	21	

1981 Martineau (50)	30 mg/kg B$_6$ + 10–15 mg/kg Mg		31 da 15 da	6 Boys; 6 girls from the Lelord study above; severely disordered with autism: bizarre responses to environment, stereotypies, aggressive and self-destructive behavior, temper tantrums, hyperesthesias, eating problems, disordered sleep; hospitalized in child psychiatric service; associated disorders of epilepsy 3/12, stunting 2/12, hydrocephalus sequelae 1/12; 50% on psychotrophic medications	12	Mean age 7 yr
1984 Jonas (48)[b]	1000 mg B$_6$ + 380 mg Mg	Placebo phase	42 da	Autism diagnosed with DSM criteria	8	
1985 Martineau (51)	Up to 1 g/kg B$_6$ or B$_6$ + 10–15 mg/kg Mg	2 Phases of no treatment; alternating treatment phases of Mg and placebo	8 wk each type of phase	37 Boys, 23 girls with autism diagnosed with DSM-III criteria; hospitalized in day-care psychiatric unit; excluded patients with gross neurological deficits, severe seizures, endocrine or systematic disease	60	Mean age 8 yr
1986 Martineau (52)	30 mg/kg pyridoxine + 15 mg/kg Mg	2 Phases of no treatment	8 mo	Autism diagnosed with DSM-III criteria: language retardation, social detachment, seclusiveness: near-normal nonverbal language age, below-average social age, excellent physical health, no developmental or neurological abnormalities, normal blood chemistry, urinalysis, and EEG	1	4 yr

Table 7 *Continued*

Study	Daily megavitamin treatment	Comparison treatment	Duration	Population	N^a	Age
1989 Martineau (53)	30 mg/kg pyridoxine + 10 mg/kg Mg	2 Phases of no treatment	14 wk	Boys with autism diagnosed with DSM-III criteria: most disturbed in impaired communication, lack of socially appropriate facial expressions/gestures, resistance to change, frustration, abnormal aggression; global DQ 30–70	6	4 y 7 mo– 8 yr
1997 Findling (54)	1 g/kg B$_6$ + 10 mg/ kg Mg	No treatment and placebo phases	10 wk	11 Boys, 1 girl diagnosed with autism using DSM-IIIR criteria; no medical or neurological disorders; no psychotropic agents within 3 mo; all lived at home	10	3–17 yr

CPRS, Children's Psychiatric Rating Scale; B$_6$, vitamin B$_6$ or pyridoxine; Mg, magnesium.
[a] All participants crossed between treatment and control conditions.
[b] Data taken from reviews (39, 41).

Table 8 Summary of Studies About Megavitamin B_6: Methods, Outcomes, Measures, and Results

Part A. Average-of-Group Results. Average status of group during megavitamin B_6 therapy compared with average status before and/or after therapy

Study and research design	Outcome of interest	Dim. of disability	Measure	Result	Clin. imp.	Statistics	LOE
1978 Rimland (49): placebo-controlled trial	Autistic behaviors	IBF	Individualized behavior checklists + teacher/parent narratives	+	Yes	$p < .05$	II-S
1980 Barthelemy (47): randomized, placebo-controlled, crossover trial	Autistic behaviors	IBF	Bretonneau II (18 items)	+	Moderate	ns	I-W
	Biochemistry: dopamine metabolism	IBF	uHVA	+			I-W
1981 Lelord (45): Part 1: open ABA trial	Biochemistry: dopamine metabolism	IBF	uHVA (gas chromatography)	+		Signif.	III-M
1981 Martineau (50): Part 1: open ABA trial[a]	Part 1: Autistic behaviors	IBF	Bretonneau II (18 items)	+	Marked	—	III-M
Part 2: open ABA trial[a]	Part 2: Biochemistry: dopamine metabolism	IBF	uHVA (gas chromatography)	+		$p < .01$	IV-W
	Electrophysiology: dopamine metabolism	IBF	AER middle latency amplitude	+			IV-W
1984 Jonas (48): placebo-controlled trial	Autistic behaviors	IBF	Bretonneau III (22 items)	+		Signif.	II-S
	Biochemistry: dopamine metabolism	IBF	uHVA	+		ns	II-S

Table 8 *Continued*

Study and research design	Outcome of interest	Dim. of disability	Measure	Result	Clin. imp.	Statistics	LOE
1985 Martineau (51): sequential controlled trials[b]	Part 1: Autistic behaviors	IBF	Behavior Summarized Evaluation	+	—	ns	II-M
Part 1: B₆ Mg/Mg	Part 2: Biochemistry: dopamine	IBF	uHVA	+		ns	II-M
	Electrophys: dopamine	IBF	EP amplitude/morphology	+		ns	II-M
Part 2: B₆ Mg/placebo	Part 2: Autistic behaviors	IBF	Behavior Summarized Evaluation	+	Marked	$p < .05$	II-M
	Biochemistry: dopamine	IBF	uHVA	+		ns	II-M
	Electrophys.: dopamine	IBF	EP amplitude/morphology	+		ns	II-M
Part 3: B₆/placebo	Part 3: Autistic behaviors	IBF	Behavior Summarized Evaluation	+		ns	II-M
	Biochemistry: dopamine	IBF	uHVA	U			II-M
1986 Martineau (52): open ABA trial	Autistic behaviors	IBF	Behavior Summarized Evaluation	+	Yes	d	III-M
	Biochemistry: dopamine metabolism	IBF	uHVA (gas chromatography)	+		d	III-M
	Electrophysiology: dopamine metabolism	IBF	EP amplitude/morphology	+[c]		d	III-M
1989 Martineau (53): open ABA trial	Electrophysiology: dopamine metabolism	IBF	AER frequency/amplitude at O site	+		$p < .05$	III-W
	dopamine metabolism	IBF	AER frequency/amplitude at C site	U			III-W

Study	Dim.	Outcome	Measure	Improved result	Worse result	Unchanged result	LOE
1997 Findling (54) placebo-controlled, crossover trial	IBF	Autistic behaviors	CPRS			ns	II-M
	IBF	Autistic behaviors	CGIS			ns	II-M
	IBF	Autistic behaviors	OCS			ns	II-M
	IBF	Autistic behaviors	Teacher Rating Scale			ns	II-M
	IBF	Autistic behaviors	Parent Rating Scale			ns	II-M

LOE, level of evidence; IBF, impairment of body function; A&P, activity and participation; +, improved result with therapy; U, unchanged result; uHVA, urinary homovanillic acid; AER, conditioned auditory evoked responses at occipital (O) and central (C) sites; EP, evoked potentials; ns, not statistically significant; Signif., significant; CPRS, Children's Psychiatric Rating Scale; CGIS, Clinical Global Impression Scale; OCS, NIMH Global Obsessive Compulsive Scale.

[a]Also contained an index healthy group.
[b]Also contained an index group comparing magnesium and placebo.
[c]Improvement after 1 mo followed by a shading off.
[d]Data plots.

Part B. Uniformity-of-Effect-Within-a-Treated Group Results

Study	Dim.	Outcome	Measure	Improved result	Worse result	Unchanged result	LOE
1981 Lelord (45): Part 1: open ABA trial	IBF	Part 1: Autistic behaviors	Bretonneau II (18 items)	15/44		29/44	III-M
Part 2: placebo-controlled, crossover trial in open-trial responders	IBF	Part 2: Autistic behaviors	Bretonneau II (18 items)	12/21			II-S

Table 9 Summary of Megavitamin B_6 Studies: Medical Complications

Study	Type of effect	No. of cases
1978 Rimland (49) $N = 16$	Increased irritability, sound sensitivity, and enuresis (resolved with addition of magnesium to B_6 administration)	Not given
1981 Lelord (45) $N = 44$	Nausea	3
	Increased excitability	3
	Increased autistic symptoms	4
1997 Findling (54) $N = 10$	Loose stools	5
	Upper respiratory infection	5

A. Rapid-Prompt Method in Children Diagnosed with Autism

1. What Is the Rapid-Prompt Method?

In January 2003, two national television stations [CBS's *60 Minutes* (55) and ABC's *Good Morning America* (56)] broadcast a story that challenges current understanding about the limitations of communication in children with autism and suggests a new educational strategy for teaching communication through writing to severely autistic, nonverbal children.

In 1999, Tito Mukhopadhyay came to the attention of the National Autistic Society in London, which brought him and his mother to a conference in the United Kingdom. Tito is reported to be a boy with severe autism who is nearly nonverbal but who writes poetry and essays in fluent English and whose written communications have provided valuable insight about his experience of autism through written answers to such questions as "Why do you flap? Why do you rock? Why can't you look me in the eyes?" In 2001, the Cure Autism Now Foundation sponsored Tito and his mother to move to the United States to involve them in the Carousel School for children with autism in Los Angeles. The Cure Autism Now Foundation and its Carousel School have been interested not only in the insights that Tito offers about autism, but also in the teaching technique his mother, Soma Mukhopadhyay, used to get him to stay on task and eventually write. They hope that other children with autism can be similarly "reached." Since coming to the United States, Tito, who is now age 14, has reportedly been examined by several university researchers in autism and is said to be severely autistic despite his unusual ability for written expression (57).

An American teacher who observed Soma Mukhopadhyay using rapid-prompt method at the Carousel School with other students was said to have described it as being "everything teachers of children with autism are trained not

Table 10 Evidence Table: Outcomes of Megavitamin B$_6$
Part A. Average-of-Group Results

Outcomes by dimensions of disability	Improved result (statistically significant)	Improved result (but not statistically evaluated)	Worse result	Unchanged and ns results ($p < .05$)
Impairment of body structures				
Impairment of body functions	• • • • •[a]	• • • • • •		• • • • • • • • • • • • •[a] • • •
Dopamine metabolism (biochemistry)	III-M (45) IV-W (50)		I-W (47) III-M (52)	I-S (48,48)
Dopamine metabolism: (electrophysiology)	III-W (53)	III-M (52) IV-W (50)		II-M (51,51,51)
Autistic behaviors	II-M (51) II-S (48,49)	III-M (50,52)		II-M (51,51) III-W (53) I-W (47) II-M (51,51,54, 54,54,54)

[a]No effect at C site but positive effect at O site.

Part B. Uniformity-of-Effect-Within-a-Treated-Group Results

Outcomes by dimensions of disability	Improved result	Worse result	Unchanged result
Impairment of body function			
Behavior	• • 15/44 III-M (45) 12/21 II-S (45)		• 29/44 III-M (45)

to do" (57). That is, teachers are currently trained to give basic directions and wait for a response because too much verbalizing has been understood to be too distracting. In contrast, Soma Mukhopadhyay talks constantly—repetitively urging, prodding, and directing. Thus, her technique is being called "rapid-prompt method." Instead of being distracting, this rapid-prompt method seems to keep the children's attention focused long enough for them to communicate. She also does not try to redirect students when they engage in stereotypic movements and fail to make eye contact. Instead, she ignores their erratic movements and wandering eyes because, according to insights gleaned from her son's writings, these behaviors appear to serve other important functions that do not interfere with learning. Tito has written that he can either see or hear, but not both simultaneously, so that he must choose one. He says that he rocks and spins because he cannot feel his body unless it is in motion.

2.   How Is It Purported to Work?

No mechanism of action has been proposed for the rapid-prompt method, but Tito's writings lend credence to a theory that autism involves scrambled brain connections and faulty sensory processing. Such theory holds that during the first years of life, children develop internal maps that involve brain regions specializing in the sense of touch and movement. By imaging the brains of higher-functioning autistic people who can stay still in scanners, researchers in the laboratory of Dr. Eric Courchesne at the University of California at San Diego were said to have found that autistic people had mixed-up brain maps (57). In normal people, for example, face recognition occurs in a well-defined brain region. In people with autism, face recognition occurs in other parts of the brain such as the frontal lobes. The same is true of maps that help plan movements. This means body maps are formed in autistic children, but they may be scrambled differently in each person.

People who lack normal body maps may not build mental models of the world that integrate sights, sounds, smells, touches, and tastes. Most people can sense sound and light even when they are separated by only a fraction of a second, but Tito cannot see light at all unless it is separated from sound by a full 3 seconds. Tito says he must choose one sensory channel at a time and prefers that to be hearing. Vision is actually painful to him. To change channels, he needs "time to prepare my eyes" or ears. "Otherwise the world is chaos" (57).

3.   What Studies Have Been Done?

No citations for any professional reports were found in the medical or educational literature with the search terms "rapid-prompt method," "Tito or Soma Mukhopadhyay." To seek information in the lay media, a search on the Internet via msn.com on February 2, 2003 yielded 114 results for websites that contained the words "Tito Mukhopadhyay"; these included a link to the Cure Autism Now website (58).

Examination of these Internet results showed, however, that all reflect the same information that originated in a *New York Times* News Service story (57) that subsequently appeared in multiple versions and venues: other newspapers, *People* magazine, and three television broadcasts. In addition, one website shows a book entitled *Beyond the Silence*, written by Tito Mukhopadhyay and published by the National Autistic Society in London (19).

4. How Much and What Kind of Evidence Is There?

The *New York Times* article stated that Soma Mukhopadhyay is testing her teaching method on a small group of children at the Carousel School in Los Angeles, but no reports or research projects (proposed or funded) were listed on the Cure Autism Now website. Cure Autism Now is a research foundation that promotes and funds research, that is associated with the Carousel School, and that sponsored the Mukhopadhyays to come to the United States. The sum total of information about this intervention is that the rapid-prompt method has been tried with a small group of students with autism, aged 9–10, at the Carousel School in Los Angeles with two outcomes that can be discerned from the stories. One anecdotally reported outcome is marked improvement in communication (i.e., written language using full sentences, complex thoughts, correctly spelled words) after 6 weeks in one boy with severe autism who is nonverbal, has unintelligible sounds, engages in self-stimulation and/or uncontrollable movements (flapping, rocking, lack of eye contact), and is diagnosed with probable mental retardation. The other anecdotally reported outcome is improvement in a small group of children with severe autism, a few of whom speak. After a year, their instructional level improved from grade 1 to grade 4 and the variety of curriculum used was expanded.

5. How Good Is This Evidence?

Though interesting, these reports are exceedingly preliminary, do not even place on the AACPDM levels of evidence classification, and do not constitute scientific evidence at any level.

V. IN THE ABSENCE OF SCIENTIFIC EVIDENCE OF EFFECTIVENESS, WHAT THEN?

Absence of evidence in support of an intervention should never be construed as proof that a treatment is not effective; rather, it may reflect areas in which research—or more meaningful research—is needed. Frequently, absence of evidence of effectiveness in existing studies is related to lack of power in a study or the lack of statistical calculations that examine whether there was adequate power to detect an effect. Moreover, even in a robust trial, the group results may obscure benefits to some individuals. Nevertheless, absence of evidence in support of an intervention does demonstrate that clinicians should be circumspect about the voracity of their treatment recommendations in the face of scarce or inconclusive evidence.

Use the evidence reports to frame clinical questions about any intervention you entertain. "What do the proponents of this intervention purport that it will do and in what time frame?" "What is the theory of the mechanism of action of this intervention?" "Is this purported outcome of greatest importance to the individual under consideration?" "What duration of treatment is reasonable to determine whether the intervention is effective?" "What valid and reliable measure(s) can be used to evaluate the outcomes in which we are interested?" "How can we control threats to the validity of the outcomes we may observe?"

Next, conduct the time-honored, but improved, "trial of therapy" to determine whether an intervention is positive or negative—for this person. David Sackett and other leading figures in evidence-based medicine have incorporated randomized controlled trial methods to create a more robust N-of-1 trial that has wide application. Guidelines for conducting such a trial are summarized in their handbook on how to teach and practice evidence-based medicine (59, p. 174).

If the N-of-1 trial does not demonstrate the intervention as effective for this individual within a reasonable period of time, or show a definite trend toward improvement, move on promptly to systematically explore other interventions that may be more beneficial.

Finally, to build more robust and extensive bodies of evidence, even these clinically based N-of-1 trials need to be replicated, outcomes aggregated and analyzed as group data, and submitted for publication to build the bodies of evidence needed for evidence-based practice.

REFERENCES

1. Butler C. AACPDM Methodology for Developing Evidence Tables and Reviewing Treatment Outcome Research. American Academy for Cerebral Palsy and Developmental Medicine. Available at: http://www.aacpdm.org.
2. World Health Organization. International Classification of Functioning, Disability and Health. World Health Organization. Available at: http://www3.who.int/icf/icftemplate.cfm?myurl = homepage.html&mytitle = Home%20Page. Accessed January 26, 2003.
3. Autism Society of America. Treatment and Education Approaches (Accessed January 17, 2003). Available at: http://www.autism-society.org/site/PageServer.

4. Schopler E. Relationship between university research and state policy: Division TEACCH—Treatment and Education of Autistic and related Communication-Handicapped Children. Pop Govern 1986; 51(4):23–32.
5. Schopler E. TEACCH. In: CR Reynolds, L Mann, eds. Encyclopedia of Special Education. Vol. 1. New York: Wiley, 1987:1536–1537.
6. Schopler E. Current and Past Research on Autistic Children and Their Families Conducted by Division TEACCH. Microfiche Accession Number ED 339 161. University of North Carolina, School of Medicine, 1991.
7. Mesibov G. An overview of Division TEACCH (Accessed February 19, 2003). Division TEACCH, University of North Carolina School of Medicine. Available at: http://www.teacch.com/aboutus.htm.
8. Cox R, Schopler E. Aggression and self-injurious behaviors in persons with autism—the TEACCH approach. Acta Paedopsychiatr 1993; 56:85–90.
9. Schopler E, Brehm S, Kinsbourne M, Reichler R. Effect of treatment structure on development in autistic children. Arch Gen Psychiatry 1971; 24:416–421.
10. Marcus L, Lansing M, Andrews C, Schopler E. Improvement of teaching effectiveness in parents of autistic children. J Am Acad Child Psychiatry 1978; 17:625–639.
11. Short A. Evaluation of short-term treatment outcome using parents as co-therapists for their own psychotic children. [Unpublished dissertation.] Chapel Hill: School of Medicine, University of North Carolina, 1980.
12. Schopler E, Mesibov G, Baker A. Evaluation of treatment for autistic children and their parents. J Am Acad Child Psychiatry 1982; 21(3):262–267.
13. Panerai S, Ferrante L, Caputo V. The TEACCH Strategy in mentally retarded childen with autism: a multidimensional assessment: pilot study. J Autism Dev Disord 1997; 27(3):345–347.
14. Ozonoff S, Cathcart K. Effectiveness of a home program intervention for young children with autism. J Autism Dev Disord 1998; 28(1):25–32.
15. Watling R, Dietz J, Kanny E, McLaughlin J. Current practices of occupational therapy for children with autism. Am J Occup Ther 1999; 53(5):498–505.
16. Ayres A, Mailloux Z. Possible pubertal effect on therapeutic gains in an autistic girl. Am J Occup Ther 1983; 37(8):535–540.
17. Vargas S, Camilli G. A meta-analysis of research on sensory integration treatment. Am J Occup Ther 1998; 53:189–198.
18. Ratey JJ, Grandin T, Miller A. Defense behavior and coping in an autistic savant: the story of Temple Grandin, PhD. Psychiatry 1992; 55(4):382–391.
19. Mukhopadhyay T. Beyond the Silence. London: National Autistic Society, 2000.
20. Gorman P. Sensory dysfunction in dual diagnosis: mental retardation/mental illness and autism. Occup Ther Ment Health 1997; 13(1):3–22.
21. Freeman B, Frankel F, Ritvo E. The effects of response contingent vestibular stimulation on the behavior of autistic and retarded children. J Autism Child Schizo 1976; 6(4):353–358.
22. Cohn E. Parent perspectives of occupational therapy using a sensory integration approach. Am J Occup Ther 2000; 55(3):285–294.

23. Reilly C, Nelson D, Bundy A. Sensorimotor versus fine motor activities in eliciting vocalizations in autistic children. Occup Ther J Res 1983; 8:187–190.

24. Stagnitti K, Raison P, Ryan P. Sensory defensiveness syndrome: a paediatric perspective and case study. Aust Occup Ther J 1999; 46:175–187.

25. Baranek G. Efficacy of sensory and motor interventions for children with autism. J Autism Dev Disord 2002; 32(5):397–422.

26. Ayres A, Tickle L. Hyper-responsivity to touch and vestibular stimuli as a predictor of positive response to sensory integration procedures by autistic children. Am J Occup Ther 1980; 34(6):375–381.

27. Case-Smith J, Bryan T. The effects of occupational therapy with sensory integration emphasis on preschool-age children with autism. Am J Occup Ther 1999; 49:645–652.

28. Linderman T, Stewart K. Sensory integrative-based occupational therapy and functional outcomes in young children with pervasive developmental disorders: a single-subject study. Am J Occup Ther 1999; 52(2):207–213.

29. Larrington G. A sensory integration based program with a severely retarded/autistic teenager: an occupational therapy case report. Occup Ther Health Care 1987; 4(2):101–107.

30. Ray T, King L, Grandin T. The effectiveness of self-initiated vestibular stimulation in producing speech sounds in an autistic child. Occup Ther J Res 1988; 8:186–190.

31. McClure M, Holtz-Yotz M. The effects of sensory stimulatory treatment on an autistic child. Am J Occup Ther 1990; 45(12):1138–1142.

32. Zissermann L. The effects of deep pressure on self-stimulating behaviors in a child with autism and other disabilities. Am J Occup Ther 1991; 46(6):547–551.

33. Field T, Lasko P, Henteleff T, Kabat S, Talpins S, Dowling M. Brief report: autistic children's attentiveness and responsivity improve after touch therapy. J Autism Dev Disord 1997; 27:333–339.

34. Edelson S, Goldberg M, Edelson M, Kerr D, Grandin T. Behavioral and physiological effects of deep pressure on children with autism: a pilot study evaluating the efficacy of Grandin's Hug Machine. Am J Occup Ther 1999; 53:145–152.

35. Watling R. Selected literature exploring the effectiveness of a sensory-based approach to the treatment of autism. Phys Occup Ther Pediatr 1998; 18(2):77–85.

36. Dawson G, Watling R. Interventions to facilitate auditory, visual, and motor integration in autism: a review of the evidence. J Autism Dev Disord 2000; 30(5):415–421.

37. Rimland B. High dosage levels of certain vitamins in the treatment of children with severe mental disorders. In: Hawkins D, Pauling L, eds. Orthomolecular Psychiatry. New York: WH Freeeman, 1973.

38. Rimland B. An orthomolecular study of psychotic children. J Orthomolec Psychiatry 1974; 3(371–377).

39. Pfeiffer S, Norton J, Nelson L, Shott S. Efficacy of vitamin B_6 and magnesium in the treatment of autism: a methodology review and summary of outcomes. J Autism Dev Disord 1995; 25(5):481–493.

40. Sankar DV. Do they have vitamin deficiencies? J Autism Dev Disord 1979; 9(1):73–82.

41. Kleijnen J, Knipschild P. Niacin and vitamin B_6 in mental functioning: a review of controlled trials in humans. Biol Psychiatry 1991; 29:931–941.

42. Tolbert L, Haigler T, Waits M, Dennis T. Brief report: lack of response in an autistic population to a low dose clinical trial of pyridoxine plus magnesium. J Autism Dev Disord 1993; 23(1):193–199.

43. Lelord G, Callaway E, Muh J, et al. Modifications in urinary homovanillic acid after ingestion of vitamin B6; functional study in autistic children. Rev Neurol (Paris) 1978; 134:797–801.

44. Barthelemy C, Garreau B, Leddet I, Ernouf D, Muh J, Lelord G. Behavioral and biological effects of oral magnesium, vitamin B_6, and combined magnesium–vitamin B_6 administration in autistic children. Magnes Bull 1981; 2:150–153.

45. Lelord G, Muh J, Barthelemy C, Martineau J, Garreau B, Callaway E. Effects of pyridoxine and magnesium on autistic symptoms—initial observations. J Autism Dev Disord 1981; 11(2):219–230.

46. Martineau J, Barthelemy C, Cheliakine C, Lelord G. Brief report: an open middle-term study of combined vitamin B_6–magnesium in a subgroup of autistic children selected on their sensitivity to treatment. J Autism Dev Disord 1988; 18:435–478.

47. Barthelemy C, Garreau B, Leddet I, et al. Biological and clinical effects of oral magnesium and associated magnesium/vitamin B_6 administration of certain disorders in infantile autism. Therapie 1980; 35:627–632.

48. Jonas C, Etienne T, Jouve J, Mariotte N. Interet clinique et biochimique de l'association vitamine B_6 + magnesium dans le traitement de l'autisme residuel a l'age adulte. Therapie 1984; 39:661–669.

49. Rimland B, Callaway E, Dreyfus P. The effect of high doses of vitamin B_6 on autistic children: a double-blind crossover study. Am J Psychiatry 1978; 135(4):472–475.

50. Martineau J, Garreau B, Barthelemy C, Callaway E, Lelord G. Effects of vitamin B_6 on averaged evoked potentials in infantile autism. Biol Psychiatry 1981; 16(7):627–640.

51. Martineau J, Barthelemy C, Garreau B, Lelord G. Vitamin B_6, magnesium, and combined B_6–Mg: therapeutic effects in childhood autism. Biol Psychiatry 1985; 20(5-467-468).

52. Martineau J, Barthelemy C, Lelord G. Long-term effects of combined vitamin B_6–magnesium administration in an autistic child: case report. Biol Psychiatry 1986; 21:511–518.

53. Martineau J, Barthelemy C, Roux S, Garreau B, Lelord G. Electrophysiological effects of fenfluramine or combined vitamin B_6 and magnesium on children with autistic behavior. Dev Med Child Neurol 1989; 31:721–727.

54. Findling R, Maxwell K, Scotese-Wojtila L, Huang J, Yamashita T, Wiznitzer M. High-dose pyridoxine and magnesium administration in children with autistic disorder: an absence of salutary effects in a double-blind, placebo-controlled study. J Autism Dev Disord 1997; 27(4):467–478.

55. CBS Television. 60 Minutes: Beyond the silence. Cure Autism Now [website]. Available at: http://www.cureautismnow.org.

56. ABC Television. Good Morning America. Cure Autism Now [website]. Available at: http://www.cureautismnow.org.

57. Blakeslee S. A rare map of autism's world. In New York Times. Cure Autism Now. Available at: http://www.cureautismnow.org.

58. Cure Autism Now. Beyond the Silence (Accessed February 2, 2003). Available at: http://www.cureautismnow.org.

59. Sackett DL, Richardson WS, Rosenberg W, Haynes RB. Evidence-Based Medicine: How to Practice and Teach EBM. New York: Churchill Livingstone, 1997.

Appendix: Prognosis in Autistic Spectrum Disorders

Chris Plauché Johnson and Vidya Bhushan Gupta

The prognosis for ASD should be considered in terms of change for the better, rather than cure. Cure is rare in ASD. Although some children, particularly those with normal intelligence, functional language, and absence of stereotypies, may not be readily recognized as autistic later in life, most continue to have at least subtle deficits in social skills. Prognosis has been shown to depend on two variables: the degree of abnormal autistic behaviors and the level of adaptive functioning in the community. Adaptive functioning is dependent on intelligence as well as on daily living abilities. Throughout the life span these two variables interact. The prognosis for any given child depends upon his/her place in the spectrum for each of these interacting trajectories. It appears that prognosis for independence as an adult may correlate better with level of adaptive functioning than with the severity of autistic behaviors (1,2,3).

- Cognitive skills (intelligence): Although prognosis is thought to be correlated with general intelligence, an isolated performance IQ score does not accurately predict outcome. Good visual memory and pattern recognition may skew results and fail to accurately reflect the child's problem solving abilities in real life. Moreover, it is difficult to measure verbal IQ accurately in younger children, especially in those without functional language. Children with mental retardation (IQ < 50) and no functional language have the poorest outcomes, despite interventions. On the other hand, one third of children with normal general intelligence and functional language tend to improve with time, such that they are able to participate fully in the community. The autistic

327

features may become barely perceptible except to the trained professional. Twenty to fifty percent may attend college as well (3,4). Early diagnosis and intensive intervention especially improves outcome in this group of children.

- Language: Children who do not develop joint attention skills by the age of 4 years or meaningful speech by 5 years have a poor prognosis (3).
- Comorbid medical and psychiatric conditions: Prognosis is worse in those with comorbid medical (tuberous sclerosis, PKU) and/or psychiatric disorders (i.e., obsessive compulsive behavior, hyperactivity, aggression, self-injurious behavior, and schizophrenia). Twenty-five to thirty-five percent of persons with autism will develop a seizure disorder. There are two peaks of onset of seizures in early childhood and ado-lescence. A seizure disorder, especially one with onset during adolesc-ence, is a poor prognostic sign.
- Gender: Generally, females with autism have a worse prognosis, but this may be due to the fact that as a group, they have lower intelligence. Additionally, fewer girls demonstrate savant skills.

In summary, prognosis should be guarded in children with subnormal intelligence and little or no functional language and cautiously optimistic in children with normal or above average intelligence and functional language. Prediction of prognosis during the preschool years is difficult since IQ test scores and the impact of intervention during this period can vary widely.

REFERENCES

1. Szatmari P. The classification of autism, Asperger's syndrome, and pervasive developmental disorder. Can J Psych 2000; 45:731–738.
2. Szatmari J, Merette C, Bryson SE, Thivierge J, Roy MA, Cayer M, Maziade M. Quantifying dimensions in autism: a factor-analytic study. Am Acad Child Adolesc Psych 2002; 41:467–474.
3. Coplan J. Counseling Parents Regarding Prognosis in Autistic Spectrum Disorder. Pediatrics 2000; 105:e65.
4. Stone WL, Ousley OY. Pervasive developmental disorders: autism. In: Wolraich ML, ed. Disorders of Development and Learning. 2nd ed, Philadelphia: Mosby-Year Book 1996, p. 379–405.
5. Committee on Educational Interventions for Children with Autism. Educating Children with Autism. National Research Council. Washington DC: National Academy of Sciences, 2001.

Index

About the Editor

VIDYA BHUSHAN GUPTA, M.D., M.P.H. is Associate Professor of Clinical Pediatrics at New York Medical College, New York, and Associate Research Scientist at the Gertrude H. Sergievsky Center, Columbia University, New York, New York. Dr. Gupta is the author, coauthor, editor, or coeditor of three books, four book chapters, and numerous scholarly articles published in journals such as *Pediatrics*, the *Journal of Clinical Epidemiology*, and *Clinical Pediatrics*. He is a Fellow of the American Academy of Pediatrics and has board certifications from the American Board of Pediatrics, Neurodevelopmental Disabilities, and Developmental–Behavioral Pediatrics. An invited expert to the 2003 American Academy of Pediatrics committee for early intervention and autism and the 2004 Pediatric Subspecialty Care/Medical Home panel organized by the U.S. Department of Health and Human Services, Dr. Gupta received the M.B.B.S. (1971) and M.D. (1976) degrees from the University of Delhi, New Delhi, India, and the M.P.H. degree (1989) from Columbia University, New York, New York.

ISBN 0-8247-5061-6

90000